Practical Hospitalist Guide to Inpatient Cardiology

Mohammed Salih

Practical Hospitalist Guide to Inpatient Cardiology

Springer

Mohammed Salih
University of Missouri
Columbia, MO, USA

ISBN 978-3-032-03239-3 ISBN 978-3-032-03240-9 (eBook)
https://doi.org/10.1007/978-3-032-03240-9

This Springer imprint is published by the registered company Springer Nature Switzerland AG
The registered company address is: Gewerbestrasse 11, 6330 Cham, Switzerland

This book is for my mother, our guiding light and everlasting hero.
For my late father, whose love and generosity have been the foundation of my life
Miss you Dad.
For my dearest wife, Rayan, the most beautiful gift God has ever placed in my hands.
And for my family, Sarora, Bamboni, Luci, and JoJo.
You are my joy, my laughter, my safe place. I could never dream of better.
Love you all.

Contents

Acute Decompensated Heart Failure (ADHF)

Contents

M. Salih, *Practical Hospitalist Guide to Inpatient Cardiology*, https://doi.org/10.1007/978-3-032-03240-9_1

The chapter provides a comprehensive overview of the clinical presentation, diagnosis, triggers, and management of acute decompensated heart failure (ADHF), a major cause of hospitalization, especially among those over 65. Key symptoms include shortness of breath, nocturnal cough, and leg swelling, with diagnostic tools such as chest X-rays and EKGs used to assess conditions such as pulmonary edema and heart arrhythmias. This chapter discusses various heart failure types categorized by ejection fraction and highlights common precipitants of ADHF such as hypertension, arrhythmias, and acute coronary syndrome. It emphasizes the importance of a thorough clinical approach, including the ABCDE assessment for unstable patients, and suggests a detailed workup including tests such as B-type natriuretic peptide (BNP) and echocardiogram (ECHO). Treatment strategies focus on diuretics, vasodilators, and supportive care, alongside addressing underlying factors like hypertension and arrhythmias. The chapter also explores specific scenarios and alternative treatments, offering a nuanced view of heart failure management.

1.1 When to Suspect and Major Etiology

- In patients presenting with symptoms such as shortness of breath (SOB), nocturnal dry or frothy productive cough, worsening leg swelling, raised jugular venous distention (JVD), basal crackles, lethargy, and potential signs of low perfusion such as lightheadedness, confusion, syncope, cyanosis, cold extremities, and decreasing urine output, diagnostic imaging and tests are crucial. A chest X-ray may reveal pulmonary edema, while an electrocardiogram (EKG) could indicate left ventricular hypertrophy (LVH), acute coronary syndrome (ACS), or atrial fibrillation (Afib). Additional findings might include acute kidney injury (AKI) and elevated B-type natriuretic peptide (BNP) levels, with an echocardiogram providing further insight into the etiology and potential severity of the condition.
- Heart failure is a leading cause of hospitalization in the United States, especially among individuals older than 65 years, with post-discharge mortality rates reaching up to 20% [1]. The types of heart failure are categorized based on ejection fraction:
  - (i) Heart failure with preserved ejection fraction (HFpEF) with EF > 50%.
  - (ii) Heart failure with reduced ejection fraction (HFrEF) with EF < 40%.
  - (iii) Heart failure with mid-range ejection fraction (HFmrEF) with EF between 41% and 49%.

Hospitalist Tip

The primary precipitants for new-onset acute decompensated heart failure (ADHF) [2]:

1. Hypertension (HTN) increases afterload, requiring the heart to exert more effort to pump. This is particularly true for heart failure with preserved ejection fraction (HFpEF) due to the noncompliant nature of the ventricles, which resist dilation or relaxation.
2. Acute arrhythmias, especially atrial fibrillation with rapid ventricular response (Afib with RVR), result in the loss of atrial kick, a crucial component in heart failure with reduced ejection fraction (HFrEF), where the heart's pumping ability is already compromised.
3. Acute coronary syndrome (ACS) is another significant factor, leading to contractility failure and potential papillary muscle rupture, with coronary artery disease (CAD) being responsible for approximately 50% of all acute-onset heart failure cases. ACS must be ruled out during triage, inpatient care, and before discharge [3]
4. Noncompliance in patients, leading to volume overload and acute decompensated chronic heart failure, is frequently due to nonadherence to dietary or medication regimens. It is important to identify patients who have recently experienced illnesses that resulted in them skipping their prescribed medications

Pearl

Additional triggers include infections/mainly pneumonia, valvular heart disease (VHD), severe anemia, hyperthyroidism, alcohol use, chemotherapy, and the use of substances such as cocaine and methamphetamines. In young patients, the most common causes of acute heart failure include cardiac sarcoidosis, various forms of myocarditis (giant cell, eosinophilic, lymphocytic), coronary artery disease from spontaneous dissection, peripartum cardiomyopathy, and takotsubo cardiomyopathy.

1.2 Clinical Approach

- The clinical presentation of heart failure includes symptoms such as shortness of breath, dry cough, orthopnea, paroxysmal nocturnal dyspnea, fatigue, weakness, lower limb edema, and abdominal discomfort with ascites. These symptoms, along with the history of recurrent admissions for acute decompensated heart failure (ADHF), suggest a need to focus on identifying underlying triggers such as syncope related to aortic stenosis, arrhythmias, medication nonadherence, excessive alcohol intake, chest pain associated with ACS, palpitations in atrial fibrillation or thyrotoxicosis, and recent flu symptoms indicating viral myocarditis. Clinical diagnosis remains paramount, with ancillary tests like X-rays and EKGs enhancing diagnostic accuracy [3].

- Key signs include raised jugular venous distention (JVD), an S3 heart sound (only prognostic), basal crackles, a displaced apex beat, pleural effusion, hepatomegaly, ascites, and lower limb edema. Identifying common precipitating triggers involves monitoring blood pressure for hypertension, checking for irregular pulses indicative of acute arrhythmias, and recognizing the clench sign for ACS, although its utility is limited [13].
- The essential workup for patients admitted with acute decompensated heart failure (ADHF) should include a complete blood count (CBC), comprehensive metabolic panel (CMP), thyroid-stimulating hormone (TSH), iron studies, cardiac enzymes or troponin levels, B-type natriuretic peptide (BNP) or N-terminal pro-b-type natriuretic peptide (NT-proBNP), electrocardiogram (EKG), chest X-ray, and possibly an echocardiogram. A pulse oximeter and arterial blood gas (ABG) analysis are crucial for determining treatment strategies based on hypoxia or respiratory failure severity. A respiratory viral panel and relevant infectious workup for myocarditis could be considered.

Pearl

Orthopnea, weight gain, and paroxysmal nocturnal dyspnea (PND) are considered reliable indicators of acute decompensated heart failure (ADHF), and it is uncommon to encounter patients with ADHF who do not exhibit any of these symptoms. Conversely, raised jugular venous distention (JVD), characterized by visible pulsation in front of the ears, is a specific sign of ADHF. However, Due to the adaptive capacity of the pulmonary lymphatic system to sustained elevations in left ventricular pressure, a significant proportion of patients with decompensated heart failure may exhibit clear lung fields on both physical examination and chest radiography; the sensitivity of rales in this context is approximately 15%. [4, 11].

Pearl

Acute right-sided heart failure often arises from left ventricular (LV) dysfunction, which is the most common cause of right ventricular (RV) dysfunction due to pressure overload and pulmonary venous hypertension. This condition is also observed in scenarios such as inferior acute coronary syndrome (ACS), massive pulmonary embolism, and right-sided acute valvular heart disease (VHD), for example, infectious endocarditis in intravenous drug users (IVDU). Shortness of breath (SOB) is the most familiar symptom of acute right-sided heart failure. Other significant clinical findings include elevated right-sided filling pressures, such as jugular venous distention and peripheral edema. Notably, the absence of pulmonary edema is a classic feature in cases where LV failure is absent. In the acute settings, give IV fluids to maintain the preload.

1

Usually, patients fit one of four clinical spectrums based on fluid status and perfusion.

Warm and dry (seen on high-output heart failure)	Cold and dry (could be seen on right ventricular infarction; should avoid nitroglycerin)
Warm and wet (considered common in inpatient settings)	Cold and wet (seen in cardiogenic shock)

Hospitalist Tip

Cold symptoms indicating potential cardiogenic shock include cool extremities, prolonged capillary refill time, peripheral cyanosis (systemic deoxygenation), narrow pulse pressure (indicating poor pulses with low and narrow systolic/diastolic blood pressure), poor mentation, and worsening kidney function or urine output. These signs serve as early warnings for cardiogenic shock, warranting immediate consultation with a cardiologist.

Pearl

In cases of unexplained new-onset acute decompensated heart failure (ADHF) where evaluations such as echocardiograms and stress testing versus left heart catheterization (LHC) are negative, it is advisable to consider advanced imaging techniques like cardiac MRI and SPECT/bone tracer cardiac scintigraphy. These tests help rule out infiltrative diseases such as sarcoidosis, myocarditis, and cardiac amyloidosis. The prevalence of cardiac amyloidosis in heart failure patients is approximately 13.7%, indicating it is not uncommon [9]. It is predominantly observed in older males and is characterized by elevated BNP levels, increased interventricular septal thickness during diastole, apical sparing, reduced left ventricular systolic function, and low voltage on EKG.

1.3 Tests to Consider for ADHF and Their Significance

Test	Clinical significance	Comments
Chest X-ray	Pulmonary edema, pleural effusion (mainly right side), vascular cephalic congestion, and heart enlargement	Heart enlargement could be absent in acute heart failure due to acute regurgitation. Also, it is not a specific sign, as it could be wide in pericardial effusion. ARDS may look similar to pulmonary edema on X-ray. Consider looking for the elevated JDV and overall fluid in ADHF. Other differential diagnoses (DD) similar to pulmonary edema include atypical pneum onia, Interstial lung disease (ILD), and cancer infiltrates.

Test	Clinical significance	Comments
EKG	Signs for ischemia, LVH, and arrhythmias. Premature ventricular contractions (PVC) and non-sustained ventricular tachycardia are common in patients with ADHF.	If EKG is totally normal, consider an alternative diagnosis [4].

Test	Clinical significance	Comments
B-type natriuretic peptide (BNP)/ NT-proBNP	It is helpful to rule out if it is below BNP <100 pg/mL, NT-proBNP <300 pg/mL [7].	It is a valuable test when your underlying cause for dyspnea is not straightforward and heart failure probability is low. It has a high negative predictive value in populations with a high prevalence of heart failure. This means if it is below the cutoff point in this population, then it is unlikely that HF will explain the dyspnea. If the patient has clear-cut heart failure symptoms and signs, a normal BNP should not misguide you. Remember, it is a clinical diagnosis in the first place. A higher BNP indicates higher mortality [6]. In patients hospitalized with acute decompensated heart failure, a significant drop in BNP at discharge combined with a BNP level below the risk threshold suggests a good prognosis for future cardiovascular events.

Test	Clinical significance	Comments
Troponin	Could be elevated even if there is no ACS in about 50% of patients [8]	If significantly elevated, consider ACS. It could be falsely elevated in AKI/CKD, stress, severe rhabdomyolysis, and sepsis. Any condition that stresses the heart may lead to troponin elevation, e.g., PE.

Test	Clinical significance	Comments
ECHO	It helps classify ADHF as HFpEF ≥50%/ HFrEF ≤40%, VHD, diastolic dysfunction with LVH, regional wall motion abnormalities in ischemic heart disease (IHD), and pericardial effusion in tamponade. Repeating TTE while inpatient may be needed if the condition changes.	Always request it if not recently done!!

Test	Clinical significance	Comments
CBC	For anemia and its correction	Significant anemia can lead to high-output cardiac failure. Other causes include obesity, hyperthyroidism, Paget disease of bone, thiamine deficiency, and arteriovenous fistula.

Test	Clinical significance	Comments
CMP and Iron studies	Electrolytes and kidney functions Especially low Na due to fluid overload. Follow levels of Mg/K in arrhythmia correction or related to diuretics side effects. AKI in cardio-renal syndrome	Low urine sodium, with urine osmolality higher than serum osmolality, is typical but not always present (hyponatremia is usually multifactorial in hospital settings). Low serum albumin correlated with higher mortality.

Test	Clinical significance	Comments
TSH	Hyperthyroidism in A-fib or hypothyroidism in pericardial tamponade and ischemic heart disease	

Test	Clinical significance	Comments
Liver function test (LFT)	Indicates ischemic liver due to hypoperfusion or increased hydrostatic pressure in the venous drainage system	Usually seen in advanced heart failure or cardiogenic shock

Test	Clinical significance	Comments
Lung US	May show B lines, but not specific	B lines highly sensitive to rule out ADHF, to almost 100%

Test	Clinical significance	Comments
Lung CT	Will show a segmental artery larger than the bronchus, peribronchial cuffing, and ground glass in the lung bases. Fluid is seen in the interlobular septa. Kerley B lines. These findings are symmetrical. Main DD: – Lymphangitic carcinomatosis (asymmetrical)	ARDS, liver failure, or nephrotic syndrome may appear similarly. CT findings must be interpreted in the proper clinical context and in relation to the underlying disease process.

Test	Clinical significance	Comments
Cardiac left heart catherization (LHC)	To rule out IHD as a culprit	Consider LHC (high IHD probability) or stress testing (intermediate probability) in all unexplained new ADHF patients before considering advanced imaging such as MRI or cardiac CT.

Test	Clinical significance	Comments
CT coronary angiography	Will show stenosis or occlusion	Could be considered when a noninvasive diagnostic test is needed, with low-intermediate probability for IHD to rule out, but would not rule out microvascular ischemia. It is a good test for acute chest pain with low-intermediate probability in the ED or patients with equivocal non-ST-segment elevation myocardial infarction (NSTEMI) [10].

Test	Clinical significance	Comments
Cardiac MRI	Has specific gadolinium enhancement in different conditions	It is mainly valuable for nonischemic causes, primarily if the clinical context supports infiltrative conditions such as sarcoidosis, hemochromatosis, Immune induced myocarditis, and amyloidosis.

Test	Clinical significance	Comments
Endomyocardial biopsy	Mainly useful for evidence of Giant Cell Myocarditis (GCM) or viral myocarditis. Does have low sensitivity for sarcoidosis	When it will influence therapy in unexplained recent-onset unexplained heart failure, new arrhythmias, or not responding to treatment. Mostly accurate following localization with MRI/PET

Pearl

Cardio-renal syndrome refers to the deterioration of kidney or heart function due to the failure or injury of the other organ, and it can present in either an acute or chronic form. In a hospital setting, acute kidney injury (AKI) frequently develops due to worsening heart failure, particularly heart failure with reduced ejection fraction (HFrEF). This condition is believed to result from sympathetic activation and venous congestion within the renal parenchyma, leading to decreased renal perfusion and prerenal AKI. It serves as an important prognostic criterion. In general, if a patient's acute kidney injury improves following diuretic therapy, it is typically appropriate to continue diuretics. This response suggests that the underlying cause of kidney injury is likely elevated venous pressure resulting in pre-renal acute kidney injury due to reduced renal perfusion.

1.4 Approaching SOB and Hypoxia for the Hospitalist (Nurse Call)

- While waiting to see the patient, instruct the nurse to monitor the patient's vital signs and pulse oximetry and perform an EKG. Upon arrival, a thorough history of shortness of breath (SOB) and associated respiratory symptoms must be conducted. Perform a focused examination of the lungs and cardiovascular system (CVS), particularly assessing for cyanosis, capillary refill, and auscultation findings. For unstable patients, follow the ABCDE approach. Check arterial blood gases (ABG) in all unstable patients and calculate the alveolar-arterial (A-a) oxygen gradient. If results are inconclusive, proceed with tests including troponin, chest X-ray, complete blood count (CBC), comprehensive metabolic panel (CMP), and computed tomography pulmonary angiography (CTPA). If all are ruled out (normal X-ray/CT/other labs), rule out shunting with bubble studies/transthoracic echocardiography (TTE). Additional laboratory tests should be ordered based on the differential diagnosis (DD). The main DD includes acute decompensated heart failure (ADHF), pneumonia, chronic obstructive pulmonary disease (COPD)/asthma, pulmonary embolism (PE), acute coronary syndrome (ACS), significant anemia, severe metabolic or respiratory acidosis (often seen in severe sepsis), pneumothorax, and rarely shunting. Less likely DDs, if the primary list is not evident, include anaphylaxis, aortic dissection, cardiac tamponade, and acute aortic regurgitation/mitral regurgitation (AR/MR).

1.5 ABCDE Approach

Approach	Assess	Manage	Monitor
A (airway)	Alert and awake	If not, protect airway with intubation, laryngeal mask airway, etc.	Check if airway is protected
B (breathing)	Brief lung exam, pulse oximeter, ABG	Give oxygen, high-flow nasal cannula (HFNC), etc. start high oxygen, then titrate low	Brief lung exam, chest X-ray, and pulse oximeter. Do Point of care Ultrasound (POCUS) if available
C (circulation)	Brief CVS exam, BP, capillary refill time	Secure peripheral lines. Fluid if hypotensive, then pressors if needed	Brief CVS exam, do EKG (keep in telemetry if suspecting arrhythmias). Echo once stable or bedside POCUS in emergency state
D (disability)	Brief CNS exam, Glascow Comma Scale (GCS), pupil size (good to assess for drug intoxication and brain stem function), and blood sugars (mimic for stroke when low)	Treat accordingly	Monitor GCS and neurological exam
E (exposure)	Head-to-toe brief assessment, looking for trauma, fractures, etc.	Treat accordingly	Reassess

1.6 Approach to Acutely Hypoxic Patient [14]

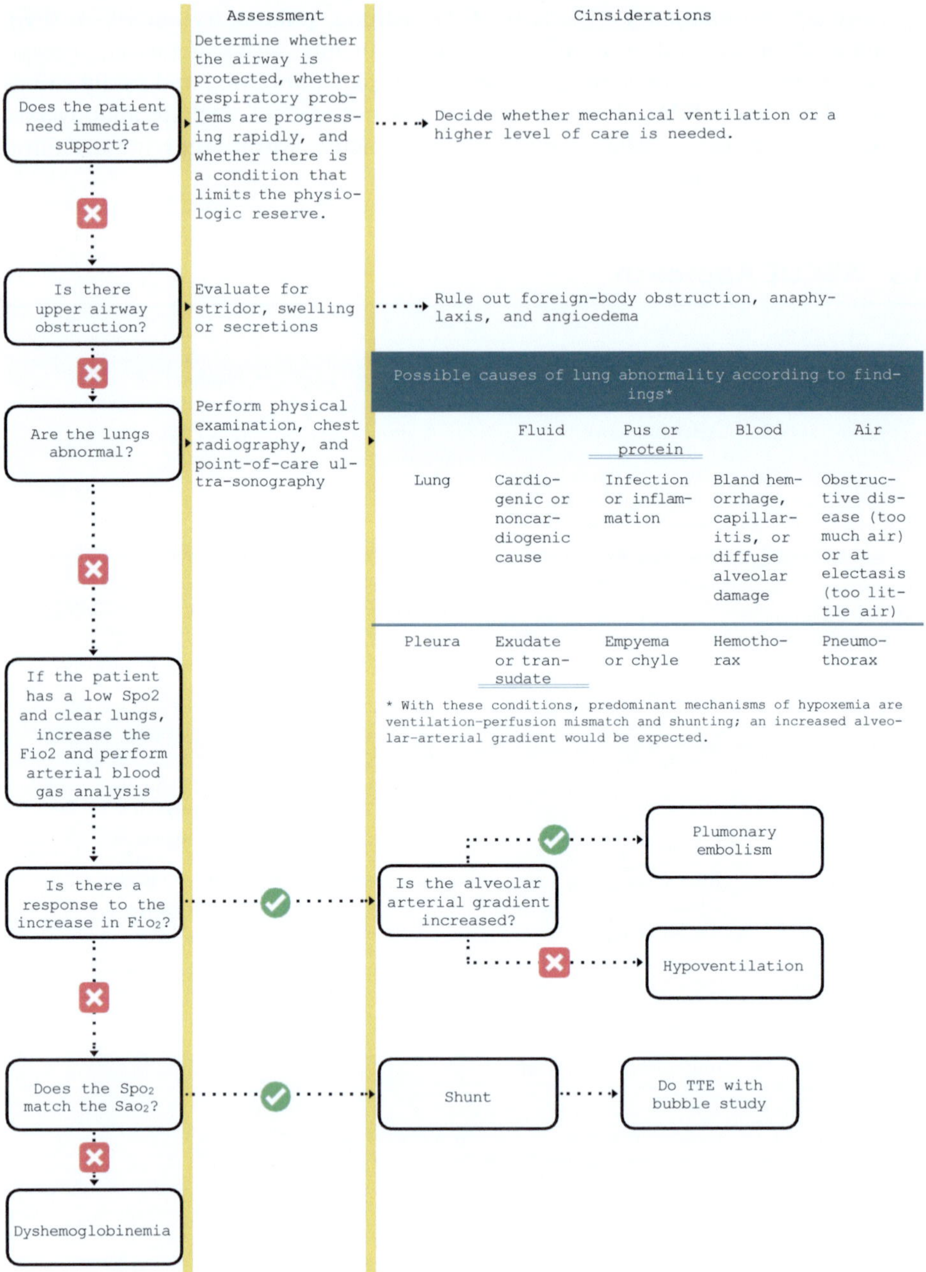

Possible causes of lung abnormality according to findings*

	Fluid	Pus or protein	Blood	Air
Lung	Cardiogenic or noncardiogenic cause	Infection or inflammation	Bland hemorrhage, capillaritis, or diffuse alveolar damage	Obstructive disease (too much air) or at electasis (too little air)
Pleura	Exudate or transudate	Empyema or chyle	Hemothorax	Pneumothorax

* With these conditions, predominant mechanisms of hypoxemia are ventilation-perfusion mismatch and shunting; an increased alveolar-arterial gradient would be expected.

1.7 Major DD of ADHF

Condition	How to differentiate
PE	Chest pain, hemoptysis. Unexplained tachycardia is common. CTPA is diagnostic. Suspect if you have a patient with SOB not improving with diuretics
COPD exacerbation	May have a productive cough, bilateral wheezes, and possible diffuse crackles. Not fluid overloaded, except in corpulmonale. POCUS is highly useful in showing A-lines with no B-lines. ADHF can present with wheeze on the exam due to airway narrowing with significant pulmonary edema. To differentiate from asthma or COPD, consider your complete picture rather than your sole finding of wheezes. Also, remember they may coexist!!
ARDS/ COVID-19	X-ray and presentation are similar. Still, they generally look sicker with significant hypoxia, not responding to diuretics or low-flow oxygen—No signs of fluid overload. The inciting factor is mostly sepsis. COVID-19 test is always reasonable in all patients presenting with unexplained SOB
Pneumonia	Fever or productive cough. Leukocytosis and X-rays show lobar/diffuse infiltration. No fluid overload. BNP could be low and helpful in routing ADHF. POCUS may help with unilateral pleural thickening, which indicates consolidation with focal B-lines. In acute SOB, absence of fever and cough is supportive of ADHF [13]
ESRD with fluid overload	Known dialysis patient with pulmonary edema usually improves with dialysis sessions and HTN control. Troponin and BNP could be falsely elevated
Advanced liver failure	Other chronic liver disease findings or history, alcoholism history, elevated LFT, jaundice, elevated PT/INR, and generalized anasarca including the scrotum. Serum ascitic albumin gradient (SAAG) is high, but total protein is usually low in ascites <2.5 g/dl
Advanced nephrotic syndrome	Significant proteinuria on random protein/creatinine ratio of over 3 grams. Generalized anasarca, including the face (uncommon in heart failure)

Pearl

Remember the above conditions may coexist!! Use your judgment if patients with a proposed diagnosis do not improve with the provisional treatment. Be mindful of your biases when the patient is not improving

1.8 Treatment Approach

- The primary treatments include diuretics, oxygen supplementation or noninvasive ventilation, vasodilators, and, if necessary, inotropes for cardiogenic shock. Addressing the underlying precipitating factors by managing hypertensive emergencies, atrial fibrillation with rapid ventricular response (RVR), and acute coronary syndrome (ACS) is essential.

1.9 Oxygenation and Ventilation [12]

- Ensure the patient maintains an oxygen saturation level above 90%. If a simple nasal cannula (NC) or mask is insufficient, consider a high-flow nasal cannula (HFNC), as meta-analyses indicate that HFNC results in a lower intubation rate than conventional oxygen therapy. Continuous positive airway pressure (CPAP) is the next step to enhance oxygenation by keeping alveoli open. Still, bilevel-positive airway pressure (BIPAP) is preferred in cases of cardiogenic pulmonary edema with hypercapnia, offering mortality benefits over oxygen alone. Intubate the patient if there is no response or if the patient worsens, especially with altered mental status.

Pearl

Avoid hyperoxygenation. The British Thoracic Society guidelines recommend a target SpO_2 range of 94 to 98% for most adult inpatients. For patients at risk for hypercapnic respiratory failure, such as those with COPD, a target range of 88 to 92% is safer to prevent oxygen-induced hypercapnia. Consider oxygen as a drug.

1.10 Diuretics

Diuretics are essential in treating heart failure if blood pressure permits (usually above 90/60), the patient is well-perfused (not cold), and not in shock. They should be initiated immediately, preferably in the emergency department. The primary loop diuretics used are furosemide, bumetanide, and torsemide (◘ Table 1.1) [17]. Gradually escalate the dose as needed. If a patient does not respond to one diuretic, switch to another, as individual responses can vary. There is no significant difference between bolus and continuous infusion diuretics, so use the latter only in patients with soft blood pressure or when dosing is difficult to titrate [18]. If the diuretic response is unclear, switch the cumulative 24-hour continuous dose to a scheduled dose twice daily. If there is no adequate response, indicated by urine sodium <50 mEq/L at 2 hours, consider increasing the dose or adding oral metolazone (often a single dose is sufficient) or spironolactone while closely monitoring electrolytes, especially potassium. If the patient was on home loop diuretics before admission, they should receive an IV dose of approximately 1 to 2.5 times the home dose divided throughout the day. For those not previously on diuretics, start with a low dose and assess volume status, blood pressure, kidney function, and symptoms every 4–6 hours after the first IV dose. If the response is brisk but transient, increase the frequency to three to four times daily. Once the patient shows improvement on IV diuretics and is nearing discharge, switch to an oral equivalent divided twice daily to ensure an adequate response before release. Consider bumetanide and torsemide for significant right-sided heart failure with bowel edema due to their better oral bioavailability and longer half-life compared to furosemide. Fluid restriction is generally unnecessary if there is a good diuretic response.

Pearl

Common issues to monitor when using diuretics include electrolyte disturbances, metabolic alkalosis, and worsening kidney function, indicated by elevated blood urea nitrogen (BUN) levels.

Hospitalist Tip

Acetazolamide is a novel adjunctive treatment for acute decompensated heart failure (ADHF) and should be used in addition to loop diuretics, not as a standalone treatment. It aids in achieving successful decongestion and can result in shorter hospital stays. Furthermore, it counteracts the metabolic alkalosis caused by diuretics by inducing metabolic acidosis. However, there is no associated mortality benefit [16].

Hospitalist Tip

The goal for urine output in patients is approximately 3–5 liters per day or achieving a negative fluid balance of around 1–2 liters per day. Fluid restriction should be set at 1.5–2 liters per day. Aim for the patient's dry weight, which is their baseline weight when asymptomatic and euvolemic, with a gradual weight loss of 1–2 pounds daily during hospitalization. Consider ultrafiltration (UF) for patients with congestion who are unresponsive to aggressive diuretic therapy or have significant worsening of AKI. But keep in mind , Plasma ultrafiltration led to more adverse events than diuretics in the AVOID-HF and CARRESS-HF trials. When volume status is unclear from exam and echocardiography, invasive hemodynamic assessment should be pursued rather than empiric fluid removal. Sometimes, it is necessary to tolerate some residual edema to avoid triggering acute kidney injury (AKI)..

1.11 Diuretic Approach [17]

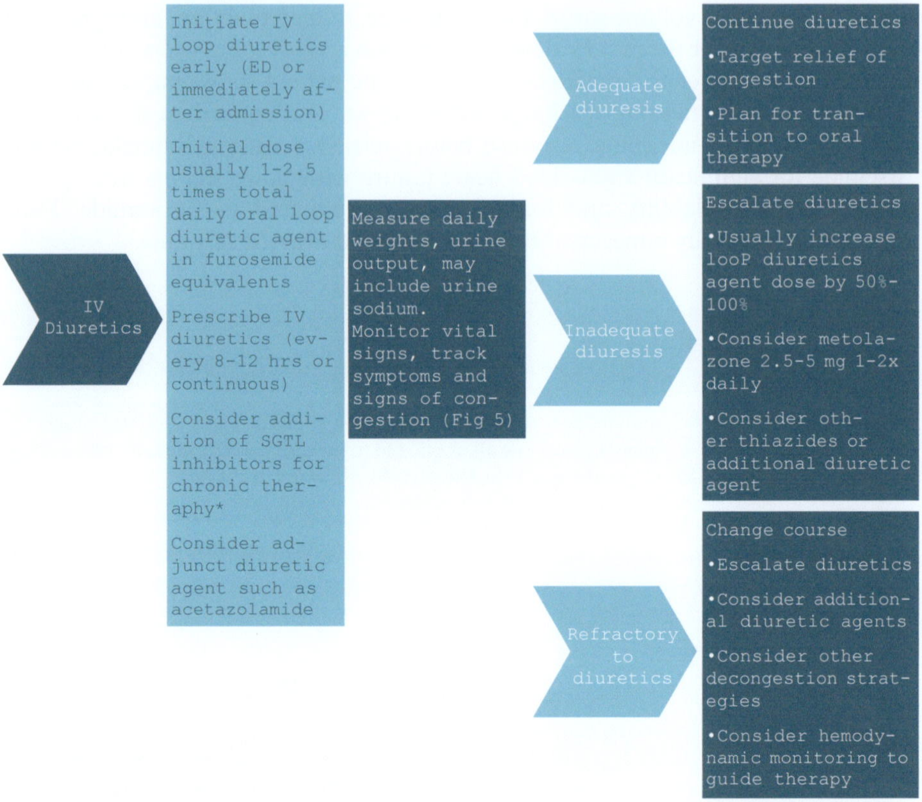

This figure has been updated to include information from recent clinical trials. When high loop diuretic doses are not effective, dual nephron blockade with the addition of either a thiazide-like diuretic or a carbonic anhydrase inhibitor (acetazolamide) can be considered. In the CLOROTIC (Safety and Efficacy of the Combination of Loop with Thiazide-Type Diuretics in Patients with Decompensated Heart Failure) trial, addition of hydrochlorothiazide to an IV loop diuretic resulted in an increased diuretic response and more weight loss without a change in patient-reported dyspnea. Metolazone can be added to the IV loop diuretic at 2.5- to 5-mg doses once or twice daily. In the ADVOR (Acetazolamide in Decompensated Heart Failure with Volume Overload) trial, acetazolamide added to a loop diuretic for 3 days exhibited a greater rate of successful decongestion and a shorter duration of hospital stay compared with placebo, with no statistically significant differences in renal safety, hypokalemia, or hypotension between groups.*If plan to continue SGLT inhibitors after discharge, determine financial feasibility. BP, blood pressure; ED, emergency department; IV, intravenous; Na, sodium; SGLT, sodium-glucose cotransporter.

1.12 Simplified Diuretic Strategy in Heart Failure [18]

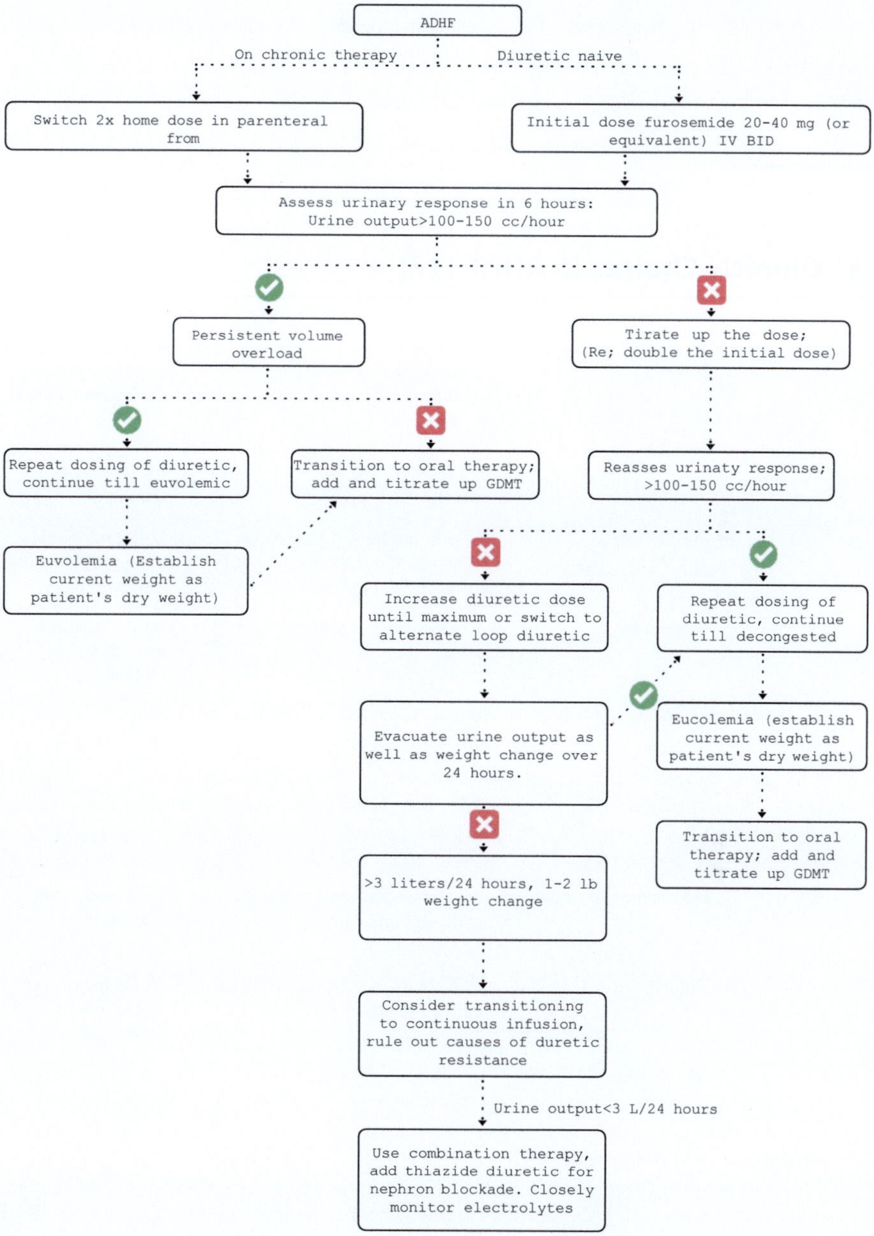

ADHF - Acute Decompensated Heart Failure
BID - Twice a day dosing

GDMT - Guideline Directed Management & Therapy
IV - Intravenous
Consider ultrafiltration; right heart catheterization for better understanding of the hemodynamics

Pearl

Adding low-dose continuous dopamine to improve diuretics is discouraged and offers no benefit [30].

1.13 Diuretic Choices in ADHF [17]

Class	Drug	Usual inpatient dosing[a] (maximum)[b]	Usual outpatient dosing (maximum)[b]
Loop diuretic agents	Bumetanide	0.5–4 mg IV 1–3 times daily (12 mg/d) OR 0.5–2 mg/h IV infusion (40 mg/h)	0.5–2 mg orally once to twice daily (10 mg/d)
	Furosemide	40–160 mg IV 1–3 times daily (200 mg/dose) OR 5–20 mg/h IV infusion (40 mg/h)	20–80 mg orally once to twice daily (600 mg/d)
	Torsemide	Not available commercially in IV form[c]	10–40 mg orally once daily (200 mg/d)
Carbonic anhydrase inhibitors	Acetazolamide	500 mg orally/IV once daily or in divided doses	N/A
Thiazide-type diuretic agents	Chlorothiazide	0.5–1 g IV once to twice daily (2 g/d)	N/A
	Hydrochlorothiazide	25–50 mg orally once to twice daily (100 mg/d)	25–50 mg orally once daily (100 mg/d)
	Chlorthalidone	12.5–25 mg orally once to twice daily (100 mg/d)	25–50 mg orally once daily (100 mg/d)
	Metolazone	2.5–5 mg orally once to twice daily (20 mg/d)	2.5–5 mg orally once daily (20 mg/d)

IV intravenous, *N/A* not applicable

[a]For patients receiving loop diuretic agents before admission, the oral dose should be changed to an intravenous dose of 1–2.5 times the home dose. For patients naïve to therapy, the lower end of the dosing interval should be used

[b]"Usual" dose ranges reflect approved product labeling and safety and efficacy results from large, randomized controlled trials. Higher ranges may be considered based on observational data and clinical experience

[c]Oral therapy may be initiated before discharge to assess patient response

1.14 Diuretics Comments in ADHF (Table 1.1)

Hospitalist Tip

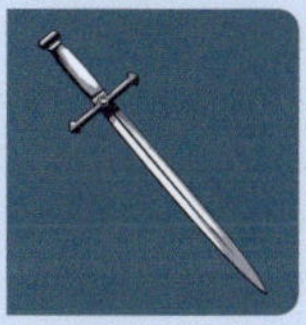

Draining the fluids may significantly improve symptoms in large symptomatic ascites or pleural effusions that do not respond to diuretics. However, it should not be done diuretics. However, it should not be done routinely.

Table 1.1 Diuretics options and their dose adjusment from IV to oral in ADHF

Diuretics	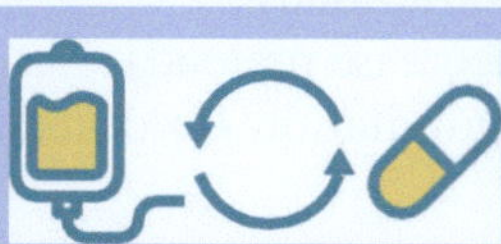	Comments
Furosemide	IV to oral dosing 1:2	After the first dose, closely monitor urine output within 4–6 hours to assess for response. The urine output goal is 100–150 ml/h
Bumetanide	IV to oral dosing 1:1	Use if not responding to furosemide. Mainly helpful on discharge with patients with significant right-sided heart failure
Torsemide	IV to oral dosing 1:1	Mainly helpful on discharge with patients with significant right-sided heart failure
Metolazone	Only oral	Added to loop if not responding well. Do not use IV chlorothiazide routinely; it is more expensive, eliminated fast, and does not have better natriuresis than metolazone
Spironolactone	Only oral	Especially if low potassium and intact kidney function. Avoid if eGFR <30, or K more than 5 mEq/L
Acetazolamide	500 mg intravenous once daily, usually for three doses	Added to standardized intravenous loop diuretics. It is helpful if the patient is not responding to the loop and is alkalotic
Ethacrynic acid	Start as 50 mg IV/day. Oral start dose is 50 mg/day	It is a loop diuretic. Used in sulfa allergy with a history of anaphylaxis; very expensive (particularly intravenous)

1.15 Vasodilators

- Vasodilators decrease preload and afterload and are utilized in patients who do not respond sufficiently to diuretics alone. They are particularly suitable for individuals with uncontrolled hypertension or those experiencing a hypertensive emergency and acute decompensated heart failure (ADHF) despite the absence of a mortality benefit (11a). The preferred drugs are nitroglycerin or nicardipine, administered as continuous infusions according to unit protocol (■ Table 1.2). The target is maintaining systolic blood pressure (SBP) below 140 mmHg. Avoid using nitroprusside or hydralazine due to significant side effects and unpredictable blood pressure responses [19]. Overall, no data suggest that IV vasodilators improve outcomes in patients hospitalized with HF [33]. In summary, vasodilators are indicated for ADHF patients experiencing the following:
  - (i) Hypertensive crisis(to decrease afterload).
  - (ii) Unresponsive to diuretics (to decrease preload).
  - (iii) Valvular heart disease with regurgitation (to decrease both preload and afterload).

Pearl

Nicardipine should be avoided in acute coronary syndrome (ACS) with acute decompensated heart failure (ADHF) because it can cause reflex tachycardia [19]. This effect reduces diastolic time, leading to diminished coronary perfusion, and increases oxygen demand.

1.16 Preferable Vasodilator Options in ADHF (■ Table 1.2) [19]

- ACE inhibitors, ARBs, potassium-sparing diuretics, and ARNIs (angiotensin receptor-neprilysin inhibitors) can usually be started or continued safely in acute decompensated heart failure (ADHF), with some limitations such as acute kidney injury (AKI), low BP, and hyerkalemia [34]. Beta-blockers should be continued if the BP and clinical picture allow [36]. The suggested approach can guide the decision on when to initiate beta-blockers (■ Table 1.3) [35]. SGLT2 inhibitors and mineralocorticoid antagonists have minimal impact on reducing blood pressure but are fundamental in guideline-directed medical therapy (GDMT). Provided there are no contraindications (such as AKI, diabetic ketoacidosis, type 1 diabetes mellitus, recent surgery, urinary tract infection/indwelling catheter, or recent infection), SGLT2 inhibitors can be started or continued in hemodynamically stable patients with an estimated glomerular filtration rate (eGFR) of at least 20 mL/min at any point during hospitalization

Table 1.2 Preferable IV Vasodilators for ADHF

Vasodilator	Dose	Comments
Nitroglycerin	5 micrograms/minute IV initially, increase by 10–20 micrograms/ minute increments every 5–15 minutes according to the response	Nitroglycerin is a valuable option in acute clinical settings due to its dual action on preload and afterload. At lower doses, it primarily reduces preload by dilating venous vessels, which decreases venous return to the heart. When administered at higher doses, particularly above 100 mcg/min, nitroglycerin exerts a more pronounced effect on arterial dilation, reducing afterload and lowering blood pressure. This pharmacological profile makes it versatile in managing various cardiovascular conditions, particularly heart failure and hypertension
Nicardipine	5 mg/h IV may increase by 2.5 mg/h every 5–15 min	Monitor HR closely. Avoid use in ACS or recent IHD

and continued upon discharge, whether the patient has heart failure with preserved ejection fraction (HFpEF) or reduced ejection fraction (HFrEF) [32]. If AKI is present, hydralazine and isosorbide dinitrate/mononitrate may be alternatives.

- In certain patients with congestive heart failure (CHF) who exhibit an ejection fraction (EF) of ≤35% and present with symptoms, the implementation of a wearable cardioverter-defibrillator (WCD), such as the LifeVest®, may prove beneficial. This is especially relevant for individuals who have been undergoing guideline-directed medical therapy (GDMT) for a duration of less than 3 months. A subsequent evaluation of the EF after this period is crucial to ascertain any improvements. If the EF remains compromised, the consideration for implantable cardioverter-defibrillator (ICD) placement becomes pertinent, potentially mitigating the risk of sudden cardiac death [37].

Pearl

ARNI (Entresto@) is known to cause symptomatic hypotension. Titrate ARNIs slowly in stable patients. They can be used for acute HFpEF or HFrEF [34, 39]. When transitioning from an ARB to an ARNI, no washout period is necessary. However, when switching from an ACE inhibitor to an ARNI, a 36-hour washout period is required to minimize the risk of angioedema associated with concurrent exposure to both agents.

Pearl

Ivabradine is approved for stable HF, LVEF ≤35%, in sinus rhythm, resting HR > 70, to reduce the risk of HF hospitalization [26].

1.17 B-Blockers Suggested Approach in ADHF (▫ Table 1.3) [35]

▫ Table 1.3 B-Blockers management Approach in ADHF

New onset ADHF, with no history of B-blockers use	May initiate during hospitalization before discharge if clinically stablestable
Tachycardia induced ADHF or HTN emergency inducedor ADHF	May initiate or titrate the dose
DHF with cardiogenic shock or SBP below 90 mmhg	Hold. Resume or start once stable
Mild to moderate ADHF (no significant pulmonary edema or hypoxia) with a patient known to be on B-blockers and stable BP. (36)	May continue home dose or adjusted to lower dose according to severity of pulmonary edema/hypoxia/BP, usually 50%.

1.18 Supportive Care

- Most patients require deep vein thrombosis (DVT) prophylaxis and a low-salt or heart-healthy diet. Hyponatremia typically resolves with diuretics and fluid restriction (less than 1.5 L) unless it is multifactorial. Salt tablets or vasopressin antagonists may be used for severe hyponatremia, but this should not be the usual practice.
- Cardio-renal syndrome (CRS) is managed with cautious escalation of diuretics, and sometimes, withholding diuresis for 1–2 days before gradually resuming can be beneficial. Nephrotoxic medications, including ACE inhibitors, ARNIs, ARBs, and aldosterone antagonists, should be withheld until kidney function improves. If all else fails, consider ultrafiltration, although evidence supporting its efficacy is not strong and maybe harmful. For patients with CRS, pulmonary artery catheterization may be indicated to guide decongestive strategies and define hemodynamics, particularly in those with worsening kidney function and/or diuretic resistance [20].
- Correct underlying anemia (especially IDA), DM, and CKD. Most patient should receive IV iron (not oral iron) until iron saturation exceeds 20%. Per the 2022 ACC/AHA/HFSA Heart Failure Guideline, IV iron therapy is reasonable (Class IIa) to improve functional status and quality of life in HFrEF patients with iron deficiency, regardless of anemia status.
- Physical therapy is recommended to improve mobility and regain functionality.
- Lastly, palliative care consultations should be considered for patients with frequent admissions.

Pearl

Patients on ARBs can transition to ARNIs directly, whereas you should wait 36 hours before switching from ACE inhibitors to ARNIs. That is due to the high risk of angioedema in the latter. Do not use ARNIs if the patient has a history of angioedema.

1.19 Discharge Planning

- Discharge should occur only when the patient nears euvolemia with oral, rather than intravenous, diuretic therapy. Consider adding or continuing SGLT2 inhibitors for all patients with heart failure, given their mortality benefits in both heart failure with reduced ejection fraction (HFrEF) and preserved ejection fraction (HFpEF). Other guideline-directed medical therapies (GDMT) should be resumed if appropriate. The patient should be closely monitored after discharge, ideally within 2 weeks. Recent guidelines recommend a model-focused discharge handoff for the patient to bring to their clinic visit [17].
- Advise the patient to avoid heavy lifting during the acute phase, limit alcohol intake, quit smoking, avoid adding salt to food, monitor daily or weekly weights, and adjust diuretic dosages accordingly by taking additional necessary doses.

1.20 Special Population

- A subset of the ADHF population may have a specialized treatment approach. The central concept is to treat the underlying cause; for example, urgent LHC is needed if the patient has STEMI or surgical repair in right-sided valvular endocarditis. The following common special situations are commonly encountered.

1.21 Hypertensive Emergency with ADHF

- Uncontrolled hypertension with a blood pressure of at least 180/110 mmHg and new-onset acute decompensated heart failure (ADHF) suggest this diagnosis.
- Aim to reduce the systolic blood pressure (SBP) to less than 140 mmHg within 1 hour [19]. Add oral guideline-directed medical therapy (GDMT) and other antihypertensives within 6–12 hours to facilitate weaning off infusions. According to AHA/ACC guidelines for patients with heart failure with reduced ejection fraction (HFrEF), ambulatory settings' primary blood pressure target should be below 130/80 mmHg. However, this may be unrealistic during inpatient care.
- Nitroglycerin and nicardipine are preferred medications for significant volume overload (◘ Table 1.4). In drier patients, after effective volume diuresis, consider switching to esmolol or metoprolol tartrate, especially in tachyphylaxis to nitroglycerin or unreasonable side effects like headaches. However, beta-blockers should be avoided initially in patients with pulmonary congestion.

1.22 Beta-Blocker Medication Option in ADHF with Hypertensive Emergency (◘ Table 1.4)

◘ **Table 1.4** Options of B-Blockers in dry patients with ADHF

Medication	Dose	Comments
Esmolol	500–1000 micrograms/kg intravenously as a loading dose, followed by 50 micrograms/kg/minute infusion	Follow institution protocol for most inputs. A good option when having ADHF (dry lung)+ HTN + Afib with RVR
Metoprolol tartrate	2.5 to 5 mg intravenously every 5 minutes according to response, maximum 15 mg/total dose	

Pearl

The non-dihydropyridine calcium channel blockers verapamil and diltiazem should not be used in HFrEF patients, as they may increase mortality. Amlodipine and nifidipine XL are fine.

Pearl

Sacubitril/valsartan is an excellent medication for HFrEF patients. It decreases mortality compared to ACE (PARA- DIGM-HF trial). It is also FDA-approved for any CHF type. A significant side effect is hypotension. It should not be given to patients with a history of angioedema, irrespective of tolerability to ARB from before. When transitioning (which you should always consider in HFrEF patients) from ACE inhibitors to sacubitril/valsartan, have a grace period of more than 36 hours due to the high risk of angioedema.

Pearl

In difficult-to-control HTN patients, consider isosorbide dinitrate–hydralazine, especially in black patients with HFrEF. They do have mortality benefits on chronic HFrEF.

Hospitalist Tip

For managing ESRD with pulmonary edema, ADHF includes ultrafiltration in stable patients or sustained low-efficiency dialysis (SLED) in critically ill patients with pressure needs. Remember that CHF, either systolic or diastolic, ACS, and arrhythmias are not uncommon in ESRD patients.

1.23 Heart Failure with Preserved Ejection Fraction (HFpEF)

- Use the H2FPEF score to assist in diagnosing heart failure with preserved ejection fraction (HFpEF), which is common in obese patients with hypertension and atrial fibrillation. An echocardiogram supports the diagnosis with findings of concentric left ventricle remodeling, left atrial dilatation, diastolic dysfunction, and pulmonary hypertension. The finding of resting PCWP >15 mm Hg or PCWP >25 mm Hg with exercise is diagnostic for HFpEF in the right clinical context [21]. B-type natriuretic peptide (BNP) levels may be falsely low, particularly in obese patients.
- Uncontrolled hypertension, hypervolemia, and arrhythmias are common triggers for acute decompensated heart failure (ADHF) in HFpEF.

In contrast, coronary artery disease (CAD) or ischemic heart disease (IHD) is less likely but should still be ruled out. Managing hypertension, using diuretics for hypervolemia, and addressing arrhythmias preferably through catheter ablation can improve cardiac hemodynamics [22].

- Only the following medications, exercise, and weight loss may improve long-term outcomes in HFpEF. These can be initiated before discharge and titrated or added gradually on an outpatient basis.
  (i) GLP-1 receptor agonists and SGLT2 inhibitors. Strong evidence to improve mortality [32].
  (ii) Aldosterone antagonists. Good evidence to shorten hospitalization, but not necessarily mortality [38].
  (iii) Entresto™. The FDA approved it for all patients with heart failure, regardless of ejection fraction. It will mainly benefit patients with EF between 45% and 55% [39].

Hospitalist Tip

Elevated diastolic dysfunction E/e', LA volume/size, RVSP, and BNP in a patient with dyspnea and normal EF should think HFpEF. However, normal BNP and echo do not rule out HFpEF.

1.24 Uncontrolled Afib with ADHF

A. Suppose a patient is hemodynamically unstable with acute decompensated heart failure (ADHF) and worsening shortness of breath (SOB) and has a heart rate greater than 150 beats per minute. Cardioversion should be performed electrically or chemically by advanced cardiovascular life support (ACLS) guidelines. Due to the high risk of thrombosis in acute atrial fibrillation (Afib), anticoagulation should be initiated with unfractionated heparin or low molecular weight heparin (LMWH). However, the priority is to perform cardioversion to stabilize the patient, which should not be delayed.

B. If the patient is stable with mild shortness of breath (SOB) and uncontrolled acute atrial fibrillation (Afib), consider rate control over rhythm control if there is uncertainty regarding thrombosis risk or the presence of a cardiac clot. Preferably, use digoxin or amiodarone in the presence of moderate to severe pulmonary edema. Avoid beta-blockers or cardiac selective calcium channel blockers (CCB) if there is concern about worsening pulmonary edema due to their adverse inotropic effects. Once the patient is more euvolemic, it is acceptable to introduce beta-blockers or cardiac selective CCB (avoid in HFrEF) (◘ Tables 1.5 and 1.6). More details in chap. 4.

1.25 Acceptable Options for Cardioversion on Hemodynamically Unstable Patients with Acute Afib (◘ Table 1.5)

◘ Table 1.5 Acceptable options for cardioversion in patients with ADHF and uncontrolled acute atrial fibrillation with rapid ventricular response, in those who are hemodynamically unstable

Modality	Dose	Comments
Direct current cardioversion/ synchronized	100–200 joules	Pre-sedate using versed 1–5 mg and fentanyl 12.5–50 mcg
Amiodarone	150 mg intravenously initially over 10 minutes, followed by 1 mg/min infusion for 6 hours, and then 0.5 mg/min infusion for 18 hours; 600–800 mg/day orally given in 2–3 divided doses up to a total loading dose of up to 10 g, followed by 200 mg once daily	

1.26 Acceptable Options for Rate Control on Hemodynamically Stable Patients with Acute Afib and ADHF (Table 1.6)

Pearl

Digoxin should be considered for ADHF with HFrEF and uncontrolled Afib (it lowers heart rate and improves contractility) or in patients resistant to standard therapy alone. It is a good option when BP is marginally low or soft, and there is no room for more diuretics or antihypertensives. However, it has no mortality benefit but reduces hospitalization [23].

Table 1.6 Acceptable options for rate control in patients with ADHF and uncontrolled acute atrial fibrillation with rapid ventricular response, in those who are hemodynamically stable

Modality	Dose	Comments
Digoxin	10.75 to 1.5 mg intravenously, as a loading dose given in divided doses on the first day, followed by a maintenance dose of 0.125 to 0.5 mg orally once daily	The use of digoxin is considered reasonable in specific scenarios, such as in patients with heart failure with reduced ejection fraction (HFrEF) and low or soft blood pressure. It is important to note that digoxin does not exert its effects immediately; it requires several hours to become effective
Amiodarone	300 mg intravenously initially over 1 hour, followed by 10–50 mg/hour infusion for 24 hours, and then 100–200 mg once daily	This lower dose is appropriate for rate control, not rhythm control. It is off-label use (not FDA approved)

1.27 Acute Right-Sided Heart Failure (RHF) [24]

- The presence of predominant left-sided heart failure is treated in the same way as pure left-sided heart failure.

Pearl

The primary goal in the setting of acute RHF is to avoid systemic hypotension to prevent sequel events such as myocardial ischemia and further hypotension.

- Treatment of predominant acute right heart failure focuses on three concepts: (1) preload optimization, (2) after load reduction, and (3) improvement of contractility. You should always consult with an intensivist and senior cardiologist, as the treatment approach is complicated, and the patient may deteriorate quickly.
  1. *Preload optimization* by adjusting volume needs is pivotal. If the patient is volume overloaded and his BP is acceptable, consider progressive diuresis of 500–1000 ml daily. However, if the patient is hypotensive, a bolus of 500 ml is given as needed until stabilization or pressors are required; that is characteristically true in acute RV infarction, where the RV output is impaired due to contractile dysfunction, but the afterload is normal; a higher preload is needed to keep the forward flow. Right heart catheterization may be necessary if volume estimation is difficult; RV diastolic filling pressure of 8–12 mmHg is optimal in RHF.
  2. *Afterload reduction*, mainly through pulmonary vasodilators, is used in conditions with high pulmonary vascular resistance (PVR). This is a problem in advanced left heart failure or primary right-sided pathology, such as corpulmonale. Choices to consider include inhaled nitric oxide (iNO), prostanoids, phosphodiesterase-5 (PDE5), endothelin receptor antagonists, and riociguat. All should be initiated in the critical care unit.
  3. *Improvement of contractility* is essential in patients who are hypotensive with severely elevated pulmonary artery pressure and signs of low cardiac output. Options include dobutamine and milrinone. If the patient remains hemodynamically unstable, mechanical support is usually needed, pending transplant eligibility if possible.

Hospitalist Tip

Treatment of RV ischemia/infarction with failure involves revascularization, adequate filling pressure, and avoidance of therapeutic agents that cause vasodilation and decreased RV filling, such as diuretics and nitrates. The initial recommendation is a volume challenge of 300–600 ml of normal saline over 10–15 min via a central line or a large-bore peripheral intravenous site. Invasive hemodynamic monitoring is preferred with cardiology input since further infusion is damaging when additional increases in the RV volume may prevent sufficient LV filling [25]. Maintain the proper atrial pressure at <18 mmHg to avoid volume overload. Pacing may be needed in advanced heart block to maintain synchrony, leading to preserving cardiac output. So remember revascularization, fluids +/– pressors or mechanical support, pacing, and avoiding vasodilators.

1.28 Cardiogenic Shock

- It is characterized by a significant reduction in cardiac output and end-organ hypoperfusion, evidenced by symptoms such as worsening altered mental status (AMS), acute kidney injury (AKI), cool extremities, prolonged capillary refill time greater than 2 seconds, and peripheral cyanosis, in a patient with systolic blood pressure (BP) below 90 mmHg. Therefore, low BP alone is not diagnostic [26]. Laboratory findings typically show elevated lactate levels, raised liver function tests (LFTs) due to ischemic liver damage, and AKI. Routine right heart invasive hemodynamic monitoring is not generally recommended, though it remains controversial [31]. It may be helpful in complex cases where the cause of shock is unclear or mixed, hemodynamics fluctuate, and volume status is challenging to optimize.
- It is vital to rule out ACS, if possible, with angiography.
- Most patients will require continuous vasopressor support in addition to addressing the underlying cause if it is reversible. These patients should be managed in a critical or cardiac intensive care unit (CICU).
- The preferred vasopressor is typically norepinephrine [27], although no definitive evidence supports the superiority of one vasopressor over another [28] (◘ Table 1.7). Other relevant options include dobutamine and milrinone. However, Initiating vasoactive agents that raise systemic vascular resistance, such as phenylephrine or vasopressin, is contraindicated in patients with cardiogenic shock with the exception of LVOT obstruction (such as HOCM or severe LVH), as dobutamine and norepinephrine can worsen obstruction by increasing LV contractility. For severe hypotension, phenylephrine can be used to raise blood pressure and reduce obstruction by increasing afterload.
- If the patient did not respond to the vasopressor, consider bridging with mechanical support such as intra-aortic balloon pump (IABP), ECMO, or Impella pending transplantation if eligible. Another consideration is to consider palliative support with a hospice comfort pathway.
- Once the patient is stable and within 24 hours of the last inotropy dose, GDMT options could be started cautiously [17].

Pearl

Inotropes should be used for the short term, expecting a definitive plan. They are not recommended for use in patients with HFpEF.

1.29 Vasopressor Options in Cardiogenic Shock (Table 1.7)

Table 1.7 Different Vasopressor options in cardiogenic shock

Vasopressor	Dose(follow institution protocol)	Comments
Norepinephrine (α1, α2 receptor agonist, less β1 receptor agonism)	12–4 mcg/min IV; start: 2.5–10 mcg/min IV, then titrate to effect; every few minutes	First line in shock
Dobutamine (β1, β2 receptor agonism)	2–20 mcg/kg/min IV	Higher doses lead to vasoconstriction, so you need higher doses in shock. Dobutamine and milrinone can cause arrhythmias and worsening of ischemia. Considered first line by many cardiologists
Milrinone (phosphodiesterase inhibition)	0.125–0.75 mcg/kg/min, usually as a constant infusion	Milrinone is an effective therapeutic agent used in the management of refractory heart failure (HF), particularly in cases characterized by low cardiac output, high PCWP, and elevated or normal pulmonary or systemic vascular resistance. It functions as a phosphodiesterase-3 inhibitor, increasing intracellular cyclic AMP and enhancing myocardial contractility and vasodilation. This dual action helps to improve cardiac output and reduce the workload on the heart, making it a critical option for patients who do not adequately respond to conventional treatments

1.30 Algorithm for Worsening ADHF with Shock [28]

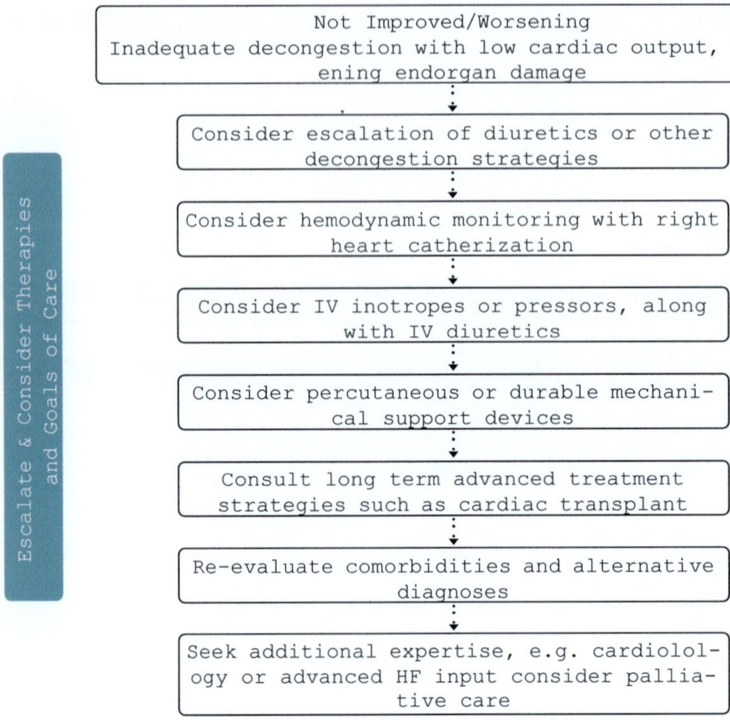

Pearl

In advanced heart failure with refractory symptoms not responding to treatment options, most patients will either need heart transplantation or mechanical circulatory support option to prolong survival. Below are very brief notes on these options. However, mechanical support does not improve mortality, and it is only transitionary regarding more definitive intervention, namely revascularization in patients with ACS [29].

A. *Heart transplantation*

- Orthotopic heart transplants lack innervation, so medications like atropine and adenosine usually will not work. They are generally indicated for selected patients with no major allosensitization. Median survival is 11–12 years after the transplant.
- Major contraindications include active drug use, active malignancy or infections, high pulmonary vascular resistance (>5–6 Wood units), advanced noncardiac conditions, lack of social support, and age above >70 years old.

- Most patients must continue on immunosuppressant agents after transplantation, including antibiotic prophylaxis with valganciclovir (if the donor or recipient is CMV+) and TMP/sulfa, so check for drug interactions while hospitalized. Common complications include rejection (new diastolic dysfunction and atrial arrhythmias), infections (CMV/HSV/pneumocystis/toxoplasma), lymphoproliferative disorder (lymphoma), and allograft vasculopathy (CAD) if at least 1 year after transplant.The gold standard for the diagnosis of cellular rejection is endomyocardial biopsy not cardiac MRI.
- Rejection may present as worsening heart failure and is of two types: either cell-mediated or antibody-mediated. If suspected, it always needs a right ventricular endomyocardial biopsy with a referral to a higher center of care. In the meantime, use high-dose steroid methylprednisolone 1 g/day for 3 days.

B. *Mechanical circulatory support*
- Indicated in advanced end-stage heart failure patients, with EF ≤25% to qualify for mechanical support. Most patients will need to continue on anticoagulation with warfarin and aspirin so that they may need bridging before any procedure. The patient may not have a pulse or BP readings (due to continuous flow). The device needs to be deactivated at the end of life, like a pacemaker-dependent patient.
- Similar contraindications to a heart transplant, except there is no specific age or weight limit.
- Major complications include infections with bacteremia, mechanical thrombus with systemic emboli with leg ischemia, RV dysfunctions, and bleeding tendency.

References

1. Alla F, Zannad F, Filippatos G. Epidemiology of acute heart failure syndromes. Heart Fail Rev. 2007;12(2):91–5.
2. Tromp J, et al. Regional differences in precipitating factors of hospitalization for acute heart failure: insights from the *REPORT-HF* registry. Jasper Tromp. 2022;24(4):645–52.
3. Nieminen MS, Brutsaert D, Dickstein K, et al. EuroHeart Failure Survey II (EHFS II): a survey on hospitalized acute heart failure patients: population description. Eur Heart J. 2006 Nov;27(22):2725–36.
4. Gillespie ND, McNeill G, Pringle T, et al. A cross-sectionalstudy of the contribution of clinical assessment and simple cardiac investigations to diagnose left ventricular systolic dysfunction in patients admitted with acute dyspnoea. BMJ. 1997;314(7085):936–40.
5. Khan NK, Goode KM, Cleland JG, et al. Prevalence of ECG abnormalities in an international survey of patients with suspected or confirmed heart failure at death or discharge. Eur J Heart Fail. 2007;9(5):491–501.
6. McDonagh TA, Metra M, Adamo M, et al. 2021 ESC guidelines for the diagnosis and treatment of acute and chronic heart failure. Eur Heart J. 2021;42(36):3599–726.
7. Fonarow GC, Peacock WF, Phillips CO, et al. Admission B-type natriuretic peptide levels and in hospital mortality in acute decompensated heart failure. J Am CollCardiol. 2007;49(19):1943–50.
8. Perna ER, Macin SM, Parras JI, et al. Cardiac troponin T levels are associated with poor short and long-term prognosis in patients with acute cardiogenic pulmonary edema. Am Heart J. 2002;143(5):814–20.

9. See ASY, Ho JS, Chan MY, Lim YC, Yeo TC, Chai P, Wong RCC, Lin W, Sia CH. Prevalence and risk factors of cardiac amyloidosis in heart failure: a systematic review and meta-analysis. Heart Lung Circ. 2022;31(11):1450–62. https://doi.org/10.1016/j.hlc.2022.08.002. Epub 2022 Sep 20. PMID: 36137915
10. CT or invasive coronary angiography in stable chest pain, the DISCHARGE Trial Group, April 2022.
11. Rybicki FJ, Udelson JE, Peacock WF, Goldhaber SZ, Isselbacher EM, Kazerooni E, Kontos MC, Litt H, Woodard PK. 2015 ACR/ACC/AHA/AATS/ACEP/ASNC/NASCI/SAEM/SCCT/SCMR/SCPC/SNMMI/STR/STS appropriate utilization of cardiovascular imaging in emergency department patients with chest pain: a joint document of the American College of Radiology Appropriateness Criteria Committee and the American College of Cardiology Appropriate use Criteria Task Force. J Am Coll Cardiol. 2016;67(7):853–79. https://doi.org/10.1016/j.jacc.2015.09.011. Epub 2016 Jan 22. PMID: 26809772
12. Markatis E, Afthinos A, Antonakis E, Papanikolaou IC. Cardiac sarcoidosis: diagnosis and management. Rev Cardiovasc Med. 2020;21(3):321–38. https://doi.org/10.31083/j.rcm.2020.03.102. [12a] McDonagh TA, Metra M, Adamo M, et al. 2021 ESC Guidelines for diagnosing and treating acute and chronic heart failure. Eur Heart J. 2021;42(36):3599–726. [12b] Ni Y-N, Luo J, Yu H, et al. Can high-flow nasal cannula reduce the rate of endotracheal intubation in adult patients with acute respiratory failure compared with conventional oxygen therapy and noninvasive positive pressure ventilation?: a systematic review and metaanalysis. Chest 2017;151:764–75. [12c] Chawla R, Dixit SB, Zirpe KG, Chaudhry D, Khilnani GC, Mehta Y, Khatib KI, Jagiasi BG, Chanchalani G, Mishra RC, Samavedam S, Govil D, Gupta S, Prayag S, Ramasubban S, Dobariya J, Marwah V, Sehgal I, Jog SA, Kulkarni AP. ISCCM guidelines for non-invasive ventilation in acute respiratory failure in adult ICUs. Indian J Crit Care Med. 2020;24(Suppl 1):S61–81. https://doi.org/10.5005/jp-journals-10071-G23186. PMID: 32205957; PM-CID: PMC7085817. PMID: 33070538
13. Basset A, Nowak E, Castellant P, Gut-Gobert C, Le Gal G, L'Her E. Development of a clinical prediction score for congestive heart failure diagnosis in the emergency care setting: the Brest score. Am J Emerg Med. 2016;34(12):2277–83. https://doi.org/10.1016/j.ajem.2016.08.023. Epub 2016 Aug 14. PMID: 27599400
14. Collins SP, Peacock WF, Lindsell CJ, Clopton P, Diercks DB, Hiestand B, Hogan C, Kontos MC, Mueller C, Nowak R, Chen WJ, Huang CH, Abraham WT, Amsterdam E, Breidthardt T, Daniels L, Hasan A, Hudson M, McCord J, Naz T, Wagoner LE, Maisel A. S3 detection as a diagnostic and prognostic aid in emergency department patients with acute dyspnea. Ann Emerg Med. 2009;53(6):748–57. https://doi.org/10.1016/j.annemergmed.2008.12.029. Epub 2009 Feb 20. PMID: 19232777
15. Marinacci LX, Simeone FJ, Lundquist AL, Kuter DJ, Mahowald GK. Case 38-2020: a 52-year-old man with cancer and acute hypoxemia. N EnglJ Med. 2020;383(24):2372–83. https://doi.org/10.1056/NEJMcpc2004991. PMID: 33296564
16. Mullens W, Dauw J, Martens P, Verbrugge FH, Nijst P, Meekers E, Tartaglia K, Chenot F, Moubayed S, Dierckx R, Blouard P, Troisfontaines P, Derthoo D, Smolders W, Bruckers L, Droogne W, Ter Maaten JM, Damman K, Lassus J, Mebazaa A, Filippatos G, Ruschitzka F, Dupont M, AD-VOR Study Group. Acetazolamide in Acute Decompensated Heart Failure with Volume Overload. N EnglJ Med. 2022;387(13):1185–95. https://doi.org/10.1056/NEJMoa2203094. Epub 2022 Aug 27. PMID: 36027559
17. 2024 ACC Expert Consensus Decision Pathway on Clinical Assessment, Management, and Trajectory of Patients Hospitalized With Heart Failure Focused Update.
18. Suri SS, Pamboukian SV. Optimal diuretic strategies in heart failure. Ann Transl Med. 2021;9(6):517. https://doi.org/10.21037/atm-20-4600. PMID: 33850914; PMCID: PMC8039650
19. Peixoto AJ. Acute severe hypertension. New England Journal of Medicine. 2019;381(19):1843–52. https://doi.org/10.1056/NEJMcp1901117. M31693807. https:/www.nejm.org/doi/full/10.1056/NEJMcp1901117
20. Lo KB, Rangaswami J. Mechanistic insights in Cardiorenal Syndrome. NEJM Evid. 2022;1(9):EVIDra2200053. https://doi.org/10.1056/EVIDra2200053. Epub 2022 Aug 23. PMID: 38319803.

21. Rush CJ, Berry C, Oldroyd KG, Rocchiccioli JP, Lindsay MM, Touyz RM, Murphy CL, Ford TJ, Sidik N, McEntegart MB, Lang NN, Jhund PS, Campbell RT, McMurray JJV, Petrie MC. Prevalence of Coronary Artery disease and coronary microvascular dysfunction in patients with heart failure with preserved ejection fraction. JAMA Cardiol. 2021;6(10):1130–43. https://doi.org/10.1001/jamacardio.2021.1825. PMID: 34160566; PMCID: PMC8223134
22. Packer DL, Piccini JP, Monahan KH, Al-Khalidi HR, Silverstein AP, Noseworthy PA, Poole JE, Bahnson TD, Lee KL, Mark DB, CABANA Investigators. Ablation versus drug therapy for atrial fibrillation in heart failure: results from the CABANA Trial. Circulation. 2021;143(14):1377–90. https://doi.org/10.1161/CIRCULATIONAHA.120.050991. Epub 2021 Feb 8. PMID: 33554614; PMCID: PMC8030730
23. Hood WB Jr, Dans AL, Guyatt GH, et al. Digitalis for treatment of heart failure in patients in sinus rhythm. Cochrane Database Syst Rev. 2014;4:CD002901.
24. Alcantara CAP, Chandra A, Morvey D, von Schwarz ER. Acute right heart failure. Right Heart Pathol. 2018:215–25. https://doi.org/10.1007/978-3-319-73764-5_10. PMCID: PMC7123149
25. Ondrus T, Kanovsky J, Novotny T, Anderson I, Spinar J, Kala P. Right ventricular myocardial infarction: from pathophysiology to prognosis. Exp Clin Cardiol. 2013;18(1):27–30.
26. Tanaka H. Effect of Ivabradine on left ventricular reverse remodeling in relatively stable heart failure outpatients with reduced ejection fraction. Circ Rep. 2024;6(5):183–6. https://doi.org/10.1253/circrep.CR-24-0034. PMID: 38736845; PMCID: PMC11081702
27. Heidenreich PA, Bozkurt B, Aguilar D, et al. 2022 AHA/ACC/HFSA guideline for the management of heart failure: a report of the American College of Cardiology/American Heart Association Joint Committee on Clinical Practice Guidelines. Circulation. 2022;145(18):e895–e1032.
28. Hollenberg SM, Warner Stevenson L, Ahmad T, Amin VJ, Bozkurt B, Butler J, Davis LL, Drazner MH, Kirkpatrick JN, Peterson PN, Reed BN, Roy CL, Storrow AB. 2019 ACC expert consensus decision pathway on risk assessment, management, and clinical trajectory of patients hospitalized with heart failure: a report of the American College of Cardiology Solution Set Oversight Committee. J Am Coll Cardiol. 2019;74(15):1966–2011. https://doi.org/10.1016/j.jacc.2019.08.001. Epub 2019 Sep 13. Erratum in: J Am Coll Cardiol. 2020 Jan 7;75(1):132. PMID: 31526538
29. Jung RG, Stotts C, Gupta A, Prosperi-Porta G, Dhaliwal S, Motazedian P, Abdel-Razek O, Di Santo P, Parlow S, Belley-Cote E, Tran A, van Diepen S, Harel-Sterling L, Goyal V, Lepage-Ratte MF, Mathew R, Jentzer JC, Price S, Naidu SS, Basir MB, Kapur NK, Thiele H, Ramirez FD, Wells G, Rochwerg B, Fernando SM, Hibbert B. Prognostic factors associated with mortality in cardiogenic shock – a systematic review and meta-analysis. NEJM Evid. 2024;3(11):EVIDoa2300323. https://doi.org/10.1056/EVIDoa2300323. Epub 2024 Oct 22. PMID: 39437131
30. Torres-Courchoud I, Chen HH. Is there still a role for low-dose dopamine use in acute heart failure? Curr Opin Crit Care. 2014;20(5):467–71. https://doi.org/10.1097/MCC.0000000000000133. PMID: 25137402
31. Osman M, Syed M, Patel B, Munir MB, Kheiri B, Caccamo M, Sokos G, Balla S, Basir MB, Kapur NK, Mamas MA, Bianco CM. Invasive hemodynamic monitoring in cardiogenic shock is associated with lower in-hospital mortality. J Am Heart Assoc. 2021;10(18):e021808. https://doi.org/10.1161/JAHA.121.021808. Epub 2021 Sep 13. PMID: 34514850; PMCID: PMC8649539
32. Gao FM, Ali AS, Bellomo R, Gaca M, Lecamwasam A, Churilov L, Ekinci EI. A systematic review and meta-analysis on the safety and efficacy of sodium-glucose cotransporter 2 inhibitor use in hospitalized patients. Diabetes Care. 2024;47(12):2275–90. https://doi.org/10.2337/dc24-0946. PMID: 39602586
33. Alexander P, Alkhawam L, Curry J, Levy P, Pang PS, Storrow AB, Collins SP. Lack of evidence for intravenous vasodilators in ED patients with acute heart failure: a systematic review. Am J Emerg Med. 2015;33(2):133–41. https://doi.org/10.1016/j.ajem.2014.09.009. Epub 2014 Sep 18. PMID: 25530194; PM-CID: PMC4344879

34. Velazquez EJ, Morrow DA, DeVore AD, Duffy CI, Ambrosy AP, McCague K, Rocha R, Braunwald E, PIONEER-HF Investigators. Angiotensin-Neprilysin inhibition in acute decompensated heart failure. N Engl J Med. 2019;380(6):539–48. https://doi.org/10.1056/NEJMoa1812851. Epub 2018 Nov 11. Erratum in: N EnglJ Med. 2019 Mar 14;380(11):1090. https://doi.org/10.1056/NEJMx190009. PMID: 30415601
35. Brennan MT, Harmouch KM, Basit J, Alraies MC. Beta-blocker usage in patients with heart failure with reduced ejection fraction during acute decompensated heart failure hospitalizations. Ochsner J. 2024;24(3):198–203. https://doi.org/10.31486/toj.24.0011. PMID: 39280877; PMCID: PMC11398626
36. Prins KW, Neill JM, Tyler JO, Eckman PM, Duval S. Effects of beta-blocker withdrawal in acute decompensated heart failure: a systematic review and meta-analysis. JACC Heart Fail. 2015;3(8):647–53. https://doi.org/10.1016/j.jchf.2015.03.008. Erratum in: JACC Heart Fail. 2015 Oct;3(10):847. PMID: 26251094; PMCID: PMC4777602
37. Al-Khatib SM, Stevenson WG, Ackerman MJ, Bryant WJ, Callans DJ, Curtis AB, Deal BJ, Dickfeld T, Field ME, Fonarow GC, Gillis AM, Granger CB, Hammill SC, Hlatky MA, Joglar JA, Kay GN, Matlock DD, Myerburg RJ, Page RL. 2017 AHA/ACC/HRS guideline for managing patients with ventricular arrhythmias and preventing sudden cardiac death: executive summary: a report of the American College of Cardiology/American Heart Association task force on clinical practice guidelines and the Heart Rhythm Society. Heart Rhythm. 2018;15(10):e190–252. https://doi.org/10.1016/j.hrthm.2017.10.035. Epub 2017 Oct 30. Erratum in: Heart Rhythm. 2018 Nov;15(11):e278-e281. https://doi.org/10.1016/j.hrthm.2018.09.026. PMID: 29097320
38. Sethi R, Vishwakarma P, Pradhan A. Evidence for aldosterone antagonism in heart failure. Card Fail Rev. 2024;10:e15. https://doi.org/10.15420/cfr.2024.10. PMID: 39588014; PMCID: PMC11588114
39. Fala L. Entresto (Sacubitril/Valsartan): first-in-class angiotensin receptor Neprilysin inhibitor FDA approved for patients with heart failure. Am Health Drug Benefits. 2015;8(6):330–4. PMID: 26557227; PMCID: PMC4636283

Acute Severe HTN

Contents

M. Salih, *Practical Hospitalist Guide to Inpatient Cardiology*, https://doi.org/10.1007/978-3-032-03240-9_2

2

This chapter delves into identifying and managing hypertensive crises, characterized by blood pressures exceeding 180/110 mmHg. It emphasizes the importance of recognizing hypertensive urgencies, often marked by mild symptoms but lacking end-organ damage, and contrasts them with hypertensive emergencies where immediate intervention is required due to potential organ damage. Common inpatient triggers include medication nonadherence, excessive IV fluids, and stress-related factors. While hypertensive urgencies might seem benign in the short term, they pose significant long-term cardiovascular risks. The chapter provides guidance on the appropriate clinical approach, highlighting the importance of accurate blood pressure measurement and the need for follow-up to ensure optimal long-term management. It also advises against the routine use of IV antihypertensive medications in non-emergent situations.

2.1 When to Suspect and Main Causes [1, 2]

- Consider the condition when BP is more than or equal to 180/110 in asymptomatic patients with mild symptoms (such as nausea, epistaxis, mild dizziness, mild headache, or non ischemic chest pain) and absence of end-organ injury. It is exceptionally common and present in up to 72% of hospital admissions.
- It is mostly a benign problem in the short term and should not trigger urgent IV BP control [3]. However, it is not harmless in the long run, as there is around 50% higher risk of cardiovascular events for patients with hypertension (HTN) urgency than patients without HTN urgency [4].
- Common inpatient hypertensive crisis precipitants include:

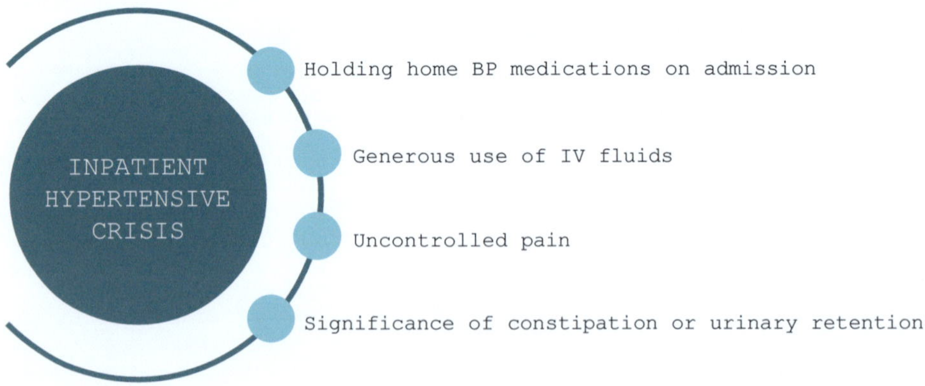

2.2 Mechanisms for Elevated BP in the Acute Care Setting [2]

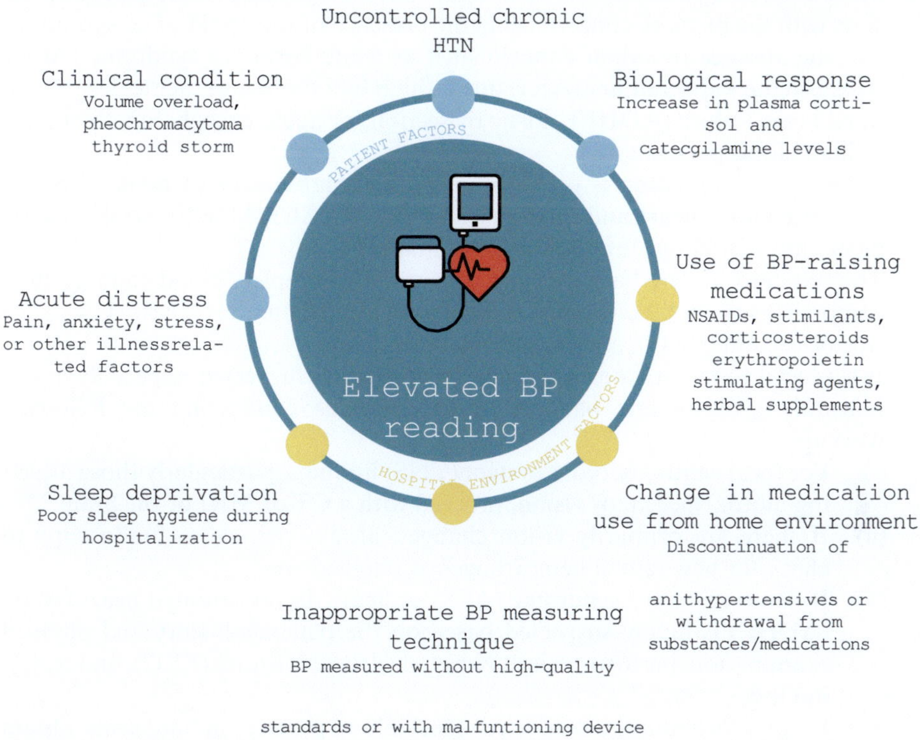

Pearl

Nonadherence to home-prescribed antihypertensive medications is the most common factor leading to a hypertensive crisis [1].

Pearl

In contrast to worse long-term cardiovascular risk, hypertensive urgencies do not appear to be associated with adverse short-term outcomes [5].

2.3 Clinical Approach

- Most frequently, a nurse will seek further advice regarding elevated blood pressure, with the primary concern being the presence of only mild or no symptoms and the absence of organ damage such as acute coronary syndrome (ACS), stroke, acute kidney injury (AKI) due to high blood pressure, acute decompensated heart failure (ADHF), aortic dissection, or acute encephalopathy linked to high blood pressure.
- A focused examination is prudent, including comparisons of bilateral pulses (for dissection), heart and lung auscultation (for ACS/ADHF), stroke assessment, and a brief eye fundoscopy examination.
- The standard of care basic workup consists of a complete blood count (CBC), comprehensive metabolic panel (CMP) with electrolytes, urinalysis (UA), electrocardiogram (EKG), and troponin levels [1].
- It is crucial to investigate end-organ damage when suspected, especially in significantly symptomatic patients, which includes conducting the following workup:
  - (i) For focal central nervous system (CNS) findings, particularly those affecting motor, speech, or vision, proceed with a CT or MRI of the brain.
  - (ii) If there are primarily vision changes, always perform a fundoscopy to check for new retinal hemorrhages or papilledema.
  - (iii) If acute coronary syndrome (ACS) or acute decompensated heart failure (ADHF) is highly suspected based on the patient's history and physical examination, perform a chest X-ray, electrocardiogram (EKG), and troponin test.
  - (iv) If aortic dissection is suspected, check blood pressure in both arms, obtain a chest X-ray, and proceed with CT angiography.
  - (v) If significant acute kidney injury (AKI) is suspected, indicated by oliguria, anuria, or uremic symptoms, proceed with a comprehensive metabolic panel (CMP), electrolyte test, and urinalysis (UA) to check for protein and blood.
  - (vi) If microangiopathic hemolytic anemia is suspected, conduct a complete blood count (CBC), lactate dehydrogenase (LDH), and haptoglobin test and examine a peripheral blood smear to identify hemolysis and thrombocytopenia.
  - (vii) If posterior reversible encephalopathy syndrome (PRESS) or reversible cerebral vasoconstriction syndrome (RCVS) is suspected, typically indicated by symptoms such as headache, visual changes, or new seizures, proceed with an MRI of the brain.

Pearl

Routine extensive workup in asymptomatic patients is not advised due to low yield [1]. Only proceed with workup based on symptoms and suspected end-organ damage of focus.

Pearl

Precipitants are likely linked to medication nonadherence by the patient, stress-related hypertension from acute conditions, or hospitalization.

Hospitalist Tip

Pseudohypertension is a term some physicians use to describe the acute rise in blood pressure due to acute medical conditions or symptoms such as severe headaches. In this case, treatment involves addressing the underlying headache or the acute medical condition.

2.4 Approach for Hypertensive Crisis [1]

2

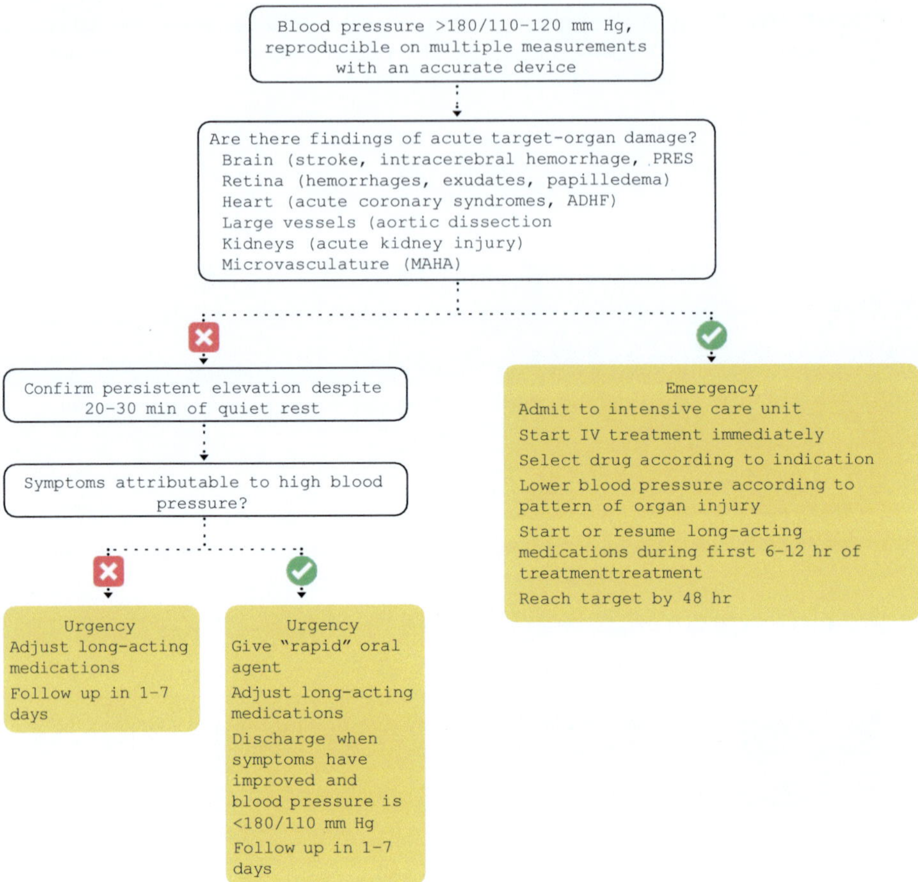

2.5 Major DD

1. **HTN emergency**
   - The patient will usually have end-organ damage.
2. **2nd HTN**
   - The patient will have features consistent with secondary HTN.

2.6 Management Approach

- Repeat the blood pressure check with a different device or manually. No urgent treatment with intravenous blood pressure medications is indicated, as using them may lead to worse outcomes and should be avoided. Instead, treat the underlying acute condition or stressor, and discontinue medications or unnecessary intravenous fluids that may induce hypertension [2]. Resume home blood pressure medication if missed during admission orders, and adjust the dose or add new medication if deemed necessary.

- The goal is to follow up with the patient shortly after discharge with their primary care provider within 1 week to adjust medication gradually, if necessary [1]. If the patient does not have a known history of hypertension but exhibits persistently elevated inpatient hypertension and concern for chronically elevated ambulatory hypertension, it may be reasonable to start oral guideline-directed blood pressure medications [2]. It will take days to weeks to fully optimize the blood pressure medications, so avoid being overly aggressive.
- Testing for secondary causes of hypertension may be reasonable for unclear, persistently elevated blood pressure [5].

Hospitalist Tip

Avoid the practice of intravenous PRN orders for antihypertensive medications, as it is harmful [2].

Hospitalist Tip

Occasionally, in patients with hypertension urgency accompanied by symptoms (but not indicative of target-organ damage) and concern for imminent end-organ injury, a focused examination is advisable. This should include comparing bilateral pulses (for dissection), heart and lung auscultation (for ACS/ADHF), and stroke assessment. Monitoring the patient while hospitalized or ensuring close follow-up with their provider within 1–7 days after discharge is acceptable. Choices for fast-acting medications include clonidine (0.1 to 0.3 mg), labetalol (200 to 400 mg), captopril (25 to 50 mg), prazosin (5 to 10 mg), or nitroglycerin 2% topical ointment (1 to 2 inches). On average, these medications can acutely lower blood pressure in about 30 min and may be administered every 30 min until the target blood pressure is achieved (usually below 180/110).

2.7 Hypertensive Emergency

2.7.1 When to Suspect

- Hypertensive emergencies are suspected when blood pressure is significantly elevated, typically exceeding 180/110 mmHg, accompanied by evidence of end-organ damage or injury [2, 6].

- Common manifestations of end-organ damage include acute coronary syndrome (ACS), aortic dissection, acute decompensated heart failure (ADHF), ischemic or hemorrhagic stroke, acute unexplained encephalopathy, microvascular injury, and acute kidney injury (AKI).

Pearl

Diffuse microvascular injury is characterized by advanced retinopathy, which may manifest as hemorrhages, exudates, or papilledema, as well as acute kidney injury (AKI), microangiopathic hemolytic anemia, or thrombocytopenia. These complications can occur individually or in combination.

2.7.2 Clinical Approach [6]

- In hypertensive emergencies, patients should be managed in a progressive care unit (PCU) or intensive care unit (ICU) setting, where close blood pressure monitoring via an arterial line and frequent vital sign checks are conducted according to hospital protocol aligned with each end-organ damage criterion.
- The initial diagnostic workup is guided by the anticipated end-organ injury, as determined by the patient's history, physical examination, and laboratory findings. Essential tests include a complete blood count (CBC), comprehensive metabolic panel (CMP), troponin, B-type natriuretic peptide (BNP), urinalysis (UA), electrocardiogram (EKG), chest X-ray, CT scan of the brain, and possibly an MRI. The selection of specific tests from this list depends on the patient's clinical presentation; for instance, CT scans and potential MRIs are crucial for patients exhibiting stroke symptoms. Remember the acronym BARKH (brain, arteries, retina, kidney, heart) to help identify and rule out target-organ damage (9).

2.7.3 Treatment Approach [2]

- Blood pressure should be monitored in conjunction with assessing underlying end-organ damage. Intravenous (IV) titratable blood pressure medications are essential, administered with an arterial line in place (9). All patients must be observed in a progressive care unit (PCU) or intensive care unit (ICU) setting. The primary objective is to reduce blood pressure, preferably following the mean blood pressure, by no more than 20 to 25% within the first hour, corresponding to the lower autoregulation physiological limit. This reduction is crucial because autoregulation mechanisms can fail if blood pressure drops below this threshold. Subsequently, blood pressure should be aimed at 160/100–110 mmHg over the next 2 to 6 h [6]. The exact rate of blood pressure reduction can vary depending on the specific end-organ damage or injury present. Long-acting oral blood pressure medications should be restarted or initiated within 6–12 h after starting IV medication to avoid the high risk of hypotension within that period. The IV blood pressure medication should be gradually tapered off within 48–72 h [2]. Patients can be discharged once hypertension is reasonably controlled for at least 24 h without the need for intravenous therapy.

2.7.4 Treatment Approaches Based on End-Organ Damage [7]

Acute target-organ damage	Timing for acute BP reduction[a]	Preferred intravenous drugs[b]
Diffuse microvascular injury ("malignant hypertension")[c]	Decrease BP by 15–25% during the first hour and to 160/100 mmHg by 2–6 h	Labetalol, nicardipine, nitroprusside
Hypertensive encephalopathy	If systolic BP is 150–220 mmHg, decrease systolic BP to 140–150 mmHg within 1 h, particularly in patients without known hypertension and those with underlying vascular abnormalities, such as aneurysms or arteriovenous malformations. In patients with large hematoma volume and evidence of increased intracranial pressure, BP management should be more liberal (keep systolic BP <180 mmHg). Lowering systolic BP below 140 mmHg maybe harmful	Labetalol, nicardipine, clevidipine, nitroprusside; avoid hydralazine
Acute ischemic stroke	If thrombolytic therapy is indicated, decrease BP to <185/110 mmHg before giving thrombolytic agents and maintain BP <180/105 mmHg for the first 24 h. If thrombolytic therapy is not indicated and there is no acute target-organ damage other than stroke, the strategy depends on BP. If BP is <220/120 mmHg, no intervention is indicated for the first 48–72 h. If BP is ≥220/120 mmHg or there is other acute target-organ damage, such as heart failure or myocardial infarction, decrease BP by 15% within 1 h	Labetalol, nicardipine, clevidipine, nitroprusside; avoid hydralazine
Acute coronary syndromes	Decrease systolic BP to <140 mmHg within 1 h; keep diastolic BP >60 mmHg	Nitroglycerin, labetalol, esmolol, metoprolol; avoid hydralazine

Acute target-organ damage	Timing for acute BP reduction[a]	Preferred intravenous drugs[b]
Acute heart failure	Decrease systolic BP to <140 mmHg within 1 h	Nitroglycerin, loop diuretics needed in most cases; avoid beta-blockers if Pulmonary edema, with wet lungs. Once patient is more dry can initiate Beta blockers
Aortic dissection	Decrease both systolic BP to <120 mmHg and heart rate to <60 beats/min within 20 min	Esmolol (or labetalol) plus one of nicardipine, clevidipine, nitroprusside, or nitroglycerin; both a beta-blocker (unless bradycardia is already present) and a vasodilator should be used

BP blood pressure

[a]Initiation, reinstatement, or adjustments of long-acting oral antihypertensive medications should take place during the first 6 to 12 h. Oral drugs are chosen on the basis of conventional guidelines. Intravenous medications can be tapered on the basis of observed blood pressure levels after the addition of oral agents

[b]Nitroprusside given its potential toxicity, it should be avoided as a first choice when other options are available

[c]Diffuse microvascular injury is identified as high-grade retinopathy (hemorrhages, exudates, or papilledema), acute kidney injury, or microangiopathic hemolytic anemia or thrombocytopenia, present alone or in combination

2.7.5 Common IV Medications used in Hypertensive Emergencies [7]

Drug	Class	Dose	Onset and offset of action	Cautions
Nicardipine	Dihydropyridine calcium channel blocker, vasodilator	5–15 mg/h IV drip; adjust by 2.5 mg/h every 5–15 min	Rapid onset (2–5 min); duration of action, 1–4 h; adjust dose more slowly (every 15 min) in patients with impaired renal or liver function	Contraindicated in patients with acute coronary ischemia (because of reflex tachycardia)

Drug	Class	Dose	Onset and offset of action	Cautions
Clevidipine	Dihydropyridine calcium channel blocker, vasodilator	1–16 mg/h IV drip; double dose every 90 s, more slowly as BP approaches goal	Rapid onset (2–4 min) and offset (5–15 min) of action	Contraindicated in patients with acute coronary ischemia (because of reflex tachycardia) and in patients with allergy to soy or eggs; may increase triglyceride levels (it is a lipid emulsion)
Labetalol	Combined non selective beta-blocker and alpha-1 blocker (IV beta-to-alpha blocking ratio, approx. 7:1)	10–20 mg IV bolus followed by drip; may repeat at same dose or double dose after 10 min before starting drip; 0.5–10 mg/min IV drip; adjust drip every 15 min; for intermittent boluses, 10–80 mg IV every 10 min (maximum cumulative dose, 300 mg)	Rapid onset (5 min) but prolonged duration of action (3–6 h, sometimes longer at higher doses)	Contraindicated in patients with wet heart failure, bradycardia or heart block, asthma or severe airway reactivity; caution in cocaine overdose
Esmolol	Selective beta-1 blocker	500–1,000 μg/kg bolus, followed by 100–300 μg/kg/min IV drip; adjust drip by 50 μg/kg/min every 5 min	Rapid onset (2–10 min) and offset (10–30 min) of action	Contraindicated in patients with wet heart failure, bradycardia or heart block, asthma, cocaine overdose
Metoprolol	Selective beta-1 blocker	2.5–5 mg IV every 5 min (maximum total dose, 15 mg), then every 4–6 h	Onset, 15 min; peak, 30–60 min; duration of action, 4–6 h; not a very potent antihypertensive	Contraindicated in patients with wet heart failure, bradycardia or heart block, asthma, cocaine overdose

2

Drug	Class	Dose	Onset and offset of action	Cautions
Nitroglycerin	Nitrate donor, mixed venous and arteriolar dilator with predominant venous effects	10–400 µg/min IV drip; adjust by 10–20 µg/min every 5–15 min	Rapid onset and offset (5–10 min) of action; with prolonged use, a higher dose may be needed for same effect	Contraindicated in patients with right ventricular infarction
Nitroprusside	Direct vasodilator with predominant arteriolar effects	0.25–10 µg/kg/min IV drip; adjust by 0.5 µg/kg/min every 5 min	Rapid onset and offset (1–2 min) of action	Contraindicated in pregnancy (risk of fetal cyanide toxicity); use with impaired renal function may lead to thiocyanate toxicity, and use in liver disease may lead to cyanide intoxication, which may occur with higher doses or prolonged infusions; may cause methemoglobinemia (dose-dependent), increased intracranial pressure
Hydralazine	Direct arterial vasodilator	5–20 mg IV every 15–20 min, then every 3–4 h (maximum dose, 20 mg per dose)	Onset and duration of action variable, depending on acetylator status; usual onset within 20 min and peak within 1 h; duration of action, 3–6 h; often demands a beta-blocker or other negative chronotropic agent to control reflex tachycardia	Use should be avoided in most cases; may worsen ischemia (owing to reflex tachycardia and possible coronary steal); unpredictable BP responses, often excessive

This table is restricted to agents mostly available in the United States.
IV intravenous

2.7.6 Common Intravenous Antihypertensive Drugs

Drug	Comment
Nicardipine	Contraindicated in patients with severe aortic stenosis or acute ACS
Hydralazine	Unpredictable, so not recommended as first line
Nitroglycerin	Best used in ACS and ADHF. Avoid using it in right ventricular infarction
Esmolol	Contraindicated in ADHF with acute pulmonary edema
Enalapril	Best used in scleroderma renal crisis
Phentolamine	Best used in pheochromocytoma, stimulant overdoses such as cocaine and amphetamine
Labetalol	Useful in overstimulation conditions

References

1. Peixoto AJ. Acute severe hypertension. N EnglJ Med. 2019;381(19):1843–52. https://doi.org/10.1056/NEJMcp1901117. PMID: 31693807
2. Bress AP, Anderson TS, Flack JM, Ghazi L, Hall ME, Laffer CL, Still CH, Taler SJ, Zachrison KS, Chang TI. American Heart Association Council on Hypertension; Council on Cardiovascular and Stroke Nursing; and Council on Clinical Cis concerned about cardiology. The Management of Elevated Blood Pressure in the Acute Care Setting: A Scientific Statement From the American Heart Association. Hypertension. 2024;81(8):e94–e106. https://doi.org/10.1161/HYP.0000000000000238. Epub 2024 May 28. PMID: 38804130
3. Patel KK, Young L, Howell EH, et al. Characteristics and outcomes of patients presenting with hypertensive urgency in the office setting. JAMA Intern Med. 2016;176:981–8.
4. Vlcek M, Bur A, Woisetschläger C, Herkner H, Laggner AN, Hirschl MM. Association between hypertensive urgencies and subsequent cardiovascular events in patients with hypertension. J Hypertens. 2008;26:657–62.
5. Carey RM, Calhoun DA, Bakris GL, et al. Resistant hypertension: detection, evaluation, and management: a scientific statement from the American Heart Association. Hypertension. 2018;72(5):e53–90.
6. Mayer SA, Kurtz P, Wyman A, et al. Clinical practices, complications, and mortality in neurological patients with acute severe hypertension: the Studying of the Treatment of Acute Hypertension Registry. Crit Care Med. 2011;39:2330–6.
7. Whelton PK, Carey RM, Aronow WS, et al. 2017 ACC/AHA/AAPA/ABC/ACPM/AGS/APhA/ASH/ASPC/NMA/PCNA guideline for the prevention, detection, evaluation, and management of high blood pressure in adults: a report of the American College of Cardiology. American Heart Association Task Force on Clinical Practice Guidelines. Hypertension. 2018;71(6):e13–e115.

Syncope

Contents

M. Salih, *Practical Hospitalist Guide to Inpatient Cardiology*, https://doi.org/10.1007/978-3-032-03240-9_3

This chapter discusses syncope, a temporary loss of consciousness due to reduced cerebral blood flow, categorizing it by underlying mechanisms: neurally mediated, cardiovascular/arrhythmogenic, and orthostatic syncope. Neurally mediated syncope, common in young individuals, often follows a vagal reflex causing vasodilation or bradycardia, while cardiovascular syncope, more serious and linked to cardiac events, can occur suddenly and without prodromal symptoms. Orthostatic syncope, prevalent among older adults, is triggered by postural changes and involves a significant drop in blood pressure. The chapter emphasizes the importance of a detailed history and examination, including EKGs, and advises against routine use of CT/MRI scans unless neurological deficits are present. Various treatment strategies are outlined based on syncope type, such as avoiding triggers for neurally mediated syncope or using medications like midodrine and fludrocortisone for orthostatic syncope.

3.1 When to Suspect and Major Etiology

- Syncope is a transient loss of consciousness resulting from reduced blood flow to the brain. Typically, consciousness is regained within a few seconds. This condition can lead to increased mortality when associated with cardiac events, particularly cardiogenic syncope. Syncope is categorized based on its underlying mechanism.
  I. Neurally mediated syncope (most common mainly in young patients)

- Syncope occurs due to a vagal reflex that induces vasodilation, bradycardia, or both, ultimately resulting in inadequate brain perfusion. Its diagnosis is symptomatic.
  II. Cardiovascular/arrhythmogenic syncope (second most common and most serious)
  III. Orthostatic syncope (third most common)

- Fall of SBP ≥20 mmHg or DBP ≥10 mmHg when changing the position to an upright posture (or sitting if cannot stand)

3.2 Common Syncope Classifications

Syncope mechanism	Clinical presentation	Comments
Neurally mediated syncope: – Vasovagal syncope (VVS; most common) – Situational syncope	– Prodromal symptoms in an upright posture, such as sweating, nausea, and an abnormal stomach feeling, frequently precede vasovagal syncope. This condition can occasionally be triggered by extreme stimuli such as pain, distressing news, or intense fear – Situational syncope is prompted by specific triggers, such as urination, defecation, sneezing, coughing, post-exertion vasodilation, neck turning, or shaving, particularly in cases of carotid hypersensitivity syncope – It is more common in younger patients	Carotid sinus syndrome predominantly affects men over 40 years of age and manifests as syncope following neck stimulation. It is diagnosed by massaging the carotid body area for a few seconds, which should be avoided in patients with a history of carotid atherosclerosis, resulting in a ventricular pause of more than 3 s and/or a drop in systolic blood pressure by more than 50 mmHg. Pacing is beneficial when bradycardia is predominant
Cardiac syncope: (a) Structural obstructive or ischemic CAD (b) Arrhythmogenic(most common cardiac syncope) [1]	Symptoms are particularly suspected if they are preceded by chest pain, shortness of breath, or exertion, which may indicate coronary artery disease, aortic stenosis, or hypertrophic obstructive cardiomyopathy, or if they occur suddenly while sitting or inactive, which is often associated with arrhythmias. Most patients do not experience prodromal symptoms. However, most cardiogenic syncope is related to significant bradycardia or a ventricular arrhythmia.	– Pulmonary embolism may cause syncope with a similar presentation to cardiac syncope. – ACS is not a common cause of syncope – Keep in mind syncope during atrial fibrillation with rapid ventricular response is uncommon
Orthostatic syncope: (A) Volume depletion (B) Loss of vascular tone: (i) Medication-induced, e.g., antihypertensive (ii) Pathological autonomic dysfunction, e.g., diabetes, Parkinson's, MS, amyloidosis, HIV, and B12 deficiency. Almost any cause of neuropathy	– Occurs when the patient changes position from sitting to standing – Mainly older adults. Associated with prodromal feeling of dizziness or lightheadedness (presyncope)	– If not explained suspect amyolid induced autonomic dysfunction

Pearl

Postural orthostatic tachycardia syndrome (POTS) manifests similarly to orthostatic syncope, characterized by an increase in heart rate of more than 30 beats per minute when moving from a recumbent to a standing position, without significant orthostatic blood pressure changes. Management includes a progressive exercise program, maintaining hydration with 2–3 liters of fluids daily, and increasing salt intake. In acute situations, treatment involves administering an intravenous fluid bolus of approximately 2 liters of saline [2].

Hospitalist Tip

Cardiogenic syncope should be suspected if it occurs during exertion or while supine, if it is accompanied by anginal chest pain, or if there is a history of cardiac diseases, conduction defects, or a family history of sudden death, particularly at a young age. An abnormal cardiac examination, a history of previous syncopal events, and being an older male patient over the age of 60 are also indicators [3]. Patients presenting with these symptoms should undergo a thorough cardiac evaluation.

Hospitalist Tip

Neurological conditions are infrequent causes of syncope and should only be considered when the clinical context includes focal neurological deficits. A critical exception is vertebrobasilar ischemia, which can manifest as syncope and must be ruled out if the patient exhibits new cranial nerve dysfunctions such as diplopia, dysphagia, dysarthria, a unique ataxic gait, and potential central vertigo. Anterior circulation strokes rarely lead to syncope and should not be readily considered.

3.3 Clinical Approach

- A detailed history is crucial since most diagnostic workups for syncope are inconclusive. Historical data should be gathered chronologically, focusing on what triggered the syncope, including events or triggers before the episode, the nature of the fall, and any post-event confusion. It is essential to ask about prodromal symptoms such as lightheadedness or tunnel vision, recent changes in medication, and blood pressure control before the event. Also, inquire about any history of diabetes, neurological or neuropathic conditions, seizures, cardiac issues, or similar past events. The most pertinent examinations include a cardiovascular system (CVS) exam, orthostatic blood pressure measurement, and a basic focused functional neurological assessment.

- All patients should undergo a 12-lead EKG to identify arrhythmogenic focus or conduction defects. Other tests have limited utility and should be ordered based on the clinical context. Inpatient telemetry has a sensitivity of about 70%, making it a reasonable option in inpatient settings if easily accessible; however, it should not be solely relied upon for diagnosis or exclusion of conditions [4].

Hospitalist Tip

CT/MRI of the brain, carotid Doppler, EEG, or CTA angiography of the neck are not typically useful in the diagnostic workup for syncope and should only be considered when focal neurological deficits, such as focal weakness or cranial nerve deficits, are present. This approach is endorsed by society guidelines, including those from the American College of Physicians (ACP) and the American Heart Association (AHA) [5].

Hospitalist Tip

The fundamental approach to syncope involves obtaining a detailed history, performing a cardiovascular system (CVS) examination, evaluating orthostatic vitals, conducting a limited neurological assessment (including checks for focal weakness and cranial nerve function), and carrying out an EKG or device interrogation. It is important to note that while orthostatic hypotension is a consideration, it does not exclude other causes of syncope, such as cardiogenic syncope.

3.4 Other Tests and Their Significance

Test	Significance	Comments
Cardiac stress test or ECHO	When suspecting cardiogenic exertional syncope	It is reasonable to consider a detailed cardiac evaluation when syncope occurs during exertion, is accompanied by anginal chest pain, or in patients with a history of cardiac diseases, conduction defects, or an abnormal cardiac exam, particularly in older patients with chronotropic incompetence

3

Test	Significance	Comments
Tilt table testing	A more thorough evaluation is strongly supported when the initial workup is inconclusive and neurally mediated syncope is suspected. It may also benefit challenging cases involving delayed orthostatic syncope, seizures, or pseudoseizure-like activity associated with syncope events. However, it should never be conducted routinely	In normal conditions, systemic vasoconstriction occurs to maintain blood pressure and brain perfusion. However, in neutrally mediated syncope, this adaptive mechanism fails, leading to increased heart contractility, stimulating mechanoreceptors, enhancing vagal stimulation and resulting in vasodilation and bradycardia

Test	Significance	Comments
Cardiac monitoring or electrophysi-ological study	When an arrhythmogenic cause of syncope is suspected, it should only be considered by a syncope specialist and not as a routine test. Different monitoring modalities are chosen based on the alleged arrhythmia frequency, such as using a loop recorder for infrequent events every few months	Arrhythmogenic syncope is suspected when there are conduction defects on an EKG, a family history of sudden death at a young age, a history of previous syncopal events, the patient is an older male over the age of 60, or if syncope occurs at rest

Test	Significance	Comments
Specialized autonomic evaluation	When the history suggests vasovagal or orthostatic syncope but orthostatic tests are negative such as inpatients with autonomic failure	

Test	Significance	Comments
CTPE protocol	This is used only when PE is highly suspected in acute settings	

3.5 Major DD

Condition	Differentiating presentation	Comments
Seizure	It is tonic-clonic in presentation, with abnormal posture, tongue biting, and prolonged postictal confusion. Amnesia of the events is important clue to seizure activity. Lactate is usually elevated in tonic clonic seizures, with mildly elevated CK	Incontinence and mild myoclonic jerks are more suggestive for seizures, but can present with syncope Syncope may have prolonged recovery if followed by major head trauma
Basilar strokes	Basilar strokes can present as syncope but are usually associated with other neurological deficits. Also, other brain stem dysfunctions are mostly present, such as diplopia, dysphagia, and dysarthria	Anterior strokes usually do not present as syncope
Significant hypoglycemia	Present like stroke with loss of consciousness	
Drug intoxication	Recent alcohol or drug intake	
Respiratory failure	Evident with recent respiratory distress before loss of consciousness	
Psychogenic	Last hours, very frequent and associated with other mood disorders	

3.6 Treatment Approach [6]

- It depends on the mechanism of the suspected syncope.
- The decision on driving restrictions depends on the mechanism of the suspected syncope. Each type of syncope has specific restrictions, so it is important to consult state laws and the most recent guidelines before determining if a patient can drive.

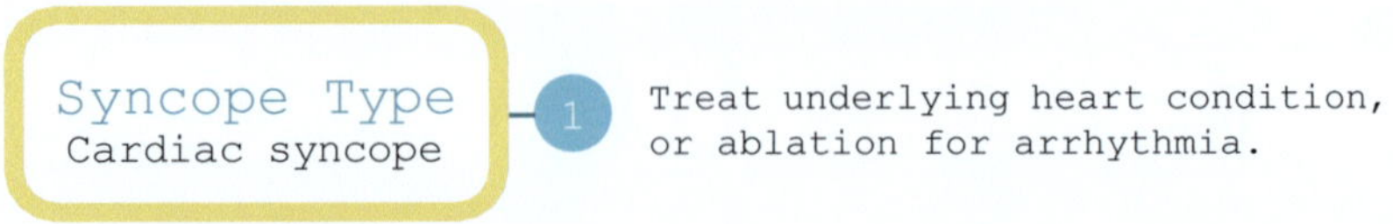

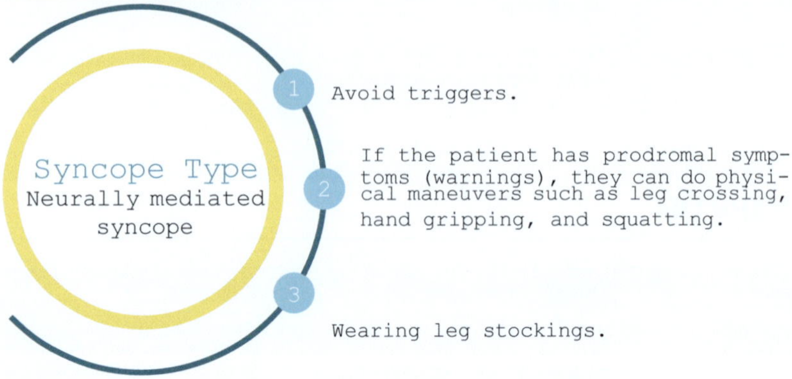

- **Comment**

The treatment options are generally the same as those for orthostatic syncope. Mostly benign, but the syncope events themselves can lead to major trauma.

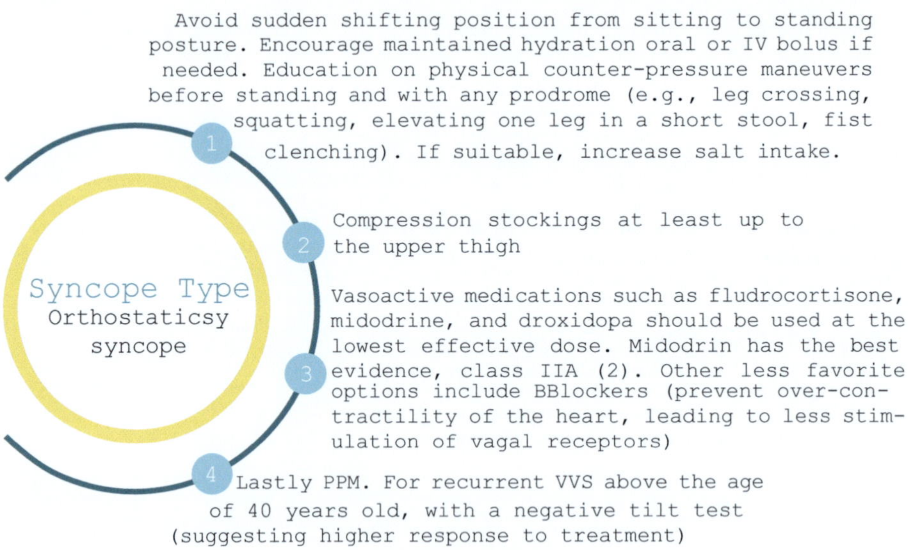

- **Comment**

- Midodrine is reasonable in patients with recurrent VVS with no history of hypertension, CHF, or urinary retention.
- Fludrocortisone might be reasonable for patients with recurrent VVS and normotensive patients.
- B-Blockers are an option if ≥42 years old with recurrent VVS [7].

Hospitalist Tip

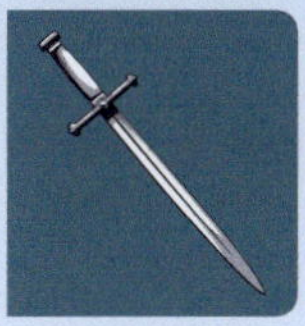

If a patient develops supine HTN at night with midodrine, consider adding oral hydralazine to be taken at bedtime. Do not take the medication after 6 pm; bed time snack may help (vasodilatation with BP drop) [8].

References

1. Soteriades ES, Evans JC, Larson MG, Chen MH, Chen L, Benjamin EJ, Levy D. Incidence and prognosis of syncope. N Engl J Med. 2002;347(12):878–85. https://doi.org/10.1056/NEJMoa012407. PMID: 12239256
2. Wells R, Spurrier AJ, Linz D, Gallagher C, Mahajan R, Sanders P, Page A, Lau DH. Postural tachycardia syndrome: current perspectives. Vasc Health Risk Manag. 2017;14:1–11. https://doi.org/10.2147/VHRM.S127393. PMID: 29343965; PMCID: PMC5749569
3. Costantino G, Sun BC, Barbic F, Bossi I, Casazza G, Dipaola F, McDermott D, Quinn J, Reed MJ, Sheldon RS, Solbiati M, Thiruganasambandamoorthy V, Beach D, Bodemer N, Brignole M, Casagranda I, Del Rosso A, Duca P, Falavigna G, Grossman SA, Ippoliti R, Krahn AD, Montano N, Morillo CA, Olshansky B, Raj SR, Ruwald MH, Sarasin FP, Shen WK, Stiell I, Ungar A, Gert van Dijk J, van Dijk N, Wieling W, Furlan R. Syncope clinical management in the emergency department: a consensus from the first international workshop on syncope risk stratification in the emergency department. Eur Heart J. 2016;37(19):1493–8. https://doi.org/10.1093/eurheartj/ehv378. Epub 2015 Aug 4. PMID: 26242712; PMCID: PMC4872282
4. Chiu DT, Shapiro NI, Sun BC, Mottley JL, Grossman SA. Are echocardiography, telemetry, ambulatory electrocardiography monitoring, and cardiac enzymes in emergency department patients presenting with syncope useful tests? A preliminary investigation. J Emerg Med. 2014;47(1):113–8. https://doi.org/10.1016/j.jemermed.2014.01.018. Epub 2014 Mar 31. PMID: 24698512
5. Hatharasinghe AT, Etebar K, Wolsky R, Akhondi H, Ayutyanont N. An assessment of the diagnostic value in syncope workup: a retrospective study. HCA Healthc J Med. 2021;2(6):423–31. https://doi.org/10.36518/2689-0216.1306. PMID: 37427395; PMCID: PMC10324800
6. Shen WK, Sheldon RS, Benditt DG, Cohen MI, Forman DE, Goldberger ZD, Grubb BP, Hamdan MH, Krahn AD, Link MS, Olshansky B, Raj SR, Sandhu RK, Sorajja D, Sun BC, Yancy CW. 2017 ACC/AHA/HRS Guide- line for Evaluating and Management Patients With Syncope: a report of the American College of Cardiology/American Heart Association Task Force on Clinical Practice Guidelines and the Heart Rhythm Society. Circulation. 2017;136(5):e60–e122. https://doi.org/10.1161/CIR.0000000000000499. Epub 2017 Mar 9. Erratum in: Circulation. 2017 Oct 17;136(16):e271- e272. doi: 10.1161/CIR.0000000000000537. PMID: 28280231
7. Sheldon RS, Morillo CA, Klingenheben T, Krahn AD, Sheldon A, Rose MS. Age-dependent effect of β-blockers in preventing vasovagal syncope. Circ Arrhythm Electrophysiol. 2012;5(5):920–6. https://doi.org/10.1161/CIRCEP.112.974386. Epub 2012 Sep 12. PMID: 22972872
8. Figueroa JJ, Basford JR, Low PA. Preventing and treating orthostatic hypotension: As easy as A, B, C. Cleve Clin J Med. 2010;77(5):298–306. https://doi.org/10.3949/ccjm.77a.09118. PMID: 20439562; PMCID: PMC2888469

Arrhythmias

Contents

M. Salih, *Practical Hospitalist Guide to Inpatient Cardiology*, https://doi.org/10.1007/978-3-032-03240-9_4

This chapter presents a structured and clinically oriented approach to electrocardiogram (EKG) interpretation and the management of key cardiac conditions. Efficient EKG analysis begins with determining heart rate using lead II, followed by rhythm evaluation to confirm sinus origin, axis determination through leads I and augmented vector foot (AVF), and identification of conduction abnormalities such as bundle branch blocks. Further analysis includes detecting chamber enlargement, ischemic changes, and segmental interval abnormalities (PR, QRS, QT, T waves) that may suggest electrolyte imbalances or structural disease. Tachyarrhythmias are classified into narrow or broad complex types, with diagnostic differentiation aided by waveform patterns and clinical context. The chapter also covers acute atrial fibrillation (AF) management, stressing rapid assessment, rhythm or rate control, and stroke prevention through appropriate anticoagulation. Inherited cardiac channelopathies, including long QT, Brugada, and catecholaminergic polymorphic ventricular tachycardia (VT), are explored with attention to genetic origins and arrhythmic risk. Preoperative considerations for patients with cardiac pacemakers are outlined, emphasizing device interrogation and perioperative planning to avoid electrical interference. Finally, cardiac heart blocks are reviewed, from first-degree to complete Atrioventricular (AV) block, with a focus on clinical presentation and pacemaker indications. Altogether, the content reinforces the integration of EKG interpretation, clinical evaluation, and individualized treatment in managing both acute and chronic cardiac conditions.

4.1 EKG Basics

4.1.1 How to Read an EKG Efficiently

1. *Rate*. This is easy to start with. Follow lead II, which is most consistent with the heart's normal axis. The number of large boxes between the R-R waves is divided by 300. If it is irregular, count the number of R waves in 10 seconds and multiply it by 6. The normal rate is between 50 and 100 beats per minute.
2. *Rhythm*. To maintain a regular sinus rhythm (conducting from the sinoatrial (SA) node), each P wave should be followed by QRS; if it is not or if it looks unusual, or a P wave is absent, it is not a sinus rhythm. The wave in sinus rhythm should always be positive in lead II if it's not suspected conduction outside the SA node, such as atrial tachycardia.

Pearl

No P wave before normal consistent QRS suggests junctional escape rhythm.

3. *Axis*: The normal P wave axis is upright in lead II. The normal QRS complex lead should be between −30 and +90 degrees. Another way is to review leads I and AVF; if both are upright, the axis is likely normal.
   - *Right axis deviation*: +90 to +180. Negative QRS deflection in lead I and positive QRS deflection in lead AVF could indicate Right Ventricular Hypertrophy (RVH), or Pulmonary Hypertension (PHT).
   - *Left axis deviation*: −30 to −90, upright QRS in lead I and negative QRS deflection in lead AVF could indicate left ventricular hypertrophy (LVH) or left anterior fascicular block (LAFB).
   - *Extreme axis deviation*: +180 to −90. Negative QRS in lead I and negative QRS deflection in lead AVF usually indicate a ventricular arrhythmia.
4. *Bundle branch block (BBB)*: A normal QRS is narrow. Check whether the QRS is wide, more than three small boxes, or more than 120 ms. If it is wide, it is either a BBB, pacemaker rhythm, nonspecific intraventricular conduction, or aberrancy (concealed pathway between the atrium and the ventricles). RBBB could be benign, according to the presentation, or indicate right heart pathology such as PHT. LBBB is almost always pathological, never benign, and indicates heart pathology. Bifascicular block = LAFB/Left Posterior Fascicular Block (LPFB) + Right Bundle Branch Block (RBBB). Trifascicular block = LAFB/LPFB + RBBB+ first-degree AV block.
5. *Presence of ischemic pattern*: Look for ST segment depression or elevation from the isoelectric line (PR line) in a specific heart location (pattern), e.g., anterior, posterior, and lateral. However, ST-segment depression or elevation could indicate other pathologies, such as BBB, LVH/RVH, or even nonheart pathology, such as brain hemorrhage rather than ischemia. Also, the absence of ST-segment changes does not rule out ischemia. In summary, ST elevation may help determine the ischemic location. However, ST depression correlates poorly with localization.
6. *Presence of atrial or ventricular hypertrophy or enlargement.*
   - *Atrial enlargement*: A tall P wave in lead II, V1 usually shows right atrial enlargement. Left atrial enlargement is evident by a bifid P wave in lead II or an increased negative deflection in lead V1. It is common in PHT.
   - *Ventricular enlargement*: RVH is evident by a tall R wave in lead V1, which is common in PHT. LVH has different criteria, including the Sokolow-Lyon criteria, in which the sum of the S wave in V1 and the R wave in V5 or V6 is greater than 35 mm, or modified Cornell criteria, in which the R wave in aVL is greater than 12 mm in amplitude. Suspect uncontrolled HTN or severe aortic stenosis (AS) in LVH.

Pearl

Common DD for LVH includes uncontrolled HTN, AS, hypertrophic obstructive cardiomyopathy (HOCM), and cardiac amyloidosis.

7. *Specific segment/wave changes*
   - *PR*: It should be less than <0.2 seconds, between three and five small boxes. If abnormally prolonged or inconsistent throughout, it indicates a heart block. If it is extremely narrow, it does suggest supraventricular tachycardia (SVT).
   - *QRS*: It should be less than 120 ms and contain three small boxes. If it is prolonged, it indicates an abnormal delay in ventricular depolarization.
   - *QT*: It is usually less than two large boxes. If it is prolonged, look for medications or electrolyte abnormalities. Long QT could lead to polymorphic VT, the same as a short QT, but it is rare.
   - *T wave*: Usually pointing in the same direction as the R wave, but not as tall. An abnormally tall or inverted T wave indicates heart irritability, possibly due to ischemia, electrolyte abnormality, stress, etc.
   - *Q wave*: It should be small and not easily visible. It suggests old ischemia if it is obvious or taller than the R waves.

Hospitalist Tip

Proper history and brief examination with an EKG will help you diagnose most of the patient's palpitation concerns. In around 40% of presentations [1], most palpitations are due to PACs or PVCs. Remember that medications or systemic and psychiatric conditions could also cause them. If symptoms are not distressing with a low cardiovascular risk profile and normal EKG, most patients could be followed on an outpatient basis without further inpatient workup.

4.2 Tachycardia Approach

4.2.1 General Concepts and Approach

- Tachycardia is defined by heart rates exceeding 100 beats per minute, with manifestations ranging from palpitations, presyncope, dyspnea, chest discomfort, and fatigue to cervical pulsations (suggestive of atrioventricular nodal reentrant tachycardia or ventricular tachycardia) and syncope. Notably, asymptomatic presentation does not preclude significant underlying pathology, and symptom severity may not correlate with condition severity.

- Historical assessment should encompass potential etiologies including anxiety disorders, cardiac arrhythmias (both brady- and tachyarrhythmias), thyroid dysfunction, stimulant/caffeine consumption, and medication effects. Comprehensive evaluation requires a detailed cardiac history, medication review, and symptom frequency assessment, as higher frequency increases diagnostic yield during short-term monitoring. A family history of sudden death may suggest inherited arrhythmogenic conditions.
- Physical examination should include a comprehensive cardiovascular and thyroid evaluation.
- Tachyarrhythmias are broadly classified as supraventricular tachycardia (characterized by narrow QRS complexes) or ventricular tachycardia (manifesting broad QRS complexes).
- Initial diagnostic evaluation should include:
  (i) Thyroid function studies (to exclude hyperthyroidism).
  (ii) Complete blood count (to assess for anemia).
  (iii) Comprehensive metabolic panel (particularly evaluating magnesium and potassium levels).
  (iv) Transthoracic echocardiography.
  (v) Electrocardiography.

Pearl

Electrocardiographic evaluation is an essential diagnostic tool for all patients with tachycardia. While transthoracic echocardiography is indicated in ventricular tachycardia and symptomatic supraventricular tachycardia to exclude structural cardiac pathology, normal echocardiographic findings do not definitively exclude significant arrhythmic conditions. Critical electrocardiographic interpretation should emphasize P wave morphology, consistency, and QRS complex duration, as these parameters provide crucial diagnostic differentiation between tachycardia classifications.

Hospitalist Tip

A patient with a normal exam, EKG, and TTE is at very low risk of serious arrhythmias.

4.2.2 Major Classifications

A. *Narrow complex tachycardia*
   1. *Regular*
      - Sinus tachycardia: Consistent P wave followed by QRS.
      - Atrioventricular nodal reentrant tachycardia (AVNRT) 60%: No clear P wave is seen or close to the QRS.
      - Atrioventricular reciprocating tachycardia (AVRT) 30%: Short PR interval and conduction through the accessory pathway.
      - Atrial tachycardia 10%/multifocal atrial tachycardia/atrial flutter: Abnormally shaped P wave.
   2. *Irregular*
      - AF: No clear P wave with asynchronous QRS waves.
      - Atrial tachycardia/multifocal atrial tachycardia/atrial flutter: Abnormally shaped P wave.

B. *Broad complex tachycardia*
   1. *Regular*
      - VT: No P wave is visible. Thromboembolism is unusual.
      - AVNRT with aberrancy (BBB or delay in ventricular conduction): P wave may be visible, with characteristic RBBB or LBBB.
      - Ventricular paced rhythms: Presence of pacer spikes.
   2. *Irregular or regular*
      - Pre-excited antidromic AVRT tachycardia (if symptomatic, usually indicates WPW syndrome): Short PR interval and presence of a delta wave.

Pearl

In the presence of a history of IHD or a family history of sudden death, broad complex tachycardia is more likely to be VT rather than SVT with aberrancy. Follow this table to help differentiate between SVT aberrancy and VT in EKG.

SVT with aberrancy	VT
Classic bundle branch block pattern (LBBB or RBBB)	Uniformity in QRS appearance throughout the leads
Either normal axis, LAD, or RAD pattern	Extreme axis deviation 180 to −90. Large R wave in AVR

SVT with aberrancy	VT
Association between P waves and the QRS waves	AV dissociation, which means no association between P waves and the QRS waves. Considered most specific sign for VT
No capture beats	Capture beats which means normal conduction out of the unusual VT pattern
No fusion beats	Fusion beats, normal sinus, and ventricular beats fuse to produce a bizarre complex

3. *Irregular*
   - Ventricular fibrillation (VF): Unstable patient/cardiac arrest, with no pulse.
   - Polymorphic VT: Different shapes and sizes of VT.
   - AF with BBB: Irregular, wide complex tachycardia with no clear P waves.

4.3 Atrial Fibrillation

4.3.1 When to Suspect a Major Etiology

- Atrial fibrillation is characterized by disorganized atrial electrical activity resulting in irregular ventricular conduction patterns. This arrhythmia is readily identifiable through electrocardiographic examination and demonstrates increasing prevalence with advancing age. Multiple modifiable and non-modifiable risk factors have been established, including tobacco use, excessive alcohol consumption, elevated body mass index, diabetes mellitus, hypertension, coronary artery disease, congestive heart failure, and obstructive sleep apnea. Acute physiological stressors, such as surgical interventions, pulmonary embolism, and critical illness, may precipitate episodes of atrial fibrillation. This cardiac dysrhythmia carries significant clinical implications, including increased risk of thromboembolic cerebrovascular events, deterioration of cardiac function with subsequent heart failure (particularly in the setting of tachycardia), and potential cognitive decline manifesting as dementia.

Pearl

Atrial fibrillation should be considered a primary diagnostic consideration in cases of cryptogenic ischemic stroke, as epidemiological studies indicate it may be the underlying etiology in approximately 20–25% of such cases [2].

Pearl

Cardiac ischemia is not a common trigger for AF.

4.3.2 Clinical Approach

- The clinical presentation of atrial fibrillation is notably variable, with many patients remaining asymptomatic, thereby contributing to its potential severity. When symptomatic, patients may present with a constellation of nonspecific manifestations including vertigo, palpitations, exertional dyspnea, thoracic discomfort, and syncopal episodes. This heterogeneous symptomatology necessitates a high index of clinical suspicion.
- Diagnostic confirmation requires electrocardiographic evidence, ranging from standard 12-lead ECG to more extensive cardiac monitoring modalities such as Holter monitors or implantable loop recorders for paroxysmal cases. A comprehensive diagnostic evaluation should include:
  1. Thyroid function studies to exclude hyperthyroidism.
  2. Complete blood count to assess for anemia.
  3. Comprehensive metabolic panel with particular attention to potassium and magnesium levels to identify potential metabolic precipitants.
  4. Transthoracic echocardiography to evaluate for structural cardiac abnormalities, including atrial thrombus, valvular heart disease, and ventricular dysfunction.
  5. Polysomnography, when clinically indicated, with a low threshold for screening for obstructive sleep apnea.
  6. Appropriate infectious disease workup based on clinical presentation.
- The primary acute complications associated with atrial fibrillation are thromboembolic cerebrovascular events and tachycardia-induced cardiomyopathy, both of which can result in significant morbidity and mortality.
- Divided according to the duration of the AF into either:
  (i) Paroxysmal AF stops spontaneously within 7 days of onset.
  (ii) Persistent AF lasts 7 days or more.
  (iii) Permanent AF refers to AF in which the physician and patient abandon attempts to maintain sinus rhythm.

Pearl

Duration of AF does not affect the treatment approach.

Hospitalist Tip

Transesophageal echocardiography (TEE) and cardiac magnetic resonance imaging (CMRI) represent the gold standard diagnostic modalities for detecting left atrial thrombi, particularly in cases of cryptogenic stroke. TEE offers superior visualization of the left atrial appendage compared to transthoracic echocardiography, while cardiac MRI provides high-resolution, multiplanar imaging with excellent tissue characterization.

4.3.3 Major DD

(i) Atrial flutter.

4.3.4 Treatment Approach for Acute AF

- It depends on urgency/hemodynamic stability:
  A. *Unstable* (ACS, ADHF, shock with blood pressure <90/60, new mental state changes with acute confusion that another reason cannot explain).
    - According to current clinical guidelines, urgent electrical or pharmacological cardioversion is the recommended class I intervention for acute management [2]. However, in cases where the onset of atrial fibrillation is either undetermined or exceeds 48 hours, there is a significant risk of thromboembolism. Therefore, immediate anticoagulation with unfractionated heparin is indicated for all patients, regardless of their CHA2DS2-VASc risk stratification score. This initial anticoagulation should be followed by a 4-week course of therapeutic anticoagulation using either low molecular weight heparin, warfarin, or direct oral anticoagulants (DOACs). The rationale for extended anticoagulation post-cardioversion stems from atrial stunning, during which impaired atrial mechanical function persists despite restoration of sinus rhythm, creating a sustained prothrombotic state. This period of increased thromboembolic risk necessitates continued anticoagulation to prevent adverse cardiovascular events.

4.3.5 Table for Acute Pharmacological Cardioversion Agents [3]

Drug: Procainamide		
Dose	**Acute monitoring**	**Drug-drug interaction (pertinent)**
15 mg/kg over 30 min (based on study protocol from RAFF2)	QRS widening, QTc prolongation, heart rate	May enhance QT-prolonging effect of concomitant QT-prolonging medications May enhance neuromuscular blocking effect of neuromuscular agents
Pharmacokinetics/ pharmacodynamics	**Major early side effects**	**Clinical considerations**
Tmax: About 60 minutes T½: 2–7 h for procainamide, 6–8 h for NAPA Primary metabolism: Hepatic via acetylation to produce N-acetyl procainamide (NAPA active metabolite) Primary clearance: Renal	Hypotension Bradycardia Ventricular tachyarrhythmia	Avoid in Brugada syndrome avoid in acute heart failure Avoid in patients allergic to ester-type local anesthetic Avoid when already hypotensive or in shock Avoid in patients with high-grade AV block or significant his-Purkinje disease Avoid in patients with LQTS, baseline prolonged QT, or on concomitant QT-prolonging medications Avoid in patients with ongoing electrolyte hypokalemia, hypomagnesemia Should be used with caution in renal disease as active metabolite NAPA is exclusively excreted renally

Drug: Flecainide		
Dose	**Acute monitoring**	**Drug-drug interaction (pertinent)**
Single dose 300 mg PO (>70 kg) 200 mg PO (≤70 kg) May not repeat in ≤24 h IV from not clinically available in the US	QRS widening, QT prolongation, PR prolongation, AV block, heart rate PO dosing does not directly cause hypotension but watch conversion pause or bradycardia which may be hemodynamically significant	Digoxin levels. May enhance bradycardiac QT-prolonging effects of concomitant medications

4

Drug: Flecainide		
Pharmacokinetics/ pharmacodynamics	**Major early side effects**	**Clinical considerations**
Tmax: 1–6 h T½: 10–17 h Primary metabolism: Hepatic, CYP2D6, CYP1A2 Primary clearance: Renal	May precipitate 1:1 conduction of atrial flutter or atrial tachycardia in the absence of AV nodal blockade Ventricular tachyarrhythmia Bradycardia with conversion AV block Negative inotropy	Avoid in structural heart disease Avoid in Brugada syndrome Avoid in ischemic heart disease Avoid in patients with high-grade AV block or significant his-Purkinje disease Avoid in patients with ongoing electrolyte abnormalities especially with concomitant hypokalemia, hypomagnesemia Should have concomitant AV nodal blockade

Drug: Propafenone		
Dose	**Acute monitoring**	**Drug-drug interaction (pertinent)**
600 mg PO (>70 kg) 450 mg PO(≤70 kg) May not repeat in ≤24 h	QRS widening, QT prolongation, PR prolongation, AV block, heart rate Watch for conversion pause or bradycardia which may be hemodynamically significant	Digoxin levels. ↓ warfarin clearance May enhance bradycardic and QT-prolonging effects of concomitant medication
Pharmacokinetics/ pharmacodynamics	**Major early side effects**	**Clinical considerations**
Tmax: 2–6 h T½: 2–10 h Primary metabolism: Hepatic, especially by CYP2D6 and CYP3A4 Primary clearance: Renal	May precipitate 1:1 conduction of atrial flutter or atrial tachycardia in the absence of AV nodal blockade Ventricular tachyarrhythmia Bradycardia with conversion AV block Heart failure exacerbation	Should have concomitant AV nodal blockade Avoid in structural heart disease Avoid in Brugada syndrome Avoid in ischemic heart disease Avoid in patients with ongoing electrolyte disarrays especially with concomitant hypokalemia, hypomagnesemia Avoid in patients with bronchospasm

Drug: Ibutilide

Dose	**Acute monitoring**	**Drug-drug interaction (pertinent)**
1 mg IV over 10 min, wait 10–20 min before infusion of second 1 mg IV over 10 minutes Strongly consider pretreating with magnesium sulfate 1–4 mg IV	Baseline K, Mg, QTc assessment Replete K and Mg before ibutilide administration QTc monitoring during and after cardioversion	Concomitant QT-prolonging drugs (including other QT-prolonging antiarrhythmic drugs) can potentiate QT prolongation and risks for torsades de pointes
Pharmacokinetics/pharmacodynamics	**Major early side effects**	**Clinical considerations**
Tmax: 30–60 minutes T½: 6–9 h Primary metabolism: Hepatic Primary clearance: Renal	QT prolongation Torsades de pointes	Avoid in patients with LQTS, baseline prolonged QT, or on concomitant QT-prolonging medications Avoid in patients with ongoing electrolyte disarrays especially with concomitant hypokalemia, hypomagnesemia, hypocalcemia

Drug: Amiodarone

Dose	**Acute monitoring**	**Drug-drug interaction (pertinent)**
150 mg IV bolus then 60 mg/h × 6 h then 30 mg/h × 18 h	QT, heart rate BP, IV preparation has been associated with hypotensive effects	Digoxin effect. Warfarin effect. Potentiate QT prolongation and risk of torsades de pointes in presence of QT-prolonging drugs
Pharmacokinetics/pharmacodynamics	**Major early side effects**	**Clinical considerations**
Tmax: 8–12 h T½: 13–103 days Primary metabolism: Hepatic, especially CYP3A4 Primary clearance: Hepatic, biliary	Hypotension (IV preparation) Bradycardia	Use with extreme caution in patients with existing bradycardia Consider alternate acute medication if patient has active issues with hepatic metabolism

B. *Stable*. Treatment consists of managing the following:

I. *Control symptoms/heart rate and risk factors*

- Management of atrial fibrillation requires a comprehensive approach addressing underlying precipitants and risk factors, including pain, hypovolemia, physiological stress, and acute decompensated heart failure (ADHF). Keep the patient on telemtry. Rate control strategies aim to achieve a target heart rate below 80 beats per minute, with acceptable parameters ranging between 60 and 110 beats per minute, tailored according to symptomatic presentation. The RACE II Trial [4] established that a lenient rate control strategy (target heart rate < 110 beats per minute) may be appropriate for patients without ADHF or symptomatic atrial fibrillation. Treatment modalities are selected based on individual clinical scenarios and adverse effect profiles.
- For patients presenting with atrial fibrillation and rapid ventricular response, first-line pharmacological interventions include:
  - (i) Intravenous beta-blockers.
  - (ii) Calcium channel blockers.
  - (iii) Amiodarone (as second-line therapy in non-responders).
- In the context of ADHF, amiodarone is considered the optimal therapeutic agent for hospitalized patients. According to current guidelines, intravenous beta-blockade, particularly esmolol, is the recommended first-line intervention for acute coronary syndrome patients [2].

Hospitalist Tip

In the context of acute decompensated heart failure (ADHF), specific antiarrhythmic agents carry contraindications. Notably, sotalol and dronedarone are specifically contraindicated due to their potential negative inotropic effects and associated increased mortality risk in this patient population. The preferred antiarrhythmic agents in ADHF are amiodarone and dofetilide, owing to their more favorable hemodynamic profiles and established safety data in patients with compromised left ventricular function [2]. However, dofetilide is not an ideal therapeutic option in patients with significant QT prolongation or impaired renal function, as these conditions increase the risk of drug accumulation and torsades de pointes.

4.3.6 Table of Acute Rate Control Agents [3]

Dose	Pharmacokinetics/ pharmacodynamics	Onset	Drug-drug interaction consideration (pertinent)	Risks
Drug: Diltiazem				
0.25 mg/kg IV bolus over 10 min (may give in 2 divided doses in elderly patients and/or those with low-end blood pressure); may repeat at 0.35 mg/kg IV	Tmax: (onset of action within minutes of administration) T½: 4–6 h	2–7 min	Use with caution with medications that may result in additive negative effects on heart rate, AV conduction, and/or cardiac contractility	Hypotension, bradycardia, negative inotropy
Drug: Metroprolol				
2.5–5 mg IV bolus slow push over 2 min; up to 3 doses	Tmax: (full onset of action within 20 minutes of administration) T½: 3–7 h	~5 minutes	Use with caution with medications that may result in additive negative effects on heart rate, AV conduction, and/or cardiac contractility	Hypotension, bradycardia, bronchospasm
Drug: Esmolol				
Initial: 50 mcg/kg/minute continuous IV infusion; titrate by 50 mcg/kg/minute every 4 minutes until goal heart rate Is attained	Tmax: (onset of action immediate with administration) T½: 9 minutes	Immediate	Use with caution with medications that may result in additive negative effects on heart rate, AV conduction, and/or cardiac contractility	Hypotension, bradycardia, bronchospasm
Drug: Digoxin				
0.25–0.5 mg IV (over several minutes), then 0.25 mg q6h; 1 mg over 24 h	Tmax: (immediate release); 4–7 h (extended release) T½: 4–10 h Primary metabolism: Hepatic Primary clearance: Renal	>1 h	Use with caution in patients with renal disease Consider reduced loading and subsequent doses in elderly patients	Bradycardia, digitalis toxicity, increase defect if hypokalemic, hypomagnesemic, or hypocalcemic

Hospitalist Tip

The posology of amiodarone demonstrates distinct protocols for rate control versus rhythm control strategies, with rate control being an off-label application. The recommended administration protocol for rate control consists of an initial intravenous loading dose of 300 mg administered over 1 hour, followed by a continuous infusion of 10–50 mg/hour for 24 hours, titrated to achieve the target heart rate [5]. In clinical practice, amiodarone is typically employed as a secondary rate-controlling agent in hemodynamically stable patients who respond inadequately to initial therapies such as metoprolol or diltiazem. Optimal management involves concurrent administration of oral rate-controlling agents (calcium channel blockers, beta-blockers, or oral amiodarone at doses of 100–200 mg daily) to facilitate the gradual reduction of the amiodarone infusion. This dual approach with concurrent oral and intravenous therapy allows for more precise titration of the amiodarone infusion while maintaining adequate rate control through the transition period. The strategy requires careful monitoring of heart rate response and potential drug interactions.

Hospitalist Tip

In patients with reduced left ventricular systolic function, non-dihydropyridine calcium channel blockers (such as diltiazem) are contraindicated due to their negative inotropic effects and associated increased mortality risk. However, dihydropyridine calcium channel blockers (such as amlodipine) maintain their safety profile in this population due to their minimal direct cardiac effects and selective action on peripheral vasculature. The class III potassium channel blockers sotalol and dronedarone are also associated with increased mortality when administered to patients with HFrEF.

Hospitalist Tip

Digoxin represents a viable therapeutic option in patients presenting with acute decompensated heart failure (ADHF) complicated by atrial fibrillation, particularly in the context of borderline blood pressure. The target therapeutic serum concentration ranges from 0.5 to 0.9 ng/mL. However, it is crucial to recognize the delayed onset of action characteristic of digoxin; its rate-controlling effects typically manifest over several hours. This pharmacodynamic profile makes digoxin suboptimal for rapid rate control in acute settings. Additionally, concomitant administration of amiodarone and digoxin can result in a significant elevation of digoxin steady-state plasma concentrations. Therefore, when these agents are coadministered, a reduction in the digoxin dosage is warranted, as is standard practice with amiodarone therapy.

Pearl

Elective cardioversion is reasonable in hemodynamically stable patients with significant symptoms who are not responding to rate control agents.

II. *Prevent strokes/thromboembolism in acute settings when the rhythm strategy is elected with medication or cardioversion* [2].

(a) *Onset ≥48 hours or unknown*

- Patients with atrial fibrillation carry an inherent thrombotic risk, independent of their CHA2DS2-VASc risk stratification score. Therefore, anticoagulation is indicated for all patients before any intervention. The choice of anticoagulant should be tailored to the patient's clinical status: unfractionated heparin is preferred for hemodynamically unstable patients, while direct oral anticoagulants (DOACs) are recommended for hemodynamically stable patients. For patients who are candidates for cardioversion (class IIa recommendation [2]), a transesophageal echocardiogram should be performed before the procedure to exclude intracardiac thrombus in hemodynamically stable patients. Following successful cardioversion, anticoagulation should be maintained for at least 4 weeks. If left atrial appendage thrombus identified, avoid cardioversion and continue anticoagulation.
- This extended anticoagulation protocol is specifically mandated in cases where the duration of atrial fibrillation is either unknown or exceeds 48 hours, regardless of the patient's CHA2DS2-VASc score. This recommendation is based on the recognized risk of delayed thromboembolism during post-cardioversion, when atrial mechanical function may remain temporarily impaired despite restoring normal electrical activity.

Hospitalist Tip

According to current clinical guidelines [2], when the precise onset of atrial fibrillation cannot be established, clinicians should operate under the conservative assumption that the arrhythmia has persisted for more than 48 hours. This scenario is particularly prevalent in the inpatient setting, where patients often present with uncertain symptom chronology or may have had an asymptomatic onset of the arrhythmia.

(b) *Onset <48 hours*

- In cases of atrial fibrillation with a documented duration of less than 48 hours, patients generally present a lower thromboembolic risk profile. However, risk stratification remains essential, as patients with elevated CHA2DS2-VASc scores (≥2 in males, ≥3 in females) require anticoagulation before cardioversion. The choice of anticoagulant should be stratified based on hemodynamic stability: unfractionated heparin is indicated for unstable patients, while direct oral anticoagulants (DOACs) are preferred for hemodynamically stable patients.
- Transesophageal echocardiography before cardioversion is not routinely indicated for these early-presenting cases due to the lower probability of existing intracardiac thrombus. However, post-cardioversion anticoagulation for at least 4 weeks is a class I recommendation [2], regardless of the patient's baseline risk score.

Hospitalist Tip

The previous approach is particularly relevant in managing patients presenting with new-onset atrial fibrillation with rapid ventricular response and no documented history of arrhythmia. The initial clinical strategy typically focuses on rate control measures; subsequently, if this approach proves inadequate and the patient remains significantly symptomatic, cardioversion becomes the next therapeutic consideration (predominantly utilizing amiodarone in hospital settings, or transesophageal echocardiography followed by electrical cardioversion when cardiology expertise is accessible). The anticoagulation algorithm then serves as a critical decision-making framework, guiding appropriate thromboprophylaxis based on the specific clinical scenario. However, keep in mind that According to the American College of Cardiology, American Heart Association, and American College of Chest Physicians, in critically ill patients with acute atrial fibrillation the decision to initiate anticoagulation for stroke prevention should be individualized, taking into account the uncertain benefit and the increased risk of bleeding in the context of acute illness. The CHA2DS2-VASc score has demonstrated limited utility in predicting the risk of acute stroke in the setting of an acute episode [2, 3].

Pearl

Subclinical AF (asymptomatic and brief, lasting less than <24 hours) will likely benefit from anticoagulation if meeting the CHA2DS2-VASc score with low bleeding risk. However, specific guidelines still need to be made on this matter [6]. Most patients will benefit from follow-up within 4 weeks. Detection of AF during hospitalization for acute illness is associated with a high rate of recurrence.

4.3.7 Table for Properties and Dosing of Parenteral Anticoagulants [3]

Primary mechanism of action	Dose	Pharmacokinetics/ pharmacodynamics	Contraindications	Clinical monitoring considerations
Drug: Heparin				
Enhances activity of antithrombin III (AT III) to inactivate thrombin, factor Xa, and factor IXa	60 to 80 units/kg IV bolus, then 12 to 18 units/kg/hour continuous IV infusion, adjusting dose to target coagulation parameter This may be the initial parenteral anticoagulation as a bridge to therapeutic oral anticoagulation with warfarin	Tmax: 20–30 min T½: 1–2 h Primary metabolism: Reticuloendothelial system	Active bleeding Severe thrombocytopenia Heparin-induced thrombocytopenia (HIT) Heparin-induced thrombocytopenia and thrombosis (HITT) Thrombocytopenia with pentosan polysulfate	Check aPTT level 6 hours after dosing or dose adjustment Titrate to target indicated coagulation parameter No specific dose modification for hepatic or renal impairment Caution with agents that may create additive bleeding risks
Drug: Enoxaparin				
Accelerating the activity of antithrombin III (AT III) which leads to inhibition of coagulationfactor Xa and factor IIa (thrombin)	1 mg/kg subcutaneously every 12 hours or 1.5 mg/kg once a day This may be the initial parenteral anticoagulation as a bridge to therapeutic oral anticoagulation with warfarin	Tmax: 3–5 h T½: 4.5–7 h Primary metabolism: Hepatic via desulfation and depolymerization Primary clearance: Renal	Active bleeding Severe thrombocytopenia Heparin-induced thrombocytopenia (HIT) Heparin-induced thrombocytopenia and thrombosis (HITT)	Caution in patients with CrCl below 30 ml/min, consider alternatives or if using with renally adjusted dose of 1 mg/kg once daily subcutaneously, consider following anti-factor Xa Dosing may be challenging in obese patients in balancing weight-based dosing and bleeding risks; monitor anti-factor Xa in obese patients, may need to adjust dose Caution with agents that may create additive bleeding risks

Primary mechanism of action	Dose	Pharmacokinetics/ pharmacodynamics	Contraindications	Clinical monitoring considerations
DALTEPARIN				
Accelerating the activity of anti-thrombin III (AT III) which leads to inhibition of coagulation factor Xa and factor IIA (thrombin)	200 units/kg subcutaneously daily or 100 units/kg every 12 hours This may be the initial parenteral anticoagulation as a bridge to therapeutic oral anticoagulation with warfarin If using in the setting of cardioversion, given need for strict therapeutic anticoagulation, the every 12 hour dosing may be preferred to the once a day dosing given range of T½	Tmax: 1–4 h T½: 3–5 h Primary clearance: Renal	History of heparin-induced thrombocytopenia (HIT) within the past 100 days or in the presence of circulating antibodies Active bleeding	Avoid in patients with CrCl below 30 ml/min Caution with agents that may create additive bleeding risks

Primary mechanism of action	Dose	Pharmacokinetics/ pharmacodynamics	Contraindications	Clinical monitoring considerations
Agratroban				
Reversibly inhibits the catalytic site of thrombin, thus neutralizing the actions of thrombin	2 mcg/kg/min continuous IV infusion Dose adjustment: Critically ill patients: Initial dose of 1 mcg/kg/min, or if significant organ dysfunction consider alternate medication or lower initial dose of 0.25 mcg/kg/min Reduce dose for patients with moderate to severe hepatic impairment or heart failure with liver congestion 0.25–0.5 mcg/kg/min To use in lieu of heparin-containing parental anticoagulant in HIT patients	Tmax: 1–3 h T½: 30–51 minutes Primary metabolism: Hepatic	Active bleeding	Monitor aPTT 2–4 h after initiation dose or dose titration, targeting 1.5 to 3 times the initial baseline value aPTT as therapeutic goal Caution with agents that may create additive bleeding risks
Bivalirudin				
Directly inhibits thrombin by binding to the catalytic site and to the anion binding, exposing circulating and clot-bound thrombin	0.15 mg/kg/hour continuous IV infusion Reduce dose for patients with renal disease To use in lieu of heparin-containing parenteral anticoagulant in HIT patients	Tmax: 2–4 minutes (infusion) T½: 25 minutes to 3.5 h pending on renal function Primary metabolism: Glomerular filtration	Active bleeding	Monitor aPTT 2–4 h after initiation dose or dose titration, targeting 1.5 to 3 times the initial baseline value aPTT as therapeutic goal Caution with agents that may create additive bleeding risk

4.3.8 Long-Term Management Plan for AF

- Treatment is focused on treating rate/rhythm and anticoagulation risk.
- Treat underlying comorbidities, HTN, and obesity with weight loss/exercise.

A. *Rate/rhythm control strategy*

  - Rate control represents a valid initial therapeutic strategy, even when rhythm control is ultimately planned. Target heart rate goals should be individualized: a strict control strategy (resting heart rate < 80 beats per minute) is appropriate for symptomatic patients or those with significant left ventricular dysfunction. A lenient approach (resting heart rate < 110 beats per minute) may suffice for asymptomatic patients with preserved left ventricular function. Rate control can be achieved through β-blockers, calcium channel blockers (contraindicated in left ventricular dysfunction), or digoxin (reserved primarily for heart failure patients). Combination therapy may be necessary for refractory cases.
  - Evidence suggests that rhythm control strategies offer superior cardiovascular outcomes [3], particularly in specific patient populations including early atrial fibrillation (within 1 year of diagnosis), younger patients (age < 50 years), heart failure with reduced ejection fraction, and individuals with multiple atherosclerotic risk factors. Rhythm control can be achieved through pharmacological intervention or catheter ablation, with or without pacemaker implantation. The "pace and ablate" strategy, involving AV nodal ablation and permanent pacing, is typically reserved for patients who have failed both conventional catheter ablation and rate control measures. Current guidelines favor catheter ablation as the preferred long-term strategy [2].
  - Emerging rhythm control interventions include the MAZE procedure, which creates strategic scarring patterns to interrupt the propagation of atrial fibrillation circuits. Additionally, left atrial appendage occlusion devices, such as the WATCHMAN, offer an alternative to long-term anticoagulation in patients with significantly elevated bleeding risk. These devices effectively reduce stroke risk by preventing thrombus formation within the left atrial appendage [7], though they typically require brief post-procedural anticoagulation (1–2 months) and possibly long-term antiplatelet therapy.
  - Rhythm control strategy failure indicators include left atrial enlargement (indicating long-standing AF). However, rhythm control is likely the best in the following scenarios:
    (i) Symptoms despite rate control.
    (ii) Tachycardia-induced cardiomyopathy (high troponin, ADHF with elevated BNP). If prolonged RVR for days.
    (iii) First attack in young patients.

Pearl

In patients with HFrEF (less than 50% EF), evidence has shown that catheter ablation of AF has favorable outcomes on mortality compared with medical therapy [8].

Pearl

AV node ablation with pacemaker implantation represents a subsequent therapeutic option for patients with atrial fibrillation who remain symptomatic despite optimized rate and rhythm control therapy (effectively preventing transmission of poorly controlled atrial rates to the ventricles, thereby managing symptoms). The implantation of a permanent pacemaker is an essential component following AV node ablation (ensuring appropriate coordination between atrial and ventricular activity). It is important to note that the majority of these patients maintain their atrial fibrillation and continue to require anticoagulation when indicated based on risk factors. This intervention should be considered a final therapeutic option, implemented only after all previous treatment strategies fail.

Pearl

Catheter ablation procedures carry significant potential complications, including thromboembolic events resulting in cerebrovascular accidents, arrhythmia recurrence, cardiac perforation leading to tamponade, and various vascular complications (including dissection, thrombosis, pseudoaneurysm formation, arteriovenous fistula development, and retroperitoneal hemorrhage). Additional serious complications include atrioesophageal fistula formation and phrenic nerve paralysis. Delayed complications may manifest, such as pulmonary vein stenosis, a rare but serious sequela presenting with right-sided heart failure symptomatology, including dyspnea and syncope.

4.3.9 Table for Long-Term Pharmacological Rhythm Control Agents [3]

Drug: Disopyramide		
Primary mechanism of action	**Pharmacokinetics/ pharmacodynamics**	**Drug-drug interaction considerations (pertinent)**
Vaughan-Williams class IA agent	Tmax: 2 h (immediate release); 4–7 h (extended release) T½: 4–10 h Primary metabolism: Hepatic Primary clearance: Renal	CYP3A4 substrate; effects may be influenced by concomitant CYP3A4 inhibitors/inducers May enhance anticholinergic and QT-prolonging effects of concomitant medications
Dose (oral)	**Contraindications**	**Clinical monitoring considerations**
CrCl 40–60 mL/min: 400 mg/day PO in divided doses (either 100 mg PO every 6 h immediate-release capsules or 200 mg PO every 12 h for extended-release capsules) CrCl 30–40 mL/min: 100 mg (immediate-release capsules) PO every 8 h CrCl 15–29 mL/min: 100 mg (immediate-release capsules) PO every 12 h CrCl <15 mL/min: 100 mg (immediate-release capsules) PO every 24 h	High-grade atrioventricular block Cardiogenic shock Long QT syndrome	Glucose levels Cr Potassium EKG

Drug: Quinidine		
Primary mechanism of action	**Pharmacokinetics/ pharmacodynamics**	**Drug-drug interaction considerations (pertinent)**
Vaughan-Williams class IA agent Inhibits the influx of sodium, increasing the recovery period after repolarization	Tmax: 6–8 h T½: 4–10 h Primary metabolism: Hepatic (extensive) Primary clearance: Renal	CYP3A4 substrate; effects may be influenced by concomitant CYP3A4 inhibitors/inducers May enhance anticholinergic and QT-prolonging effects of concomitant medications

Drug: Quinidine		
Dose (oral)	**Contraindications**	**Clinical monitoring considerations**
Immediate release: Initial dosing of 200 mg PO every 6 h Extended release: Initial dosing of 324 mg every 8 to 12 h, may cautiously uptitrate to effect to dosing of 648 mg every 8 to 12 h	High-grade atrioventricular block or intraventricular conduction defect in the absence of pacemaker Cardiogenic shock Long QT syndrome G6PD deficiency	Inhibits CYP2D6 and P-gp May enhance anticholinergic and QT-prolonging effects of concomitant medications

Drug: Flecainide		
Primary mechanism of action	**Pharmacokinetics/ pharmacodynamics**	**Drug-drug interaction considerations (pertinent)**
Vaughan-Williams class IC agent Inhibits fast sodium channels; significantly slows his-Purkinje conduction and causes QRS widening; shorten action potential of Purkinje fibers	Tmax: 1–6 h T½: 10–17 h Primary metabolism: Hepatic, CYP2D6, CYP1A2 Primary clearance: Renal	Metabolized by CYP2D6; use caution with inhibitors of CYP2D6 − Digoxin levels. May enhance bradycardic and QT-prolonging effects of concomitant medications
Dose (oral)	**Contraindications**	**Clinical monitoring considerations**
500 mg–200 mg every 12 h	Cardiogenic shock Sick sinus syndrome, bradycardia, or high-grade atrioventricular block without pacemaker	Avoid use in patients with coronary artery disease or significant ventricular remodeling or hypertrophy Monitor QRS width (also consider dynamic assessment with treadmill stress testing) Should have concomitant AV nodal blockade

Drug: Propafenone		
Primary mechanism of action	**Pharmacokinetics/ pharmacodynamics**	**Drug-drug interaction considerations (pertinent)**
Vaughan-Williams class IC agent Inhibits fast sodium channels; significantly slows his-Purkinje conduction and causes QRS widening; shorten action potential of Purkinje fibers	Tmax: 2–6 h T½: 2–10 h Primary metabolism: Hepatic, especially by CYP2D6 and CYP3A4 Primary clearance: Renal	Metabolized by CYP2D6; use caution with inhibitors of CYP2D6 – Digoxin levels. May enhance bradycardic and QT-prolonging effects of concomitant medications
Dose (oral	**Contraindications**	**Clinical monitoring considerations**
Immediate release: 150–300 mg every 8 h Extended release: 225–425 mg every 12 h	Acute bronchospasm Brugada syndrome Cardiogenic shock Heart failure Hypotension Sick sinus syndrome, bradycardia, or high-grade atrioventricular block without pacemaker	Avoid use in patients with coronary artery disease Avoid use in patients with heart failure and/or left ventricular dysfunction or significant ventricular remodeling or hypertrophy Monitor QRS width (also consider dynamic assessment with treadmill stress testing) Should have concomitant AV nodal blockade

Drug: Amiodarone		
Primary mechanism of action	**Pharmacokinetics/ pharmacodynamics**	**Drug-drug interaction considerations (pertinent)**
Vaughan-Williams class III agent Exact mechanism unknown; inhibits adrenergic stimulation; prolongs action potential, and decreases AV conduction and sinus node function	Tmax: 8–12 h T½: 13–103 days Primary metabolism: Hepatic, especially by CYO3A4	Moderate CYP3A4/2C9/1A4 inhibitor; monitor medications substrates in these pathways May enhance bradycardic and QT-prolonging effect of concomitant medications

Drug: Amiodarone		
Dose (oral)	**Contraindications**	**Clinical monitoring considerations**
400 to 1200 mg/day in divided doses up to a total of 8–10 g; then 100 mg to 200 mg once daily	Cardiogenic shock Iodine hypersensitivity Use with caution in patient with sick sinus syndrome, bradycardia, or high-grade atrioventricular block without pacemaker	Monitor thyroid function tests, pulmonary function tests, liver function tests Should have ophthalmology follow-up given potential for ocular changes

Drug: Dofetilide		
Primary mechanism of action	**Pharmacokinetics/ pharmacodynamics**	**Drug-drug interaction considerations (pertinent)**
Vaughan-Williams class III agent Selective blockade of the Ikr channel, prolongs action potential; prolongs effective refractory period	Tmax: 2–3 h T½: 8–10 h Primary metabolism: Hepatic Primary clearance: Renal	Substrate of CYP3A4; avoid potent CYP3A4 inhibitors May enhance the QT-prolonging effect of medications that prolong QT intervals; consider therapeutic alternatives
Dose (oral)	**Contraindications**	**Clinical monitoring considerations**
Individualize dosage (125 mcg, 250 mcg, 500 mcg capsule initially) based on CrCl and QTc Calculate CrCl using the Cockcroft-gault equation Inpatient initiation with close monitoring per manufacturer protocol	CrCl <20 mL/minute Prolonged QT Torsades de pointes Long QT syndrome	Monitor CrCl, potassium, magnesium ECG (QTc, heart rate; bradycardia may potentiate proarrhythmic risks of QT prolongation)

4

Drug: Dofetilide		
Primary mechanism of action	**Pharmacokinetics/ pharmacodynamics**	**Drug-drug interaction considerations (pertinent)**
Vaughan-Williams class III agent Exact mechanism unknown; inhibits sodium and potassium channels; prolongs action potential	Tmax: 4 h T½: 13–19 h Primary metabolism: Hepatic (extensive) Primary clearance: Fecal	Moderate inhibitor of CYO3A, 2D6, P-gp – Digoxin levels. – Risk of myopathy with simvastatin therapy. – Cilostazol serum concentration. – Colchicine serum concentration. – Edoxaban serum concentration. May enhance bradycardic and QT-prolonging effect of concomitant medications
Dose (oral)	**Contraindications**	**Clinical monitoring considerations**
400 mg twice daily	Heart failure Persistent atrial fibrillation Significant bradycardia, sick sinus syndrome, or high-grade atrioventricular block without pacemaker QT prolongation Amiodarone-induced liver/ lung toxicity	Discontinue class I or III antiarrhythmics or strong CY3A4 inhibitors prior to initiating dronedarone therapy ECG Heart failure symptoms Cr, potassium, magnesium Liver function INR, in patients on warfarin

Drug: Sotalol		
Primary mechanism of action	**Pharmacokinetics/ pharmacodynamics**	**Drug-drug interaction considerations (pertinent)**
Vaughan-Williams class III agent Racemic mixture of isomers: Block Ikr and b-receptors	Tmax: 4 h T½: 12 h Primary clearance: Renal (unchanged)	May enhance the QT prolonging effect of medications that prolong QT intervals; can potentiate risks for torsades de pointes; consider therapeutic alternatives Use with extreme caution in patients with renal disease

Drug: Sotalol		
Dose (oral)	**Contraindications**	**Clinical monitoring considerations**
Calculate CrCl using the Cockcroft-gault equation CrCl >60 mL/min: 80 mg twice daily to start, may uptitrate with monitoring of clinical response and QTc. While maximum dosing is 160 mg twice daily, maximal clinical response often seen with dose at 120 mg twice daily CrCl 40–60 mL/min: Extended dosage interval to every 24 h CrCl <40 mL/minute: Avoid	Bronchospasm Cardiogenic shock, decompensated heart failure QT prolongation CrCl <40 mL/minute Hypokalemia, hypomagnesemia Significant bradycardia without pacemaker	Avoid abrupt discontinuation; 36 h between dosage adjustments to allow steady state Monitor QTc, renal function, electrolytes as part of long-term monitoring

Pearl

Rapid infusion of amiodarone may induce hypotension.

Hospitalist Tip

Class 1c antiarrhythmic medications are exclusively indicated for patients with symptomatic paroxysmal atrial fibrillation who demonstrate no evidence of structural heart disease. For patients with documented structural cardiac pathology, including heart failure or ischemic heart disease, class III antiarrhythmic agents are the preferred therapeutic option, particularly in cases with minimal drug-drug interactions. With normal QTc and kidney function, dofetilide is the best choice from all antiarrhythmic medications. Amiodarone emerges as the optimal choice in the hospital setting for patients with impaired renal function or concurrent heart failure. Before initiating amiodarone therapy, a comprehensive baseline evaluation should include electrocardiography, thyroid function tests, liver function studies, chest radiography, and ophthalmologic examination (when feasible).

Hospitalist Tip

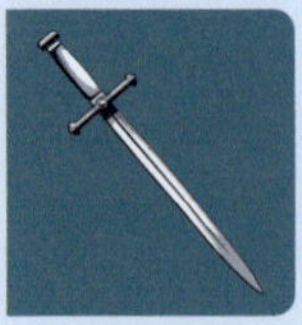

The initiation of sotalol or dofetilide necessitates rigorous inpatient monitoring with continuous telemetry and sequential electrocardiographic assessments for a minimum of 3 days or five doses, owing to the significant risk of QT interval prolongation (Not to exceed 500 msec). This risk happens because, certain class III antiarrhythmic agents, including sotalol, dofetilide, and ibutilide, demonstrate a reverse use-dependent effect on cardiac repolarization. This property is characterized by a prolongation of repolarization time and the refractory period at slower heart rates. Clinically, this results in QT interval prolongation during bradycardia, thereby increasing the risk of torsades de pointes (TdP). Regular monitoring and appropriate correction of serum creatinine, potassium, and magnesium levels are essential therapy components. These agents are considered preferred long-term therapeutic options due to their favorable chronic toxicity profile compared to amiodarone, except in patients predisposed to electrolyte abnormalities. Given the complexity of managing these medications and their potential risks, cardiology consultation is advisable for clinicians who lack specific training or experience in their administration.

B. *Anticoagulation strategy* [2].

- Thromboembolic prophylaxis is crucial, particularly in patients with multiple comorbidities. Risk stratification is accomplished through the CHA2DS2-VASc scoring system, with anticoagulation indicated for men scoring ≥2 or women scoring ≥3, as endorsed by the American College of Cardiology and American Heart Association. Direct oral anticoagulants (DOACs) are generally preferred over warfarin due to their reduced bleeding risk profile. However, warfarin remains the sole approved option for patients with moderate to severe mitral stenosis or mechanical valve prostheses, as DOACs have demonstrated increased thrombotic risk in these populations.
- For patients requiring both post-percutaneous coronary intervention dual antiplatelet therapy (DAPT) and anticoagulation for atrial fibrillation, the preferred strategy involves dual therapy with clopidogrel (or ticagrelor) plus a DOAC, rather than triple therapy, due to lower bleeding risk. These patients should avoid medications that increase bleeding risk, such as NSAIDs, and should receive prophylactic proton pump inhibitor therapy. Notably, aspirin monotherapy is insufficient for stroke prevention in atrial fibrillation.
- The WATCHMAN left atrial appendage closure device is indicated for patients with contraindications to long-term anticoagulation due to elevated bleeding risk [2]. Bleeding risk assessment utilizing the HAS-BLED score (≥3 indicating high risk) helps guide therapeutic decision-making. Evidence from randomized trials is limited regarding anticoagulation strategies for patients with atrial fibrillation who have recurrent bleeding and a limited life expectancy. In these situations, clinicians must weigh the potential stroke prevention benefits against the heightened bleeding risk and the patient's overall symptom burden, especially when the likelihood of achieving meaningful long-term benefit is reduced.

- For subclinical atrial fibrillation (duration <24 hours), anticoagulation may be beneficial in patients meeting specific criteria: elevated thrombotic risk score, history of stroke/transient ischemic attack, and low bleeding risk [9]. However, this decision requires careful consideration of the bleeding risk-benefit ratio [6]. An individualized approach, incorporating patient preferences and specialist consultation, is recommended for optimal outcomes.

Pearl

Successfully implementing rhythm control strategies does not alter anticoagulation requirements in patients with atrial fibrillation. The decision to anticoagulate should continue to be guided by the patient's CHA2DS2-VASc risk stratification score, independent of restoring and maintaining sinus rhythm. This approach acknowledges that even patients who achieve apparent rhythm control may experience subclinical or asymptomatic recurrences of atrial fibrillation, maintaining their thromboembolic risk profile.

Pearl

In patients with valvular heart disease complicated by atrial fibrillation, direct oral anticoagulants (DOACs) are the preferred anticoagulation strategy over warfarin, with specific exceptions. Warfarin remains the exclusive anticoagulant option in cases involving mechanical prosthetic valves, rheumatic heart disease, or significant mitral stenosis. In the particular context of hypertrophic obstructive cardiomyopathy with concurrent atrial fibrillation, anticoagulation is mandatory regardless of the CHA2DS2-VASc risk score, with DOACs being the preferred agent, though warfarin remains an acceptable alternative.

Pearl

Clinical evidence demonstrates that rivaroxaban monotherapy is noninferior to combination therapy with rivaroxaban plus aspirin in patients with concurrent stable coronary artery disease (without prior percutaneous coronary intervention) and atrial fibrillation [10]. Furthermore, the monotherapy approach confers a more favorable bleeding risk profile.

4

4.3.10 Table for Properties and Dosing of Oral Anticoagulants [3]

Vitamin K antagonist		
Drug	**Dose**	**Consideration**
Warfarin	PT/INR adjusted to indication (oral)	Contraindicated in known bleeding complications
Medication classification	**Clinical monitoring and dose adjustment**	**Drug-drug interaction considerations (pertinent)**
Vitamin K antagonist	Monitor vitamin K-containing foods Frequent PT/INR in the beginning until INR 2–3 is achieved (INS 2.5–3.5 for patients with concomitant mechanical mitral valve)	Numerous: Monitor CYP3A4, 2C19, 1A2 *CYP2C9 inhibitors *CYO3A4 inhibitors
Primary mechanism of action	**Pharmacokinetics/pharmacodynamics**	**Reversal agents**
Inhibits vitamin K-dependent clotting factors II, VII, IX, X and proteins C and S	Tmax: 4 h T½: ~40 h Primary metabolism: Hepatic, extensive	– Vitamin K (dose/route dependent on INR/clinical situation). – Fresh frozen plasma (FFP). – 4-factor prothrombin complex concentrate (4F-PCC).

Direct oral anticoagulant (DOAC)		
Drug	**Dose**	**Consideration**
Dabigatran	150 mg twice daily (oral)	Contraindicated in known bleeding complications Contraindicated in mechanical heart valves
Medication classification	**Clinical monitoring and dose adjustment**	**Drug-drug interaction considerations (pertinent)**
Direct thrombin inhibitor (DTI)	Reduce dose to 75 mg twice daily if CrCl 15–30 mL/minute Not recommended if CrCl <15 mL/minute Reduce dose to 75 mg twice daily if coadministered with dronedarone or systemic ketoconazole in patients with CrCl 30–50 mL/min	Monitor strong P-glycoprotein inhibitors/inducers (particularly dronedarone and ketoconazole, see dose adjustment; avoid coadministration with rifampin)

Direct oral anticoagulant (DOAC)		
Drug	**Dose**	**Consideration**
Primary mechanism of action	**Pharmacokinetics/pharmacodynamics**	**Reversal agents**
Competitively inhibits direct thrombin (includes free and clot-bound thrombin)	Tmax:1 to 2 h T½: 12–17 h, longer in elderly and in patients with renal impairment Primary metabolism: P-glycoprotein (P-gp) primary clearance: Renal	– Idarucizumab. – Consider activated 4-factor prothrombin complex concentrate (4F-PCC) if idarucizumab is unavailable.

Drug	Dose	Consideration
Rivaroxaban	20 mg once daily (oral)	Known bleeding complications Avoid in mechanical valve
Medication classification	**Clinical monitoring and dose adjustment**	**Drug-drug interaction considerations (pertinent)**
Direct XA inhibitor	Reduce dose to 15 mg once daily if CrCl 15–50 mL/minute Avoid if CrCl <15 mL/minute Avoid coadministration with P-gp and CYP3A4 inhibitor	Monitor strong P-glycoprotein inhibitors/inducers CYP3A4 inhibitors
Primary mechanism of action	**Pharmacokinetics/pharmacodynamics**	**Reversal agents**
Directly inhibits free factor Xa and prothrombinase activity	Tmax: 2–4 h T½: 5–9 h (11–13 h elderly) Primary metabolism: P-glycoprotein CYP primary clearance: Renal	– Andexanet alpha. – Consider activated 4-factor prothrombin complex concentrate (4F-PCC) if andexanet alpha is unavailable.

Drug	Dose	Consideration
Apixaban	5 mg twice daily (oral)	Known bleeding complications Avoid in mechanical valve
Medication classification	**Clinical monitoring and dose adjustment**	**Drug-drug interaction considerations (pertinent)**
Direct XA inhibitor	Reduce dose to 2.5 mg twice daily if any 2 of the following 3 criteria are met: Cr ≥1.5 mg/dL, ≥80 years of age, body weight ≤60 kg Reduce dose to 2.5 mg twice daily if coadministration with CYP3A4 inhibitors Not recommended in patients with severe hepatic impairment (child-Pugh C)	CYP3A4 and P-glycoprotein inhibitors/inducers

Drug	Dose	Consideration
Primary mechanism of action	**Pharmacokinetics/pharmacodynamics**	**Reversal agents**
Directly inhibits free factor Xa and prothrombinase activity	Tmax: 3–4 h T½: 8–15 h Primary metabolism: Hepatic (especially CYP3A4), also P-glycoprotein Primary clearance: Biliary (73%); renal (27%)	– Andexanet alpha. – Consider activated/inactivated 4-factor prothrombin complex concentrate (4F-PCC) if andexanet alpha is unavailable.

Drug	Dose	Consideration
Edoxaban	60 mg once daily (oral)	Known bleeding complications Avoid in mechanical valve
Medication classification	**Clinical monitoring and dose adjustment**	**Drug-drug interaction considerations (pertinent)**
Direct XA inhibitor	Calculate CrCl using the Cockcroft-gault equation Reduce dose to 30 mg once daily if CrCl 15–50 mL/minute Reduce dose to 30 mg once daily if ≥65 years of age AND at least one of the following: Weight ≤60 kg, concomitant use of potent P-gp inhibitor (e.g., verapamil, quinidine), CrCl 30–50 mL/min Avoid if CrCl <15 mL/minute Avoid in patients with CrCl <95 mL/minute Avoid in patients with moderate to severe liver impairment (child-Pugh class B and C)	CYP3A4 and P-glycoprotein inhibitors/inducers
Primary mechanism of action	**Pharmacokinetics/pharmacodynamics**	**Reversal agents**
Directly inhibits free factor Xa and prothrombinase activity	Tmax: 1–2 h T½: 10–14 h Primary metabolism: CYP3A4,hydrolysis, P-gp substrate Primary clearance: Renal (50%)	– Andexanet alpha. – Consider activated/inactivated 4-factor prothrombin complex concentrate (4F-PCC) if andexanet alpha is unavailable.

Hospitalist Tip

In patients with end-stage renal disease (ESRD), anticoagulation options are limited to apixaban or warfarin due to their more favorable pharmacokinetic profiles. Other direct oral anticoagulants (DOACs) are contraindicated in this population due to their substantial renal clearance, which could lead to drug accumulation and increased bleeding risk in dialysis-dependent patients. Another important note to keep in mind is that High fall risk alone should not be a reason to withhold anticoagulation in patients at elevated risk for thromboembolic events. In Most patients, the risk of thrombosis is higher. Evidence suggests the risk of bleeding would only outweigh the stroke prevention benefit if a patient were to experience approximately hundreds of falls per year.

Pearl

Warfarin and DOACs have multiple drug interactions and may need dose adjustments or even discontinuation. Please check for drug interaction before use; a good one is the Epocrates@ app.

4.3.11 Atrial Flutter

- Atrial flutter is characterized by rapid atrial rates approaching 300 beats per minute, manifesting as distinctive flutter waves with a characteristic sawtooth pattern on electrocardiography. When the diagnosis is uncertain, administration of atrioventricular nodal blocking agents can unmask the underlying flutter wave morphology. Patients with atrial flutter frequently demonstrate resistance to rate control strategies, though these agents may be employed as temporary measures using protocols similar to those for atrial fibrillation management. Given the limited efficacy of pharmacological rate control, the preferred definitive treatment approach involves rhythm control through catheter ablation. Regarding thromboprophylaxis, the anticoagulation strategy parallels atrial fibrillation's, utilizing identical risk stratification and treatment algorithms.

4.4 SVT

4.4.1 General Concepts

- Supraventricular tachycardia encompasses all tachyarrhythmias originating superior to the atrioventricular node, though clinicians predominantly encounter atrioventricular nodal reentrant tachycardia (AVNRT, 60%) and atrioventricular reciprocating tachycardia (AVRT, 30%) [11]. The condition typically affects younger populations, presenting with characteristic paroxysmal symptoms including sudden-onset palpitations, cervical pulsations, lightheadedness, profound fatigue, dizziness, chest discomfort, and dyspnea. These manifestations characteristically demonstrate abrupt resolution. Episodes exhibit variable duration, ranging from seconds to minutes. While syncope and hemodynamic compromise can occur, these severe presentations are uncommon. The subjective patient experience often involves significant distress. Physical examination may reveal diagnostic cannon waves in the cervical vessels.

- Diagnostic evaluation encompasses thyroid function studies to exclude hyperthyroidism, complete blood count to assess for anemia, comprehensive metabolic panel for electrolyte assessment, transthoracic echocardiography, and continuous cardiac monitoring. While typically manifesting as narrow complex tachycardia, QRS duration may exceed 120 milliseconds, resulting in a wide complex presentation.

4.4.2 Sinus Tachycardia (ST)

- Sinus tachycardia is characterized by regular P wave morphology with a ventricular rate exceeding 100 beats per minute. This physiologic response typically occurs secondary to underlying conditions, including anemia, pyrexia, hypovolemia, circulatory shock, infectious processes, and psychological stress. Management should focus on identifying and treating the precipitating etiology rather than suppressing the appropriate compensatory tachycardia with chronotropic agents such as beta-blockers, as this adaptive response represents a normal physiological mechanism.
- Two unusual types of ST to remember include:
  A. Inappropriate sinus tachycardia (IST) represents a distinct clinical entity characterized by persistent sinus tachycardia without identifiable physiological triggers, accompanied by distressing symptomatology, particularly palpitations. The condition demonstrates a predilection for middle-aged female patients and varies in symptomatic presentation. While spontaneous resolution frequently occurs over time, persistent cases may warrant pharmacological intervention with beta-adrenergic blocking agents or ivabradine, a selective inhibitor of the sinoatrial node's funny current (If).

Pearl

Before concluding IST, rule out secondary causes mentioned above in the general concept.

B. Postural orthostatic tachycardia syndrome (POTS) manifests as position-dependent sinus tachycardia, primarily occurring with assumption of upright posture. Diagnostic criteria include an increment in heart rate of 30 beats per minute from baseline or acceleration to rates exceeding 120 beats per minute within 10 minutes of standing. Initial management encompasses volume status optimization, utilization of compression garments, and structured exercise rehabilitation under physical therapy supervision. For cases refractory to conservative measures, pharmacological intervention may include beta-adrenergic blockade or ivabradine administration. Additional therapeutic options, though less commonly employed, include fludrocortisone, selective serotonin reuptake inhibitors, midodrine, and pyridostigmine.

4.4.3 Atrioventricular Nodal Reentrant Tachycardia (AVNRT)

- Atrioventricular nodal reentrant tachycardia (AVNRT) is more prevalent than atrioventricular reciprocating tachycardia (AVRT) [11]. Its electrocardiographic characteristics include a shortened PR interval and narrow QRS complexes, with P waves typically obscured within the QRS complex due to simultaneous atrial and ventricular activation at rapid rates.
- This arrhythmia predominantly affects young female patients without underlying structural cardiac abnormalities and generally carries a benign prognosis. Paroxysmal onset, distinctive superior cervical palpitations, and acute sensation of malaise characterize the clinical presentation.
- Treatment according to the stability of the patient.
  (a) *Unstable*. Follow the ACLS algorithm, with possible need for cardioversion.
  (b) *Stable*. Initial management of AVNRT prioritizes vagal maneuvers as first-line intervention, followed by pharmacological options including adenosine, beta-adrenergic blocking agents, and calcium channel blockers in the acute setting. For patients experiencing recurrent episodes, catheter ablation represents the definitive therapeutic strategy. Despite the generally benign nature of narrow complex tachycardia in hemodynamically stable patients, the immediate availability of resuscitation equipment remains a crucial safety requirement during therapeutic interventions.

Pearl

The long-term therapeutic approach for supraventricular tachycardia generally does not necessitate chronic administration of atrioventricular nodal blocking agents or antiarrhythmic medications. Instead, catheter ablation emerges as the preferred definitive management strategy, offering superior outcomes and eliminating the need for long-term pharmacological therapy in most affected patients.

4.4.4 AVRT

- The problem is an accessory pathway that may or may not pass through normal conduction through the A-V node. Typically, it requires an evaluation by a cardiologist, which may include electrophysiology testing. It is either:
  (i) Orthodromic (narrow complex AVRT/concealed pathway) conduction through the A-V node. More than 90% of the AVRT. A short PR interval may be the only clue.
  (ii) Antidromic (wide complex AVRT) conduction through the accessory pathway. Its short PR interval activates the ventricles faster than AV conduction, and the QRS complex shows slow-rising, slurred waves due to premature ventricular depolarization (preexcitation). WPW (AVRT + symptoms) is the most common form that is clinically known and symptomatic. WPW can lead to VT through accessory pathway conduction, especially when the rate is fast, which is particularly concerning when AF is present (a common occurrence in WPW). The most common tachycardia with WPW is either AF or AVNRT [12].
- Usually diagnosed through prolonged monitoring, stress tests, or electrophysiology (EP) studies.
- Treatment according to the stability of the patient.
  (a) *Unstable*. Follow the ACLS algorithm, with possible need for cardioversion [12].
  (b) *Stable*. For narrow QRS presentations, initial interventions include vagal maneuvers, followed by pharmacological therapy with adenosine, beta-adrenergic blockers, or calcium channel blockers. Wide QRS complex atrioventricular reciprocating tachycardia necessitates treatment with procainamide or ibutilide. In cases of recurrent AVRT, catheter ablation represents the definitive therapeutic approach. Despite the typically stable presentation of narrow complex tachycardia, immediate access to resuscitation equipment remains essential during therapeutic interventions. Current guidelines [12] recommend catheter ablation as first-line therapy for highly symptomatic patients with Wolff-Parkinson-White syndrome.

Pearl

Wolff-Parkinson-white syndrome demonstrates distinctive electrocardiographic characteristics: Abbreviated PR interval with delta wave morphology and QRS duration variability contingent upon the conduction pathway (normal duration via AV node, prolonged via accessory pathway). Concurrent atrial fibrillation in WPW syndrome carries the risk of deterioration to ventricular fibrillation, manifesting as irregular, wide complex tachycardia on electrocardiography, device interrogation, or continuous cardiac monitoring. Procainamide and ibutilide are appropriate pharmacological interventions in hemodynamically stable symptomatic patients awaiting definitive catheter ablation. Beta-adrenergic blockers, calcium channel blockers, digoxin, adenosine, and amiodarone are contraindicated due to their potential to precipitate ventricular tachycardia or fibrillation, particularly in antidromic or antegrade conduction patterns [12]. Hemodynamic instability necessitates immediate electrical cardioversion. Incidental discovery of an asymptomatic WPW pattern on electrocardiography generally does not warrant specific intervention, though cardiology consultation or follow-up is considered reasonable practice [12].

Hospitalist Tip

Adenosine administration is contraindicated in two specific clinical scenarios: Wolff-Parkinson-white syndrome with concurrent atrial fibrillation (due to the risk of precipitating ventricular tachycardia or fibrillation via accessory pathway conduction) and in cardiac transplant recipients (as denervated cardiac tissue demonstrates heightened sensitivity to the drug's chronotropic effects, potentially resulting in severe bradyarrhythmia) [13].

4.4.5 Atrial Tachycardia (AT)

- Atrial tachycardia (AT), while potentially indicative of structural cardiac disease, can occur in its absence. The diagnostic hallmark includes P waves with morphology distinct from those originating from the sinoatrial node. Clinical suspicion should arise when narrow complex supraventricular tachycardia demonstrates resistance to adenosine administration. Initial evaluation should include transthoracic echocardiography to exclude underlying cardiac dysfunction. Management typically begins with intravenous beta-adrenergic blockade or calcium channel blockers, with catheter ablation reserved as a second-line intervention for persistent cases [12].

- Multifocal atrial tachycardia (MAT), a distinct variant of AT, is characterized by three or more distinct P-wave morphologies with ventricular rates exceeding 100 beats per minute. This arrhythmia typically signifies severe underlying pulmonary pathology. Treatment prioritizes addressing hypoxemia, respiratory failure, and the primary pulmonary condition. Second-line therapy involves calcium channel blockade, particularly with diltiazem, while catheter ablation represents a third-line intervention [12].

4.4.6 Premature Atrial Contractions (PAC)

- Atrial ectopy represents an arrhythmia originating from atrial myocardial tissue outside the sinoatrial node. While frequently encountered and generally benign, significant atrial ectopy may serve as a precursor to atrial fibrillation. Most cases do not warrant therapeutic intervention; however, management typically involves rate control with beta-adrenergic blocking agents or calcium channel blockers when symptomatic.

4.5 VT

4.5.1 General Concepts

- Wide complex tachycardia originates in tissue distal to the atrioventricular node, resulting in characteristic QRS complex prolongation. Epidemiological data indicate that ventricular tachycardia (VT) represents the predominant form of wide complex tachycardia, accounting for approximately 80% of cases [14]. The clinical presentation typically manifests as syncope or, in severe cases, sudden cardiac death.
- Comprehensive evaluation requires several essential components, including a detailed assessment of acute coronary syndrome history, review of medications associated with QT interval prolongation, and investigation of family history, particularly focusing on sudden cardiac death. Additionally, management necessitates thorough cardiovascular examination and diagnostic studies including electrocardiography, transthoracic echocardiography, and comprehensive electrolyte analysis with particular attention to potassium and magnesium levels.

4.5.2 PVC (Premature Ventricular Contractions)

- Premature ventricular contractions represent a form of non-sustained ventricular tachycardia with a duration of less than 30 seconds. This arrhythmia, with a prevalence of 50%–75%, is frequently discovered incidentally and typically bears minimal clinical significance [15]. While some patients may report cervical pulsations, the condition often remains asymptomatic. Common precipitating factors include alcohol consumption, caffeine intake, sleep deprivation, thyroid dysfunction, and anemia. The condition demonstrates increased prevalence in patients with underlying structural cardiac disease, coronary artery disease, and uncontrolled hypertension. Symptomatic manifestations, when present, are typically subtle, including palpitations, dizziness, or perceived missed beats.

- Diagnostic evaluation is generally unnecessary unless PVCs are suspected as the underlying etiology of serious complications such as syncope, sudden cardiac arrest, chest pain, or cardiac dysfunction. These complications manifest only when the PVC burden exceeds 10%–20% of total cardiac beats or 10,000 premature ventricular contractions daily, emphasizing the importance of daily telemetry review. The inpatient evaluation protocol includes thyroid function studies, complete blood count, comprehensive metabolic panel, electrolyte analysis, echocardiography, and continuous telemetry monitoring. Outpatient polysomnography may be indicated, and cardiac magnetic resonance imaging can assist in identifying ablation-amenable scar tissue when conventional diagnostic modalities prove inconclusive [16].
- It is noteworthy that the majority of PVCs do not originate from ischemic heart disease; therefore, in the absence of clinical suspicion, extensive ischemic evaluation is not warranted.
- Treatment is indicated with ablation if [17]:
  1. Asymptomatic with high burden >10%–25% of all beats or 10,000 PVCs per day.
  2. Symptomatic or cardiomyopathy (unlikely unless burden >10% of all beats or 10,000 PVCs per day).
- Initial management of premature ventricular contractions focuses on addressing underlying etiologies, correcting electrolyte derangements, and restricting caffeine consumption during hospitalization. These conservative measures often prove sufficient for symptom resolution. When pharmacological intervention is indicated for PVC suppression, first-line therapeutic options include beta-blockers or cardiac-selective calcium channel blockers (with the latter contraindicated in patients with systolic dysfunction). For cases refractory to initial therapy, second-line treatment involves antiarrhythmic medications, with amiodarone being the preferred agent in the inpatient setting. In cases of persistent symptomatology or significant cardiac dysfunction despite medical management, catheter ablation emerges as the optimal therapeutic strategy.

Hospitalist Tip

Routine antiarrhythmic therapy is mostly not indicated in asymptomatic PVC.

4.5.3 Ventricular Tachycardia (VT)

- Ventricular tachycardia is characterized by a persistent, accelerated rhythm with QRS complex duration of 120 milliseconds or greater on electrocardiography. This arrhythmia typically produces significant symptomatology and carries potential lethal consequences when sustained (duration exceeding 30 seconds). The morphological classification distinguishes between monomorphic and polymorphic variants, each with distinct therapeutic implications and prognostic significance.

Pearl

Absence of symptoms does not rule out sustained VT, but it is less likely.

Hospitalist Tip

Consider ACS or medications that prolong QT whenever you encounter a VT.

- It is mostly seen in patients with structural heart disease, especially IHD 90% (scar tissue is a good conductor for VT) [14], in which case it could rapidly progress to VF. It is two types based on underlying heart conditions:
  A. *Structural heart disease-induced VT*. Ventricular tachycardia commonly occurs in the context of underlying cardiac pathologies, including ischemic heart disease, heart failure, cardiac infiltrative disorders, amyloidosis, and arrhythmogenic right ventricular cardiomyopathy. Comprehensive diagnostic evaluation encompasses electrocardiography with potential ischemic workup, transthoracic echocardiography, coronary angiography, cardiac magnetic resonance imaging (particularly valuable in detecting sarcoidosis and myocardial scarring), and technetium-99 m pyrophosphate scintigraphy for cardiac amyloidosis assessment. Various precipitating factors may trigger episodes, including electrolyte disturbances, physiological stressors, and numerous pharmacological agents (including antiarrhythmics, chemo-

therapeutic agents, anticonvulsants, antidepressants, mood stabilizers, and antipsychotic medications).

B. *Idiopathic ventricular tachycardia (no underlying heart disease)*. Idiopathic ventricular tachycardia predominantly affects middle-aged individuals and represents a generally benign arrhythmia characterized by intermittent palpitations in the absence of structural cardiac abnormalities. While mortality is rare, the condition warrants clinical attention. Episodes are frequently precipitated by periods of psychological stress. Diagnostic evaluation may necessitate implantable loop recorder placement when clinical suspicion exists. Analogous to premature ventricular contractions, a ventricular tachycardia burden exceeding 10% of total cardiac activity is associated with the development of cardiomyopathy [18].

- Important differentials to consider include:
  (i) *SVT with aberrancy (BBB)*
  (ii) *Preexcited antidromic tachycardia (if symptomatic, usually indicates WPW syndrome)*
  (iii) *Ventricular paced rhythms*
  (iv) *Artifact*. A short burst of a wide QRS complex, squared off at both ends, which does not appear typical for a QRS. The patient is asymptomatic at the time of presentation.

Pearl

Electrophysiologic studies serve as a valuable diagnostic tool in cases where the diagnosis of ventricular tachycardia remains uncertain or requires differentiation from other arrhythmic conditions, particularly supraventricular tachycardia with aberrant conduction. Given the complexity of interpretation and therapeutic implications, consultation with an electrophysiology specialist is strongly recommended for optimal diagnostic and management strategies.

Pearl

An irregular wide complex tachycardia pattern is more suggestive of Wolff-Parkinson-White syndrome with concurrent atrial fibrillation rather than ventricular tachycardia. Management should follow WPW protocols, with the critical caveat that atrioventricular nodal blocking agents, including beta-blockers and calcium channel blockers, are contraindicated. In hemodynamically stable patients presenting with symptomatic arrhythmia, procainamide is the preferred therapeutic agent.

- Treatment mainly focuses on treating the underlying causes and hemodynamic stability:
  (a) *Hemodynamically unstable or cardiac arrest.* Follow the ACLS algorithm.
  (b) *Hemodynamically stable.*
- Initial management focuses on addressing precipitating factors and normalizing electrolyte abnormalities, particularly magnesium, potassium, and calcium levels, before initiating antiarrhythmic therapy. In the inpatient setting, amiodarone represents the preferred antiarrhythmic agent, though sotalol and dofetilide remain viable alternatives.
- Early cardiology consultation is essential for evaluating the need for ablation procedures and cardiac catheterization to exclude ischemic etiology.
- Secondary prevention strategies vary according to clinical context. Patients who experience cardiac arrest due to ventricular tachycardia typically require implantable cardioverter-defibrillator (ICD) placement, with or without concurrent ablation. The latter is particularly indicated in post-myocardial infarction ventricular tachycardia [19], given the unacceptable risk of recurrent cardiac arrest. Similarly, patients with sustained ventricular tachycardia and underlying structural heart disease, which typically results in permanent myocardial scarring, are candidates for device therapy. In contrast, idiopathic ventricular tachycardia is amenable to catheter ablation, with beta-blockers serving as first-line therapy, and cardiac-selective calcium channel blockers as alternative agents. Notably, ICD placement is generally unnecessary in idiopathic ventricular tachycardia due to its low risk of precipitating hemodynamic compromise or cardiac arrest [18].
- Beta-blocker therapy remains a cornerstone of secondary prevention across all variants of ventricular tachycardia.

Hospitalist Tip

A fundamental principle in managing wide complex tachycardia is to presume ventricular tachycardia (VT) until definitively proven otherwise. This conservative approach is justified by epidemiological data demonstrating that VT represents the predominant form of wide complex tachycardia and carries significantly greater morbidity and mortality if misdiagnosed. Management should strictly adhere to advanced cardiac life support (ACLS) protocols, ensuring standardized, evidence-based treatment approaches for these potentially life-threatening arrhythmias.

Pearl

Implantable cardioverter-defibrillator (ICD) placement is indicated for primary prevention of sudden cardiac death from ventricular tachycardia or ventricular fibrillation in patients meeting specific criteria: Left ventricular ejection fraction less than or equal to 35%, New York heart association (NYHA) functional class II or III heart failure symptomatology, and completion of at least 3 months of guideline-directed medical therapy (GDMT) [18].

4.6 Bradycardia

4.6.1 General Concepts

- Bradycardia is defined by a heart rate below 50 beats per minute. Symptomatology primarily reflects compromised cardiac output, including syncope, lightheadedness, dyspnea, and fatigue. The etiology may be external to cardiac tissue or intrinsic to the cardiac conduction system, involving the sinoatrial node, atrioventricular node, or Purkinje fibers.
- A comprehensive historical assessment should encompass medication review, documentation of pre-existing conditions, including hypothyroidism, cardiac pathology, sleep apnea, elevated intracranial pressure, and athletic participation history.
- Initial diagnostic evaluation requires electrocardiography, electrolyte analysis, and thyroid function studies. When intrinsic cardiac disease is suspected, transthoracic echocardiography is indicated. In cases of diagnostic uncertainty, extended cardiac monitoring or ambulatory electrocardiography may be warranted for definitive diagnosis.

4.6.2 Sinus Bradycardia

- Sinus bradycardia represents a predominantly benign condition frequently observed in athletes, elderly individuals (due to age-related sinoatrial node fibrosis), during vagal stimulation (including coughing, emesis, defecation, and micturition), and nocturnal sleep. Benign etiologies typically demonstrate appropriate chronotropic response during exercise testing.
- Common pathological causes encompass pharmacological agents (beta-blockers, cardiac calcium channel blockers, clonidine, amiodarone, digoxin, opioids, intensive care sedatives including propofol, and donepezil), endocrine dysfunction (hypothyroidism), elevated intracranial pressure (associated with hypertension and altered consciousness), obstructive sleep apnea, and structural cardiac pathologies, both ischemic (particularly right-sided) and non-ischemic (including infiltrative disorders such as amyloidosis, hemochromatosis, and sarcoidosis).
- Therapeutic intervention is generally unnecessary except in cases of hemodynamic compromise (without a specific heart rate threshold), which should follow Advanced Cardiac Life Support protocols. Otherwise, management focuses on addressing underlying etiologies or discontinuing causative medications. Symptomatic sinus bradycardia without a reversible cause necessitates permanent pacemaker implantation. Additional specific indications for pacing are noted in current guidelines [20]:
  (i) Symptomatic sinus node dysfunction at rest.
  (ii) Symptomatic chronotropic incompetence.
  (iii) Symptomatic tachy-brady syndrome.

Hospitalist Tip

In all patients with bradycardia, review the medication list very cautiously to uncover a possible correlation with the bradycardia.

4.6.3 Sick Sinus Syndrome (SSS)/Sinus Node Dysfunction, or Tachy-Brady Syndrome

- Sick sinus syndrome is characterized by sinoatrial node dysfunction manifesting as unpredictable alternation between bradycardia and tachycardia. This condition predominantly affects elderly populations, typically resulting from age-related fibrotic changes. While often asymptomatic, symptomatic cases generally require permanent pacemaker implantation. A diagnostic hallmark includes chronotropic incompetence, evidenced by inadequate heart rate response to physical exertion (failure to reach 80% maximum predicted HR with exercise). The syndrome frequently manifests with episodes of atrial fibrillation followed by prolonged compensatory pauses on electrocardiography, reflecting impaired spontaneous depolarization. The workup for SSS includes assessing for underlying diseases such as sleep apnea, assessing for structural heart disease, and stress testing if symptoms occur with exercise, to assess for chronotropic incompetence.
- The condition may be iatrogenic or secondary to underlying cardiac pathology. Current epidemiological data indicate that sick sinus syndrome represents one of the principal indications for permanent pacemaker implantation in the geriatric population when symptomatic [21].

Hospitalist Tip

A common scenario for SSS is an older patient with paroxysmal AF who develops a prolonged pause after termination of AF, accompanied by symptoms on telemetry.

Pearl

The most common indications for permanent pacemaker implantation are SSS and high-grade atrioventricular (AV) block [22].

4.6.4 AV Block

- Atrioventricular block may be iatrogenic or secondary to underlying cardiac pathologies. Symptomatic manifestations typically emerge at heart rates below 40 beats per minute. Exercise stress testing can assist in differentiating between low-grade and high-grade atrioventricular (AV) block. In cases of Mobitz type I AV block, the increase in sympathetic tone induced by exercise typically enhances AV nodal conduction, which may result in resolution of the block.
- The condition is classified into first-degree, second-degree, or third-degree (complete heart block). The bundle branch block morphology on baseline electrocardiography is often a diagnostic indicator.
  - I. First-degree atrioventricular block is characterized by prolonged AV conduction with PR intervals exceeding 200 milliseconds. While previously considered benign, it correlates with increased mortality risk and atrial fibrillation development. This conduction delay commonly manifests during sleep or in association with beta-adrenergic or calcium channel blockade.
  - II. Second-degree block presents in two variants:
    - (a) Mobitz type 1 demonstrates progressive PR interval prolongation culminating in a dropped QRS complex.
    - (b) Mobitz type 2 exhibits intermittent non-conducted P waves with consistent PR intervals and improves with sympathetic activation. This variant frequently progresses to complete heart block, with deterioration during sympathetic stimulation.
  - III. Third-degree (complete) heart block is characterized by complete dissociation between atrial and ventricular activity, manifesting as non-conducted P waves with an independent, slow ventricular escape rhythm.
- Treatment depends on:
  - (a) Hemodynamically unstable. Follow ACLS.
  - (b) Hemodynamically stable. Management of atrioventricular block primarily focuses on addressing reversible underlying etiologies. However, permanent pacemaker implantation is indicated in specific scenarios, including complete heart block and Mobitz type 2 second-degree atrioventricular block, regardless of symptom status. Additional indications for permanent pacing include atrial fibrillation with pauses exceeding 3 seconds and selected cases of bifascicular block meeting specific clinical criteria.

Hospitalist Tip

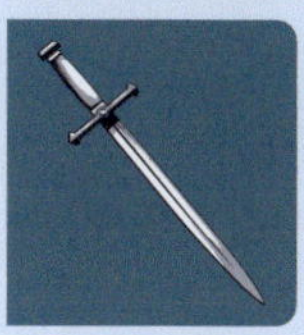

Do not routinely consult for pacemaker placement for:
- (i) Asymptomatic first-degree or Mobitz I block
- (ii) Any reversible AV block (e.g., drugs, OSA).
- (iii) Asymptomatic, physiologic AV block (e.g., during sleep, vagal response).

4.7 Cardiac Channelopathies

4.7.1 Clinical Approach [23]

- Inherited cardiac channelopathies should be considered in the differential diagnosis when evaluating young to middle-aged patients without prior cardiac history who present with acute cardiac manifestations, including syncope, presyncope, significant dizziness, or cardiac arrest. Family history often reveals unexplained deaths, particularly among young first-degree relatives.
- These conditions share the potential for premature, unexplained, sudden cardiac death (SCD) as a presenting feature. Each syndrome demonstrates distinct triggering factors that warrant specific investigation. Initial diagnostic evaluation encompasses electrocardiography and transthoracic echocardiography. Additional imaging modalities may be indicated based on clinical context, including left heart catheterization (particularly valuable in spontaneous monomorphic ventricular tachycardia), cardiac computed tomography, and magnetic resonance imaging.
- When initial diagnostic studies prove unremarkable and echocardiography demonstrates preserved ejection fraction, electrophysiological studies may be warranted, conducted under cardiologist supervision following a 48-hour antiarrhythmic medication washout period. Genetic testing, guided by electrophysiology specialists, can influence therapeutic decision-making, especially in long QT syndromes.
- Given these conditions' complexity and potential severity, management should be deferred to cardiac electrophysiology specialists rather than attempted independently. Particular emphasis should be placed on the critical nature of exertional syncope or seizures, which warrant thorough evaluation before being deemed benign.

Pearl

Sudden cardiac arrest demonstrates multiple potential etiologies, including congestive heart failure, acute coronary syndromes, hypertrophic obstructive cardiomyopathy, non-sustained ventricular arrhythmias, advanced renal dysfunction, significant electrolyte derangements, and obstructive sleep apnea. The diagnostic approach should be tailored to individual clinical presentation and risk factors, with investigation protocols designed to identify and address these underlying pathophysiological mechanisms.

Hospitalist Tip

In all patients with unexplained sudden cardiac arrest, basic workup should include EKG, coronary angiography/ischemic workup, TTE, and possible cardiac MRI.

- Management of cardiac arrhythmias frequently centers on trigger avoidance without necessitating implantable cardioverter-defibrillator (ICD) placement. This approach applies to several conditions, including asymptomatic Wolff-Parkinson-White syndrome, ventricular fibrillation or polymorphic ventricular tachycardia occurring within 48 hours of acute coronary syndrome, drug-induced or electrolyte-mediated arrhythmias, and ablatable arrhythmias in structurally normal hearts. Cardiology consultation remains mandatory for all cases requiring ICD placement or ablation procedures. Beta-adrenergic blockade represents fundamental therapy across the spectrum of cardiovascular pathologies. It is crucial to recognize that while ICD therapy prevents sudden cardiac death, it does not address the underlying pathophysiology, necessitating comprehensive investigation and management of the primary cardiac condition.

Pearl

Most patients with inherited cardiac channelopathies do not require an implantable cardioverter-defibrillator (ICD).

Pearl

Common class I indications for ICD placement *before discharge from the hospital* include [23]:

(i) Sustained VT (>30 seconds).
(ii) Unexplained SCD, irrespective of EF.
(iii) CHF with EF less than 35% for at least 3 months, compared to previous echo (if the patient has an interventricular conduction delay of 150 or more, they will benefit from additional CRRT).

- *The most common ones are listed below*:
  I. *Brugada syndrome*
  - Brugada syndrome is characterized by distinctive ST-segment elevation in leads V1–V3, with potential progression to ventricular fibrillation and cardiac arrest. The electrocardiographic pattern typically manifests as an incomplete right bundle branch block in the anterior leads. Ventricular tachycardia/fibrillation episodes predominantly occur during rest or nocturnal periods, with known triggers including psychological stress, pyrexia, specific medications (including tricyclic antidepressants and propofol), and substance use (alcohol/cannabis). A comprehensive list of precipitating medicines is available at ▶ https://www.brugadadrugs.org/.
  - The condition demonstrates male predominance, typically presenting in young adults with syncope or sudden cardiac death. Diagnostic probability assessment utilizes the Shanghai score system [24].
  - Management strategy encompasses trigger avoidance and cardiology consultation for consideration of implantable cardioverter-defibrillator placement or ablation procedures in symptomatic patients or survivors of sudden cardiac death. ICD implantation is not universally indicated, particularly in asymptomatic individuals. For hospitalized patients with known Brugada syndrome, management priorities include aggressive antipyretic therapy and avoidance of arrhythmogenic medications [25]. Beta-blockers can increase ST-segment elevation and are therefore contraindicated. Quinidine therapy may be beneficial in reducing ICD shock events in patients with existing devices or when ICD therapy is contraindicated or impractical [26].

  II. *Long QT syndromes (LQT)*
  - Long QT syndrome represents one of the most prevalent inherited channelopathies, encompassing multiple genotypic variants. The condition is defined by QTc interval prolongation (exceeding 480 milliseconds) without secondary causes. The prolongation is most readily identifiable in lead II or V5, with intervals exceeding 500 milliseconds being highly specific for the syndrome and warranting electrophysiology consultation [27]. This threshold also serves as a critical parameter for discontinuing QT-prolonging medications.
  - Clinical presentation typically includes exertional syncope or sudden cardiac death. The syndrome demonstrates notable associations with seizure disorders and, in the juvenile variant, congenital deafness.
  - Specific genotypes correlate with distinct triggering factors, potentially precipitating polymorphic ventricular tachycardia and subsequent cardiac arrest.
  - Diagnostic evaluation mandates exclusion of secondary acquired causes, particularly medication effects and electrolyte disturbances (specifically potassium and magnesium abnormalities).

- Management encompasses multiple strategies: discontinuing causative medications, electrolyte normalization, and beta-blockade [28]. In congenital long QT syndrome (LQTS), arrhythmias are primarily triggered by adrenergic stimulation rather than by bradycardia. Therefore, beta-blocker therapy remains beneficial, as its protective effects outweigh the potential risks of bradycardia. Among available agents, nadolol and propranolol are preferred due to their non-selective, long-acting adrenergic blockade and minimal intrinsic sympathomimetic properties. In acquired long QT syndrome (LQTS), such as that caused by medications or electrolyte abnormalities, bradycardia frequently serves as a precipitating factor for torsades de pointes. Thats why In acute settings, in cases of torsades de pointes that are refractory to magnesium therapy, QTc interval shortening may be achieved by increasing the heart rate through temporary pacing or intravenous administration of isoproterenol. Trigger avoidance, particularly extreme physical exertion and psychological stressors, is essential. Implantable cardioverter-defibrillator placement is typically indicated for patients with major symptomatology (syncope or aborted sudden cardiac death) or asymptomatic individuals with QT intervals exceeding 500 milliseconds, implemented under cardiologist guidance [27]. In refractory cases, left cardiac sympathetic denervation represents a potential last-resort intervention. All suspected instances warrant electrophysiology consultation for comprehensive evaluation and definitive diagnosis.

Pearl

The most implicated medications include antibiotics (macrolides and fluoroquinolones), antipsychotics, antiarrhythmics, and antidepressants. For a comprehensive list of drugs, visit this website: ► https://crediblemeds.org/

Pearl

Short QT syndrome (less than 330–360 ms) is the opposite of long QT with VT/VF arrhythmias. Suspect it if the QT is immediately attached to the QRS without any delay in the EKG. It does lead to sudden cardiac death.

III. *Catecholaminergic polymorphic VT (CPVT)*

- Catecholaminergic polymorphic ventricular tachycardia is characterized by stress-induced premature ventricular contractions or bidirectional ventricular tachycardia, precipitated by physical exertion or emotional stress. The condition typically manifests as exercise-induced syncope or sudden cardiac death, notably in the presence of normal cardiac structure on echocardiography. This channelopathy predominantly affects young individuals.
- Therapeutic management encompasses multiple modalities: primary intervention with beta-adrenergic blockade (preferentially nadolol or propranolol), second-line therapy with flecainide, implantable cardioverter-defibrillator placement in selected cases, and systematic avoidance of known triggering factors [29].

Pearl

CPVT should be suspected in exertional syncope, with EKG findings of exertion-induced PVC/VT. Baseline EKG and TTE are usually normal.

IV. *Arrhythmogenic right ventricular cardiomyopathy (ARVC)*

- Arrhythmogenic right ventricular cardiomyopathy (ARVC) is characterized by myocardial replacement with adipose tissue in the right ventricular wall, with familial inheritance documented in 30% of cases.
- The diagnostic criteria encompass specific cardiac magnetic resonance imaging findings (including right ventricular wall motion abnormalities, aneurismal formation, and fatty infiltration) and characteristic electrocardiographic features (T-wave inversion in right precordial leads V1–3, epsilon waves, and paroxysmal ventricular tachycardia), often accompanied by positive family history. The condition demonstrates age-variable presentation across the lifespan and may progress to heart failure. Exercise typically serves as an arrhythmogenic trigger.
- Management of ARVC with concurrent ventricular tachycardia necessitates a dual approach of implantable cardioverter-defibrillator placement and catheter ablation. During the pre-implantation period, beta-adrenergic blockade is indicated, with consideration of antiarrhythmic therapy (sotalol or amiodarone) for persistent arrhythmias. Discharge counseling should emphasize the avoidance of excessive physical exertion and psychological stressors.

4.8 Cardiac Devices

4.8.1 ICD/Automated Implantable Cardioverter-Defibrillator (AICD)

- Implantable cardioverter-defibrillators (ICDs) serve a fundamental therapeutic purpose: terminating potentially lethal ventricular arrhythmias, specifically sustained ventricular tachycardia (VT) and ventricular fibrillation (VF). This life-saving intervention represents a critical advancement in the prevention of sudden cardiac death through automated detection and termination of malignant ventricular arrhythmias.

Pearl

Subcutaneous implantable cardioverter-defibrillators (S-ICDs) are distinguished by their capability to deliver defibrillatory shocks without providing pacing functionality, owing to their anatomical distance from cardiac tissue, precluding effective sensing of cardiac electrical activity. These devices offer particular utility in specific patient populations, including those with compromised vascular access, recent bacteremia, or elevated risk of vascular infection-related complications. This alternative approach to defibrillator therapy provides a valuable option for patients in whom traditional transvenous systems may be contraindicated.

Pearl

Thick and long white right ventricular leads in chest X-ray indicate defibrillator function.

- *It is indicated in either of the following*:
  A. *Primary prevention* (high risk of ventricular arrhythmias/sudden cardiac death, but has not happened yet).
     (i) Most cardiac patients inherit congenital arrhythmia syndromes (Brugadas, prolonged QT congenital syndromes, ARVC, etc.). Suppose they meet the specific indications for ICD placement.
     (ii) Symptomatic (NYHAII-III) CHF with ischemic or non-ischemic cardiomyopathy, EF $\leq 35\%$.
     (iii) HOCM with high-risk features (► Chap. 11).

B. *Secondary prevention* (patients had an event and would like to prevent further ones): expected survival of >1 year for all patients.
   (i) Patients with stable, sustained, unexplained (no reversible factor) VT.
   (ii) Any unstable VT leads to sudden cardiac death or significant hemodynamic compromise.
   (iii) Previous unexplained sudden cardiac death.
   (iv) Inducible sustained VT with recent myocardial infarction within 40 days. VF or polymorphic VT within 48 h of ACS usually does not need ICD placement, as it will resolve spontaneously.
   (v) EF of ≤40% with non-sustained VT.

- Major complications associated with implantable cardioverter-defibrillators (ICDs) primarily manifest in oversensing and undersensing phenomena. Oversensing occurs when the device misinterprets non-pathological electrical activity (most commonly atrial fibrillation with rapid ventricular response) as ventricular tachycardia or fibrillation, resulting in inappropriate shock delivery. This situation necessitates immediate intervention through magnet application over the device. Conversely, undersensing represents failure to detect and respond to genuine ventricular arrhythmias, potentially withholding necessary therapy. Device infection represents another significant complication (detailed in ▶ Chap. 7). Both oversensing and undersensing scenarios warrant prompt cardiology consultation with device interrogation. In cases of suspected oversensing, adherence to Advanced Cardiac Life Support protocols for ventricular tachycardia/fibrillation is mandatory until definitively excluded through device interrogation and clinical correlation.

Pearl

Implantable cardioverter-defibrillator (ICD) placement is generally contraindicated in patients with a projected life expectancy of less than 1 year. This therapeutic decision requires a multidisciplinary approach involving cardiology consultation and implementation of shared decision-making principles with patients and their families. This approach acknowledges the complex interplay between potential therapeutic benefits, quality of life considerations, and limited life expectancy, emphasizing the importance of patient-centered care in advanced cardiac disease management.

Pearl

Device interrogation is accomplished by applying an external reader over the generator to retrieve functional data. Device identification is facilitated by patient-specific device cards and electronic applications capable of identifying device manufacturers through radiographic imaging. The interrogation typically generates a multi-page report summarizing principal findings on the initial page. For hospitalist practitioners, priority review should focus on the executive summary, with particular attention to several critical parameters:

(i) Battery status and longevity.
(ii) Programmed pacing mode.
(iii) Degree of pace dependence.
(iv) Programmed lower rate limit.
(v) Defibrillator therapy parameters (in ICDs).
(vi) Rate responsiveness characteristics.
(vii) Device response to magnet application.

4.8.2 Cardiac Resynchronization Therapy (CRT)

- Cardiac resynchronization therapy (CRT) represents a specialized pacing modality designed to optimize biventricular synchrony, enhancing cardiac output in heart failure patients with demonstrated mortality benefit. These devices typically incorporate multiple therapeutic functions, including defibrillation capability and anti-bradycardia pacing support. Radiographic visualization reveals a characteristic three-lead configuration, comprising right atrial and bilateral ventricular leads, which function cooperatively to achieve coordinated cardiac mechanical synchrony.
- *The main indications are*:
  (i) Symptomatic CHF in sinus rhythm with EF ≤35% and a prolonged QRS complex of >150 ms with or without LBBB.
  (ii) Symptomatic CHF with EF ≤35% and LBBB.

Pearl

Cardiac resynchronization therapy (CRT) facilitates the optimization of guideline-directed medical therapy (GDMT) for chronic heart failure by improving hemodynamic parameters, specifically cardiac output and blood pressure. This enhancement in cardiovascular function enables more aggressive titration of evidence-based pharmacological interventions, optimizing therapeutic outcomes in patients with advanced heart failure.

4.8.3 PPM (Transvenous/Leadless)

- Permanent pacemakers (PPM) primarily prevent bradyarrhythmia and asystole by detecting subthreshold heart rates and subsequent delivery of electrical stimulation, resulting in mechanical capture of designated cardiac chambers. Device implementation may be permanent or temporary, based on clinical indications.
- The nomenclature of pacemaker systems follows a standardized three-letter code: the first letter designates chamber pacing capability, the second indicates sensing function, and the third describes the device's response mode (either inhibition or triggering) to sensed native cardiac activity. For instance, in dual-chamber systems (DDD), atrial sensing without ventricular sensing triggers ventricular pacing while inhibiting atrial pacing. The DDD configuration, offering comprehensive functionality, represents the predominant pacemaker type in clinical practice.
- Electrocardiographic manifestations of pacing include characteristic vertical spikes preceding chamber activation. Ventricular pacing produces prolonged QRS complexes with left bundle branch block morphology. Sensing functions, while operational, do not generate visible electrocardiographic signatures. In VVI mode, ventricular pacing produces wide QRS complexes with inhibition during normal atrioventricular conduction, while atrial activity remains dissociated due to the absence of atrial sensing or pacing capabilities.
- Contemporary practice increasingly utilizes leadless pacing systems, which are fully intracardiac and may be imperceptible on physical examination, though visible radiographically. Dual-chamber leadless systems (exemplified by the Abbott AVEIR DR device) demonstrate a distinctive radiographic appearance with separate atrial and right ventricular components.

Hospitalist Tip

Pacing indicates depolarization but not necessarily mechanical capture and contraction. Feeling and listening for a heartbeat or pulse is vital when the ventricles are paced. Place the patient on a pulse oximeter to confirm pulse wave and oxygenation.

Pearl

In the presence of LBBB morphology with paced ventricles, it is not easy to diagnose acute ischemia. Use any of the modified Sagarbosa criteria to diagnose acute ischemia:

A. Concordant ST elevation $\geq$1 mm in $\geq$1 lead.
B. Concordant ST depression $\geq$1 mm in $\geq$1 lead of V1–V3.
C. Proportionally excessive discordant STE in $\geq$1 lead, anywhere with $\geq$1 mm STE, as defined by $\geq$25% of the depth of the preceding S wave.

- *The main indications are*:
  (i) Unexplained symptomatic sinus bradycardia or SSS. It is vital to rule out secondary causes before considering PPM.
  (ii) High-grade AV block (complete heart block, Mobitz type 2 second-degree AV block, even if asymptomatic).
- *Common PPM malfunctions*:
  (i) *Failure to capture*. The spikes are present but do not follow depolarization (missed P wave or QRS complex) and mechanical capture. As a result, the patient's heart rate will be slow. This could be due to device problems, mainly the leads, but other physiological or pathological causes preventing the heart from depolarizing normally, such as ischemic cardiac tissue, also need to be ruled out.
  (ii) *Pacemaker output failure*. Failure of the generator to generate spikes, resulting in bradycardia. A malfunction of the generator, battery, or lead is most likely.
  (iii) *Undersensing*. Failure to sense will lead to unusual duplicate waves or asynchronicity, mostly due to lead or battery issues.
  (iv) *Oversensing*. It will appear as missed-paced beats or bradycardia due to oversensing other tissues rather than the heart, leading to inhibition of appropriate delivery.
  (v) *Pacemaker-related tachycardia*. Inappropriately paced tachycardia.
  (vi) *Pacemaker-related cardiomyopathy*. Long-term pacing complications.

4.8.4 Implantable Loop Recorders (ILRs)

- Implantable loop recorders (ILRs) are subcutaneously placed continuous cardiac monitoring devices typically positioned in the left anterior chest wall. They are detectable through both palpation and radiographic imaging.
- These devices are primarily indicated for patients with suspected paroxysmal or infrequent arrhythmic events requiring extended monitoring periods.
- Magnetic resonance imaging does not significantly compromise device function or data integrity.
- The implantation site warrants protection from surgical interventions, as electromagnetic interference may disrupt data acquisition and storage capabilities.

4.8.5 Management Approach for Cardiac Device Concerns

- Device malfunction evaluation necessitates a systematic approach, including electrocardiography and manufacturer-specific device interrogation (Boston Scientific, Biotronic, Medtronic, St. Jude Medical). A comprehensive assessment should include a complete metabolic panel, electrolyte analysis, thyroid function studies, transthoracic echocardiography, and chest radiography to evaluate lead integrity and positioning. Medication review is essential, and clinical presentation may warrant ischemic evaluation. Cardiology or electrophysiology consultation is indicated for significant concern regarding device dysfunction, applicable across permanent pacemakers, implantable cardioverter-defibrillators, and cardiac resynchronization therapy devices.

- In emergent situations involving pacemaker malfunction with hemodynamic compromise, magnet application over the generator converts the device to a predetermined fixed-rate/asynchronous mode (AOO, VOO, or DOO, representing atrial, ventricular, or dual-chamber asynchronous pacing, respectively) or prevents defibrillator discharge. Magnet removal should occur once the clinical situation permits. Continuous monitoring of pulse and oxygen saturation is mandatory to confirm mechanical capture. Prophylactic placement of transcutaneous pacing and defibrillation pads is recommended. Immediate electrophysiology or cardiology consultation is essential.

Pearl

Magnet application requires judicious consideration and should be restricted to situations of absolute necessity. Device-specific responses to magnetic fields vary considerably, with some defibrillators maintaining unaltered pacing function during magnet application. Furthermore, electromagnetic interference during surgical procedures may result in pacing inhibition despite magnet placement. This variability necessitates cardiology consultation for appropriate device reprogramming both pre- and post-procedurally. While some devices emit characteristic audible signals confirming magnet recognition and mode conversion, this feature is not universal across all devices. This heterogeneity in device response underscores the importance of thorough familiarity with specific device characteristics and appropriate specialist consultation before magnet utilization.

4.8.6 Managing Cardiovascular Implantable Devices (CIDs) During Perioperative Care [30, 31]

- Perioperative management of cardiac devices requires comprehensive information acquisition, including device identification (via device card) or manufacturer consultation, to determine device specifications, indication, dependency status, magnetic resonance imaging compatibility, and procedure-specific considerations. Essential preparatory measures include:
  (i) Device site demarcation.
  (ii) Pre-procedure verification of magnet response when indicated.

(iii) Cardiology clearance and device programming optimization.
(iv) Continuous telemetry monitoring throughout the procedure.
(v) Prophylactic placement of transcutaneous pacing/defibrillation pads.

- Post-procedural management mandates device re-interrogation and restoration of original programming parameters under cardiologist supervision, ensuring appropriate device function and optimal patient safety.

Pearl

If magnet use is anticipated during the procedure, the magnet must be continuously applied directly to the CID without contaminating the sterile field. When the magnet is no longer detected, the device will return to its prior settings [30].

Hospitalist Tip

Most, but not all, contemporary devices are considered MRI-compatible. However, always check if the device is MRI-compatible before sending it for an MRI scan. Some devices will need to be switched to MRI mode. All patients should be monitored by tele and pulse oximeter at the time of the MRI.

Hospitalist Tip

Avoiding central line access on the ipsilateral side of a CID may reduce the risk of vascular stenosis, arrhythmia, and infection.

A. *ICD/ICD + pacemaker*: Preoperative management of implantable cardioverter-defibrillators (ICDs) requires mandatory deactivation of tachyarrhythmia detection functions. In cases of concurrent pacemaker dependency, device reprogramming is necessary as magnet application may not consistently modify pacing parameters. Cardiology expertise is essential for appropriate device reprogramming, as pacing typically converts to asynchronous mode. During periods of ICD therapy deactivation, external defibrillation capability must be maintained through transcutaneous pad placement to address potential ventricular arrhythmias or pacing requirements. For subcutaneous ICDs, proper magnet positioning is confirmed by an R-wave synchronous auditory signal. Absence of this confirmatory tone necessitates device reprogramming [31].

Pearl

If a device programmer is not available to turn the ICD "off" and the procedure is urgent, a magnet may be placed over the pulse generator during the procedure. Always check with your cardiology service.

B. *Pacemakers, including leadless devices*:
- For pacemaker-dependent patients undergoing procedures with anticipated electromagnetic interference (EMI) superior to the umbilicus, cardiology consultation for pre- and postoperative device reprogramming is mandatory. Procedures performed inferior to the umbilicus in non-dependent patients carry minimal risk of device interference, though cardiology consultation remains advisable.
- Leadless pacemaker management requires specific consideration. These devices remain susceptible to EMI-induced inappropriate sensing and pacing failure. Device-specific responses vary significantly: Abbott AVEIR VR and DR systems demonstrate predictable magnet responses (converting to asynchronous pacing modes—VOO, AOO, or DOO—at predetermined rates based on battery voltage, with automatic restoration of baseline settings upon magnet removal). Conversely, Medtronic Micra VR and AV devices require electrophysiology specialists to manually reprogram them.
- Implantable loop recorders present minimal perioperative risk from EMI exposure. However, device interrogation should be performed pre- and post-procedurally, with potential reprogramming necessary if significant EMI exposure (such as electrocautery) is anticipated.

4.8.7 Transvenous CIED Perioperative Approach [31]

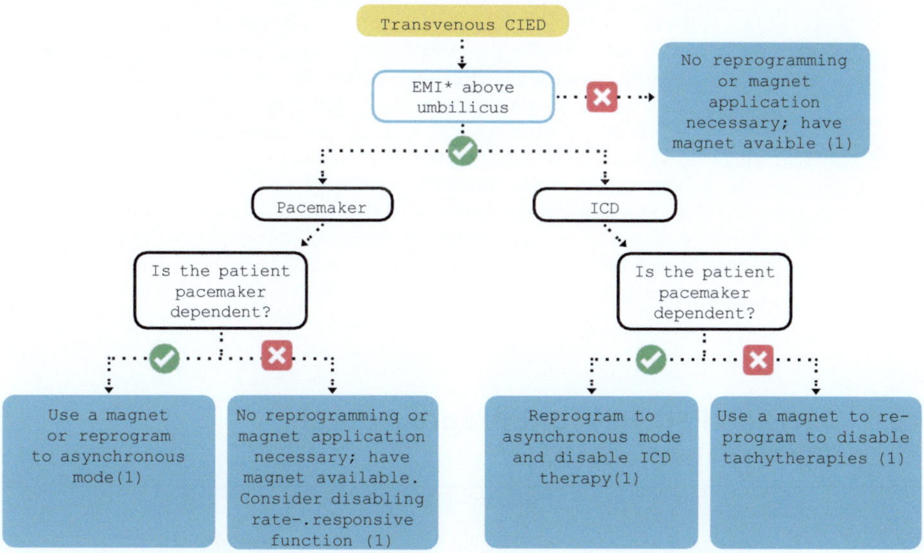

4.8.8 Nontransvenous Device Perioperative Approach [31]

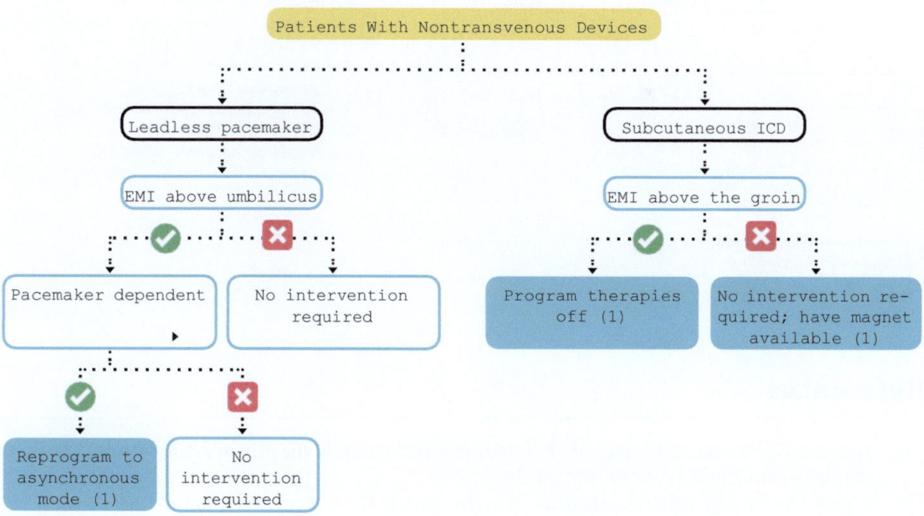

Pearl

During surgical procedures, electrocautery-induced electromagnetic interference (EMI) can significantly impact cardiac device function through multiple mechanisms: pacemaker inhibition, inappropriate tracking resulting in maximal tracking rate tachycardia, or delivery of unnecessary defibrillator shocks due to misinterpretation of EMI as cardiac electrical activity. These complications are significant in pacemaker-dependent patients, where device dysfunction could result in severe hemodynamic compromise. This potential for device-EMI interaction necessitates routine cardiology or electrophysiology consultation for appropriate device programming or deactivation before any surgical intervention.

4.8.9 Decision Pathway for Intraprocedural CID Management [32]

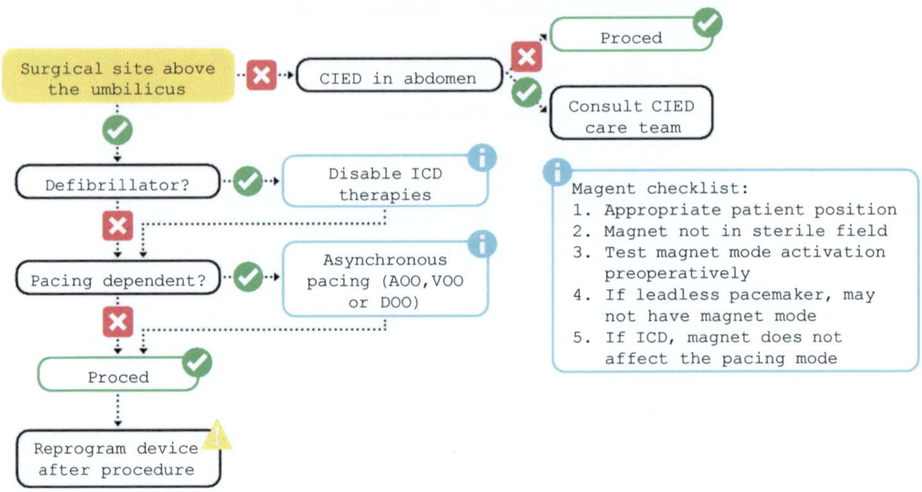

References

1. Wexler RK, Pleister A, Raman SV. Palpitations: evaluation in the primary care setting. Am Fam Physician. 2017;96(12):784–9. PMID: 29431371
2. Joglar JA, Chung MK, Armbruster AL, Benjamin EJ, Chyou JY, Cronin EM, Deswal A, Eckhardt LL, Goldberger ZD, Gopinathannair R, Gorenek B, Hess PL, Hlatky M, Hogan G, Ibeh C, Indik JH, Kido K, Kusumoto F, Link MS, Linta KT, Marcus GM, McCarthy PM, Patel N, Patton KK, Perez MV, Piccini JP, Russo AM, Sanders P, Streur MM, Thomas KL, Times S, Tisdale JE, Valente AM, Van Wagoner DR, Peer Review Committee Members. 2023 ACC/AHA/ACCP/HRS guideline for the diagnosis and management of atrial fibrillation: a report of

the American College of Cardiology/American Heart Association Joint Committee on Clinical Practice Guidelines. Circulation. 2024;149(1):e1–e156. https://doi.org/10.1161/CIR.0000000000001193. Epub 2023 Nov 30. Erratum in: Circulation. 2024 Jan 2;149(1):e167. https://doi.org/10.1161/CIR.0000000000001207. Erratum in: Circulation. 2024 Feb 27;149(9):e936. https://doi.org/10.1161/CIR.0000000000001218. Erratum in: Circulation. 2024 Jun 11;149(24):e1413. https://doi.org/10.1161/CIR.0000000000001263. PMID: 38033089; PMCID: PMC11095842

3. Chyou JY, Barkoudah E, Dukes JW, Goldstein LB, Joglar JA, Lee AM, Lubitz SA, Marill KA, Sneed KB, Streur MM, Wong GC, Gopinathannair R, American Heart Association Acute Cardiac Care and General Cardiology Committee, Electrocardiography and Arrhythmias Committee, and Clinical Pharmacology Committee of the Council on Clinical Cardiology, Council on Cardiovascular Surgery and Anesthesia, Council on Cardiopulmonary, Critical Care, Perioperative and Resuscitation, Council on Cardiovascular and Stroke Nursing; and Stroke Council. Atrial fibrillation occurring during acute hospitalization: a scientific statement from the American Heart Association. Circulation. 2023;147(15):e676–98.
4. Van Gelder IC, Groenveld HF, Crijns HJ, Tuininga YS, Tijssen JG, Alings AM, Hillege HL, Bergsma-Kadijk JA, Cornel JH, Kamp O, Tukkie R, Bosker HA, Van Veldhuisen DJ, Van den Berg MP, RACE II Investigators. Lenient versus strict rate control in patients with atrial fibrillation. N Engl J Med. 2010;362(15):1363–73. https://doi.org/10.1056/NEJMoa1001337. Epub 2010 Mar 15. PMID: 20231232
5. Florek JB, Lucas A, Girzadas D. Amiodarone. [Updated 2023 Nov 12]. In: StatPearls [Internet]. Treasure Island (FL): StatPearls Publishing; 2025 Jan-. Available from: https://www.ncbi.nlm.nih.gov/books/NBK482154/
6. Healey JS, Lopes RD, Granger CB, Alings M, Rivard L, McIntyre WF, Atar D, Birnie DH, Boriani G, Camm AJ, Conen D, Erath JW, Gold MR, Hohnloser SH, Ip J, Kautzner J, Kutyifa V, Linde C, Mabo P, Mairesse G, Benezet Mazuecos J, Cosedis Nielsen J, Philippon F, Proietti M, Sticherling C, Wong JA, Wright DJ, Zarraga IG, Coutts SB, Kaplan A, Pombo M, Ayala-Paredes F, Xu L, Simek K, Nevills S, Mian R, Connolly SJ, ARTESIA Investigators. Apixaban for stroke prevention in subclinical atrial fibrillation. N Engl J Med. 2024;390(2):107–17. https://doi.org/10.1056/NEJMoa2310234. Epub 2023 Nov 12. PMID: 37952132
7. Holmes DR Jr, Kar S, Price MJ, Whisenant B, Sievert H, Doshi SK, Huber K, Reddy VY. Prospective randomized evaluation of the Watchman left atrial appendage closure device in patients with atrial fibrillation versus long-term warfarin therapy: the PREVAIL trial. J Am Coll Cardiol. 2014;64(1):1–12. https://doi.org/10.1016/j.jacc.2014.04.029. Erratum in: J Am Coll Cardiol 2014 Sep 16;64(11):1186. PMID: 24998121
8. AlTurki A, Proietti R, Dawas A, Alturki H, Huynh T, Essebag V. Catheter ablation for atrial fibrillation in heart failure with reduced ejection fraction: a systematic review and meta-analysis of randomized controlled trials. BMC Cardiovasc Disord. 2019;19(1):18. https://doi.org/10.1186/s12872-019-0998-2. PMID: 30646857; PMCID: PMC6332840
9. Shoamanesh A, Field TS, Coutts SB, Sharma M, Gladstone D, Hart RG, Boriani G, Wright DJ, Sticherling C, Birnie DH, Gold MR, Erath JW, Kutyifa V, Mian R, Benz AP, Granger CB, McIntyre WF, Connolly SJ, Nielsen JC, Alings M, Rivard L, Lopes RD, Healey JS, ARTESiA Study Investigators. Apixaban versus aspirin for stroke prevention in people with subclinical atrial fibrillation and a history of stroke or transient ischaemic attack: subgroup analysis of the ARTESiA randomised controlled trial. Lancet Neurol. 2025;24(2):140–51. https://doi.org/10.1016/S1474-4422(24)00475-7. PMID: 39862882
10. Bainey KR, Welsh RC, Connolly SJ, Marsden T, Bosch J, Fox KAA, Steg PG, Vinereanu D, Connolly DL, Berkowitz SD, Foody JM, Probstfield JL, Branch KR, Lewis BS, Diaz R, Muehlhofer E, Widimsky P, Yusuf S, Eikelboom JW, Bhatt DL, COMPASS Investigators. Rivaroxaban plus aspirin versus aspirin alone in patients with prior percutaneous coronary intervention (COMPASS-PCI). Circulation. 2020;141(14):1141–51. https://doi.org/10.1161/CIRCULATIONAHA.119.044598. Epub 2020 Mar 17. Erratum in: Circulation. 2020 Jun 9;141(23):e905. https://doi.org/10.1161/CIR.0000000000000847. PMID: 32178526

11. Kotadia ID, Williams SE, O'Neill M. Supraventricular tachycardia: an overview of diagnosis and management. Clin Med (Lond). 2020;20(1):43–7. https://doi.org/10.7861/clinmed.cme.20.1.3. PMID: 31941731; PMCID: PMC6964177
12. Page RL, Joglar JA, Caldwell MA, Calkins H, Conti JB, Deal BJ, Estes NA 3rd, Field ME, Goldberger ZD, Hammill SC, Indik JH, Lindsay BD, Olshansky B, Russo AM, Shen WK, Tracy CM, Al-Khatib SM; Evidence Review Committee Chair‡. 2015 ACC/AHA/HRS guideline for the management of adult patients with supraventricular tachycardia: executive summary: a report of the American College of Cardiology/American Heart Association Task Force on Clinical Practice Guidelines and the Heart Rhythm Society. Circulation. 2016;133(14):e471–505. https://doi.org/10.1161/CIR.0000000000000310. Epub 2015 Sep 23. Erratum in: Circulation. 2016 Sep 13;134(11):e232–3. https://doi.org/10.1161/CIR.0000000000000447. PMID: 26399662.
13. Gupta AK, Shah CP, Maheshwari A, Thakur RK, Hayes OW, Lokhandwala YY. Adenosine induced ventricular fibrillation in Wolff-Parkinson-White syndrome. Pacing Clin Electrophysiol. 2002;25(4 Pt 1):477–80. https://doi.org/10.1046/j.1460-9592.2002.00477.x. PMID: 11991373
14. Garner JB, Miller JM. Wide complex tachycardia – ventricular tachycardia or not ventricular tachycardia, that remains the question. Arrhythm Electrophysiol Rev. 2013;2(1):23–9. https://doi.org/10.15420/aer.2013.2.1.23. PMID: 26835036; PMCID: PMC4711501
15. Koester C, Ibrahim AM, Cancel M, Labedi MR. The ubiquitous premature ventricular complex. Cureus. 2020;12(1):e6585. https://doi.org/10.7759/cureus.6585. PMID: 32051798; PMCID: PMC7001138
16. Ghannam M, Yokokawa M, Liang JJ, Cochet H, Jais P, Dabagh GS, Latchamsetty R, Jongnarangsin K, Morady F, Bogun F. Clinical significance of myocardial scar in patients with frequent premature ventricular complexes undergoing catheter ablation. Heart Rhythm. 2021;18(1):20–6. https://doi.org/10.1016/j.hrthm.2020.07.030. Epub 2020 Jul 25. PMID: 32721479
17. Panizo JG, Barra S, Mellor G, Heck P, Agarwal S. Premature ventricular complex-induced cardiomyopathy. Arrhythm Electrophysiol Rev. 2018;7(2):128–34. https://doi.org/10.15420/aer.2018.23.2. PMID: 29967685; PMCID: PMC6020182
18. Al-Khatib SM, Stevenson WG, Ackerman MJ, Bryant WJ, Callans DJ, Curtis AB, Deal BJ, Dickfeld T, Field ME, Fonarow GC, Gillis AM, Granger CB, Hammill SC, Hlatky MA, Joglar JA, Kay GN, Matlock DD, Myerburg RJ, Page RL. 2017 AHA/ACC/HRS guideline for management of patients with ventricular arrhythmias and the prevention of sudden cardiac death: executive summary: a report of the American College of Cardiology/American Heart Association task force on clinical practice guidelines and the Heart Rhythm Society. Heart Rhythm. 2018;15(10):e190–252. https://doi.org/10.1016/j.hrthm.2017.10.035. Epub 2017 Oct 30. Erratum in: heart rhythm. 2018 Nov;15(11):e278-e281. https://doi.org/10.1016/j.hrthm.2018.09.026. PMID: 29097320
19. Sapp JL, Tang ASL, Parkash R, Stevenson WG, Healey JS, Gula LJ, Nair GM, Essebag V, Rivard L, Roux JF, Nery PB, Sarrazin JF, Amit G, Raymond JM, Deyell M, Lane C, Sacher F, de Chillou C, Kuriachan V, Abdel-Wahab A, Nault I, Dyrda K, Wilton S, Jolly U, Kanagasundram A, Wells GA, VANISH2 Study Team. Catheter ablation or antiarrhythmic drugs for ventricular tachycardia. N Engl J Med. 2024; https://doi.org/10.1056/NEJMoa2409501. Epub ahead of print. PMID: 39555820
20. Kusumoto FM, Schoenfeld MH, Barrett C, Edgerton JR, Ellenbogen KA, Gold MR, Goldschlager NF, Hamilton RM, Joglar JA, Kim RJ, Lee R, Marine JE, McLeod CJ, Oken KR, Patton KK, Pellegrini CN, Selzman KA, Thompson A, Varosy PD. 2018 ACC/AHA/HRS guideline on the evaluation and management of patients with bradycardia and cardiac conduction delay: a report of the American College of Cardiology/American Heart Association task force on clinical practice guidelines and the Heart Rhythm Society. J Am Coll Cardiol. 2019;74(7):e51–e156. https://doi.org/10.1016/j.jacc.2018.10.044. Epub 2018 Nov 6. Erratum in: J Am Coll Cardiol. 2019 Aug 20;74(7):1016-1018. doi: 10.1016/j.jacc.2019.06.048. PMID: 30412709
21. Jensen PN, Gronroos NN, Chen LY, Folsom AR, deFilippi C, Heckbert SR, Alonso A. Incidence of and risk factors for sick sinus syndrome in the general population. J Am Coll Cardiol.

2014;64(6):531–8. https://doi.org/10.1016/j.jacc.2014.03.056. PMID: 25104519; PMCID: PMC4139053

22. Dalia T, Amr BS. Pacemaker Indications. [Updated 2023 Aug 14]. In: StatPearls [Internet]. Treasure Island (FL): StatPearls Publishing; 2025 Jan-. Available from: https://www.ncbi.nlm.nih.gov/books/NBK507823/
23. Al-Khatib SM, Stevenson WG, Ackerman MJ, Bryant WJ, Callans DJ, Curtis AB, Deal BJ, Dickfeld T, Field ME, Fonarow GC, Gillis AM, Granger CB, Hammill SC, Hlatky MA, Joglar JA, Kay GN, Matlock DD, Myerburg RJ, Page RL. 2017 AHA/ACC/HRS guideline for management of patients with ventricular arrhythmias and preventing sudden cardiac death: executive summary: a report of the American College of Cardiology/American Heart Association task force on clinical practice guidelines and the Heart Rhythm Society. Circulation. 2018;138(13):e210–71. https://doi.org/10.1161/CIR.0000000000000548. Erratum in: Circulation 2018 Sep 25;138(13):e415-e418. https://doi.org/10.1161/CIR.0000000000000615. PMID: 29084733
24. Kawada S, Morita H, Antzelevitch C, Morimoto Y, Nakagawa K, Watanabe A, Nishii N, Nakamura K, Ito H. Shanghai score system for diagnosis of Brugada syndrome: validation of the score system and reclassification of the patients. JACC Clin Electrophysiol. 2018;4(6):724–30. https://doi.org/10.1016/j.jacep.2018.02.009. Epub 2018 Mar 28. PMID: 29929664
25. Manohar S, Dahal BR, Gitler B. Fever-induced Brugada syndrome. J Investig Med High Impact Case Rep. 2015;3(1):2324709615577414. https://doi.org/10.1177/2324709615577414. PMID: 26425637; PMCID: PMC4586913
26. Shen T, Yuan B, Geng J, Chen C, Zhou X, Shan Q. Low-dose quinidine effectively reduced shocks in Brugada syndrome patients with an implantable cardioverter defibrillator: a Chinese case series report. Ann Noninvasive Electrocardiol. 2017;22(1):e12375. https://doi.org/10.1111/anec.12375. Epub 2016 Aug 23. PMID: 27550400; PMCID: PMC6931864
27. Goldenberg I, Moss AJ. Long QT syndrome. J Am Coll Cardiol. 2008;51(24):2291–300. https://doi.org/10.1016/j.jacc.2008.02.068. PMID: 18549912
28. Went TR, Sultan W, Sapkota A, Khurshid H, Qureshi IA, Jahan N, Tara A, Win M, Wiltshire DA, Kannan A, Ruo SW, Alfonso M. A systematic review on the role of Beta-blockers in reducing cardiac arrhythmias in long QT syndrome subtypes 1-3. Cureus. 2021;13(9):e17632. https://doi.org/10.7759/cureus.17632. PMID: 34646680; PMCID: PMC8485362
29. Baltogiannis GG, Lysitsas DN, di Giovanni G, Ciconte G, Sieira J, Conte G, Kolettis TM, Chierchia GB, de Asmundis C, Brugada P. CPVT: arrhythmogenesis, therapeutic management, and future perspectives. A brief review of the literature. Front Cardiovasc Med. 2019;6:92. https://doi.org/10.3389/fcvm.2019.00092. PMID: 31380394; PMCID: PMC6644488
30. Neelankavil JP, Thompson A, Mahajan A. Managing cardiovascular implantable electronic devices (CIEDs) during perioperative care. Anesth Patient Saf Found Newsl. 2013;28(2):29–35.
31. Thompson A, Fleischmann KE, Smilowitz NR, de Las Fuentes L, Mukherjee D, Aggarwal NR, Ahmad FS, Allen RB, Altin SE, Auerbach A, Berger JS, Chow B, Dakik HA, Eisenstein EL, Gerhard-Herman M, Ghadimi K, Kachulis B, Leclerc J, Lee CS, Macaulay TE, Mates G, Merli GJ, Parwani P, Poole JE, Rich MW, Ruetzler K, Stain SC, Sweitzer B, Talbot AW, Vallabhajosyula S, Whittle J, Williams KA Sr, Peer Review Committee Members. 2024 AHA/ACC/ACS/ASNC/HRS/SCA/SCCT/SCMR/SVM guideline for perioperative cardiovascular management for noncardiac surgery: a report of the American College of Cardiology/American Heart Association joint Committee on clinical practice guidelines. Circulation. 2024;150(19):e351–442. https://doi.org/10.1161/CIR.0000000000001285. Epub 2024 Sep 24. Erratum in: Circulation. 2024 Nov 19;150(21):e466. https://doi.org/10.1161/CIR.0000000000001298. PMID: 39316661
32. Wan EY, Rogers AJ, Lavelle M, Marcus M, Stone SA, Ottoboni L, Srivatsa U, Leal MA, Russo AM, Jackson LR 2nd, Crossley GH; American Heart Association Electrocardiography and Arrhythmias Committee of the Council on Clinical Cardiology; Council on Cardiovascular and Stroke Nursing; Council on Cardiovascular Surgery and Anesthesia; and Council on Peripheral Vascular Disease. Periprocedural management and multidisciplinary care pathways for patients with cardiac implantable electronic devices: a scientific statement from the American Heart Association. Circulation. 2024;150(8):e183–96. https://doi.org/10.1161/CIR.0000000000001264. Epub 2024 Jul 10. PMID: 38984417

Cardiac Ischemia

Contents

M. Salih, *Practical Hospitalist Guide to Inpatient Cardiology*, https://doi.org/10.1007/978-3-032-03240-9_5

This chapter provides a practical, evidence-based framework for hospitalists to diagnose and manage acute coronary syndrome (ACS), emphasizing rapid risk stratification, appropriate use of troponin testing, ECG interpretation, and guideline-directed medical therapy. It outlines the diagnostic criteria for ACS subtypes—unstable angina, non-ST-segment elevation mycocardial infarction (NSTEMI), and STEMI—highlighting the importance of integrating clinical presentation with dynamic ECG changes and serial troponin trends. A key focus is distinguishing between **acute myocardial injury** and **type 2 myocardial infarction (MI)**: while both conditions may present with troponin elevation, type 2 MI is defined by a mismatch in oxygen supply and demand (e.g., sepsis, anemia, tachyarrhythmia) with clinical evidence of ischemia, whereas nonischemic acute myocardial injury (e.g., myocarditis and renal failure) lacks ischemic symptoms or ECG changes. The chapter stresses the importance of context and comorbidities in diagnosis, guiding hospitalists on when to involve cardiology, pursue invasive evaluation, or opt for conservative management. Ultimately, the goal is to improve outcomes through accurate diagnosis, risk-appropriate treatment, and timely disposition planning.

5.1 When to Suspect and Major Etiology

- Impaired coronary blood flow leads to ischemic cardiac dysfunction. Usually, the diagnosis is based on probability rather than definitive certainty. The primary clinical manifestation is anginal chest pain, which is typically exacerbated by exertion and relieved by rest or nitroglycerin. However, it may also be asymptomatic (silent ischemia) or present as sudden cardiac death.
- Several clinical findings increase the likelihood of acute coronary syndrome (ACS), with the most significant being intermittent anginal chest pain (likelihood ratio [LR] 5.8), new ischemic electrocardiogram (ECG) changes, diaphoresis, a history of myocardial infarction (MI), the presence of arcus senilis, age over 70 years, an ear lobe crease, and new pulmonary crackles [1]. In patients aged 65 years and younger, nonatherosclerotic causes of myocardial infarction are relatively common, particularly among women. Reported etiologies include atherothrombosis (67%), supply–demand mismatch (23%), spontaneous coronary artery dissection (SCAD, 4%), coronary embolism (2%), vasospasm (1%), and myocardial infarction with nonobstructed coronary arteries (MINOCA, 3%) [33].
- ACS is classified into the following categories:
  A. STEMI
    - Characterized by ST-segment elevation on ECG and typically associated with elevated troponin levels.
    - ST-segment depression in anterior leads with tall R waves is considered equivalent to posterior wall STEMI.
    - Another STEMI equivalent is new-onset left bundle branch block (LBBB), which strongly suggests infarction in the left anterior descending (LAD) or left circumflex (LCX) artery territory.

B. Non-ST-segment elevation myocardial infarction (NSTEMI)
   - Defined by the absence of ST-segment elevation on ECG but with elevated troponin levels.

C. Unstable angina
   - A newly occurring or worsening pattern of anginal pain that occurs at rest, without troponin elevation.
   - Frequently underdiagnosed as non-ACS due to the absence of ECG changes or troponin elevation. Clinicians should remain vigilant, as it may still present with clinical features suggestive of ACS.

Pearl

Not all patients with ACS present with classic symptoms; some may exhibit mild or atypical chest pain. Up to 45% of myocardial infarctions (MIs) are silent or unrecognized, yet their mortality rates are comparable to recognized MIs [2]. This is particularly common among elderly individuals, especially women, and diabetic patients with neuropathy. Clinical judgment should be guided by the overall clinical context, premorbid risk factors, and the probability of ACS based on the patient's presentation.

Hospitalist Tip

The likelihood of ACS is lower in patients with a normal ECG, pleuritic chest pain, localized pain with specific pointing signs, chest wall tenderness, and age younger than 40 years [4]. However, if ACS remains a concern, serial ECGs should be performed to monitor for evolving changes.

Pearl

Patients with a history of radiation therapy are at an elevated risk for ischemic events due to an increased propensity for atherosclerotic disease, even at a younger age [14]. Radiation exposure is also associated with an increased risk of valvular calcification.

5.2 Unusual DD of ACS

(i) Spontaneous coronary artery dissection (SCAD) is a rare but important cause of acute coronary syndrome (ACS) in young pregnant or postpartum female patients. Diagnosis is confirmed through left heart catheterization (LHC). Management is primarily supportive, including aspirin and beta-blockers. For any young female patient presenting with elevated troponin levels and ischemic changes on ECG, prompt cardiology consultation is essential to guide further evaluation and treatment.

(ii) Coronary artery vasospasm (Prinzmetal/variant angina). Coronary vasospasm, also known as variant or Prinzmetal's angina, is more common in postmenopausal women and smokers and is often triggered by cold exposure or emotional stress. It presents as severe paroxysmal chest pain that is relieved by nitroglycerin. Diagnosis is confirmed via coronary angiography with intracoronary nitroglycerin administration, which demonstrates improved coronary flow. Management includes long-acting nitrates, calcium channel blockers (CCBs), smoking cessation, and statin therapy. Non-selective beta-blockers should be avoided as they may theoretically exacerbate vasospasm by blocking β2-mediated vasodilation.

(iii) Stress cardiomyopathy (Takotsubo cardiomyopathy). In a patient presenting with new-onset acute decompensated heart failure (ADHF), reduced left ventricular ejection fraction (LVEF), elevated troponin, and ischemic ECG changes but with a negative left heart catheterization (LHC), Takotsubo cardiomyopathy should be considered. This condition mimics STEMI but lacks obstructive coronary lesions on angiography and is often triggered by physical or emotional stressors. Key differential diagnoses include Prinzmetal's angina and stimulant-induced myocardial injury. Diagnosis is confirmed via echocardiography, which typically reveals apical ballooning with basal myocardial sparing. Management includes beta-blockers and ACE inhibitors/ARBs, which have supportive evidence for ongoing use. Diuretics should be administered for volume overload as needed.

Pearl

Type I MI is ACS caused by plaque rupture. Type 2 MI is demand ischemia leading to ACS. Note that MI in percutaneous coronary intervention (PCI) settings is called type IV MI; in CABG settings, it is called type V MI.

5.3 Stable CAD for the Hospitalist

- For patients admitted with unexplained progressive shortness of breath (SOB) over weeks, particularly when chest X-ray and echocardiography findings are non-significant, ischemic heart disease (IHD) should be considered. The most common presentation of IHD is stable angina, characterized by reproducible chest discomfort precipitated by exertion or stress and relieved by rest or nitroglycerin. However, this symptom alone may not reliably differentiate between cardiac and non-cardiac chest pain [5]. Stable angina typically presents with a chronic and consistent severity over time and may be triggered by cold weather or postprandial states. Other possible symptoms of IHD include jaw or arm discomfort, unexplained SOB, and epigastric discomfort, which are more frequently observed in elderly patients, women, and individuals with diabetes. Troponin levels are usually within the normal range or at the patient's baseline. In all cases, ACS should first be ruled out before proceeding with further evaluation.
- Patients suspected of having coronary artery disease (CAD) are categorized into low-, intermediate-, and high-probability groups based on clinical presentation and risk factors. High-probability patients are typically older males with significant atherosclerotic risk factors, including smoking, hypertension, hyperlipidemia, diabetes, CKD, and obesity. Low-probability patients have minimal or no risk factors, while intermediate-probability patients have some but not all risk factors, making the likelihood of CAD uncertain. This intermediate group benefits the most from further testing. Low-probability patients do not require additional testing and should be reassured. Intermediate-probability patients benefit from stress testing, with a pharmacologic vasodilator nuclear stress test being the preferred option, as most patients cannot exercise, and alternative tests may be less convenient, time-consuming, or cost-effective. A dobutamine stress echocardiogram is a reasonable second option, offering additional valvular assessment without radiation exposure. If the stress test is positive, further evaluation with coronary angiography or adjusted medical therapy is warranted. High-probability patients are more likely to require diagnostic coronary angiography and the initiation of appropriate treatment or intervention; that is especially true if the patient has newly reduced LV systolic function or clinical heart failure. Lastly, the Coronary artery calcium score is reserved as a risk assessment tool to guide long-term medical management, but has no role in the evaluation of acute chest pain.

Pearl

High-risk coronary anatomy is defined as patients with obstructive stenosis, such as ≥50% left main stenosis or anatomically significant three-vessel disease (≥70% stenosis). Fractional flow reserve testing is used to assess the degree of hemodynamic severity of fixed coronary stenosis. an FFR of ≤0.80 supports percutaneous coronary intervention [6].

Hospitalist Tip

Stress testing should be avoided in patients who are acutely ill, such as those with sepsis, active pain from acute coronary syndrome (ACS), or symptomatic severe aortic stenosis (AS). Additionally, patients with acute myocarditis should not undergo stress testing, as it may provoke arrhythmias. These conditions present significant risks, and stress testing could worsen the clinical status or lead to serious complications.

Hospitalist Tip

In hospital settings where there is a questionable concern for acute coronary syndrome (ACS), particularly in patients with low to intermediate probability of CAD, coronary CT angiography is a highly sensitive and valuable tool with a high negative predictive value for ruling out significant acute coronary artery disease [8]. If coronary CT angiography (CCTA) is available, it should be utilized, especially in patients with acute chest discomfort and low probability of CAD, due to its ability to rule out significant coronary pathology accurately. The 2021 Multisociety Guideline for the Evaluation and Diagnosis of Chest Pain recommends both coronary computed tomographic angiography (CCTA) and stress testing as appropriate first-line modalities for the initial assessment of patients with suspected coronary artery disease. The presence of a coronary stent and a high burden of coronary calcification diminish the specificity and diagnostic accuracy of coronary computed tomographic angiography (CCTA)

5.4 Contraindications for Specific Stress Testing Modalities [6]

Vasodilator pharmacological stress imaging	Significant arrhythmias (e.g., VT, second- or third-degree atrioventricular block), significant hypotension (SBP <90 mm Hg), known or suspected bronchoconstrictive or bronchospastic disease or use of dipyridamole or methylxanthines (e.g., aminophylline, caffeine) within 12 h
Exercise stress testing (with or without imaging)	Inability to exercise
Dobutamine stress echocardiography	Critical aortic stenosis, hemodynamically significant LVOT obstruction

- Treatment for stable angina/coronary cardiac disease (CCD) focuses on managing the underlying risk factors. Smoking cessation is essential for all patients. Eating healthy, maintaining mental health, having a low salt intake, and exercising are vital. Aspirin should be prescribed to all patients; if allergic, clopidogrel is an alternative. Prasugrel and ticagrelor have not been studied in stable angina without vascular intervention, so they should be avoided unless there is a prior history of acute coronary syndrome (ACS) or percutaneous coronary intervention (PCI). For patients who have had a vascular intervention, dual antiplatelet therapy (DAPT) should be continued indefinitely if tolerated. Additional management includes lipid-lowering medications, blood pressure control (target <130/80 mmHg), diabetes management, sleep apnea control with continuous positive airway pressure (CPAP), and obesity management. Anti-anginal medications typically include beta-blockers (BB) on a scheduled daily basis, with calcium channel blockers (CCB) used if BBs are contraindicated or not tolerated. Sublingual nitroglycerin can be used as needed for acute symptom relief. Beta-blockers should be titrated according to symptoms, with a target heart rate of 55–60 beats per minute. If symptoms persist, consider adding CCBs or long-acting nitrates. Ranolazine, which may prolong the QT interval and cause drug-drug interactions, is a last resort with continued symptoms despite the use of beta-blockers or who cannot use acceptable doses of beta-blockers before considering angiography and potential revascularization. There are two options:
  A. **Coronary artery bypass grafting (CABG)** is primarily indicated in patients with left main coronary artery disease and multivessel disease, especially when combined with left ventricular dysfunction, complex disease, or diabetes. CABG has demonstrated mortality benefits compared to PCI. All patients undergoing CABG will benefit from DAPT for at least 12 months [9].
  B. **PCI** is recommended for patients with medically refractory angina [10] and those with ≥70% non–left main disease or ≥50% left main disease. However, PCI does not improve survival in patients with stable CAD. In stable CAD, PCI is used primarily for symptom relief, not for mortality reduction, compared to guideline-directed medical therapy (GDMT) [11].

Pearl

Do not take prescribed phosphodiesterase inhibitors within 24 h of long-acting nitrates, and do not prescribe nitrates for 24 h after the use of sildenafil or 48 h after tadalafil due to the risk of significant hypotension.

Hospitalist Tip

The duration of dual antiplatelet therapy (DAPT) following percutaneous coronary intervention (PCI) in patients with stable angina depends on the type of stent used. For drug-eluting stents (DES), DAPT should be continued for at least 6 months, as there is a higher risk of thrombosis. The recommended duration for bare-metal stents (BMS) is at least 1 month. If the patient is at higher thrombotic risk (previous MI), DAPT may need to be extended, potentially up to 3 years [6]. However, in patients at high bleeding risk, DAPT can be shortened to 1–3 months, with continuation of the P2Y12 inhibitor only. If the patient requires anticoagulation therapy, after 1 month of triple therapy (aspirin, P2Y12 inhibitor, and anticoagulant), warfarin or a direct oral anticoagulant (DOAC) can be used in conjunction with clopidogrel, but DOACs should not be used in patients with mechanical heart valve prostheses [6]. This approach also applies after an acute coronary syndrome (ACS) event. Understanding these guidelines is crucial when managing patients admitted for elective surgery requiring clearance, as the minimum DAPT duration must be followed without interruption. For stable CAD patients without PCI who also have atrial fibrillation (AF), anticoagulation monotherapy has been shown to reduce nonfatal major bleeding and clinically relevant nonmajor bleeding without increasing the risk of ischemic events [12, 13]. Also, keep in mind that Prasugrel and Ticagrelor are P2Y12 inhibitors that have been studied in acute coronary syndromes, but not in patients with Stable CAD.

Hospitalist Tip

To reduce thrombotic events in patients with high thrombotic risk, low bleeding risk, or significant peripheral vascular disease (PVD), low-dose rivaroxaban (2.5 mg twice daily) may be added to their regimen [3]. If the patient is already on dual antiplatelet therapy (DAPT), switch to clopidogrel combined with rivaroxaban, as this combination can offer additional protection against thrombosis while minimizing bleeding risks [3].

Hospitalist Tip

In patients with CCD who have type 2 diabetes, the use of either an SGLT2 inhibitor or a GLP-1 receptor agonist, with proven cardiovascular benefit, is recommended to reduce the risk of major adverse cardiovascular events (MACE).

Pearl

For cholesterol-lowering therapy, initiate a high-intensity statin to lower LDL cholesterol levels effectively. If LDL remains elevated above 70 mg/dL, consider adding ezetimibe to reduce LDL levels further. If the LDL is still not adequately controlled, PCSK9 inhibitors may be introduced as a next step. In cases where triglycerides remain elevated above 150 mg/dL, adding icosapent ethyl (an omega-3 fatty acid) should be considered to help lower triglyceride levels and reduce cardiovascular risk.

5.5 Approaching Chest Pain for the Hospitalist (Nurse Call)

- When evaluating a patient with chest pain, first ask the nurse to check the patient's vitals and EKG. It is important to note that a normal EKG does not rule out acute coronary syndrome (ACS). Upon arrival, take a detailed history of the pain, including its onset, character, duration, and associated symptoms, particularly shortness of breath (SOB) and other features suggestive of ACS. Conduct a focused physical examination, including a cardiovascular exam (often normal in early ACS) and an abdominal exam (to rule out conditions that mimic chest pain). Follow the ABCDE approach for managing unstable patients. If the diagnosis remains inconclusive, proceed with troponin levels and a chest X-ray to help rule out aortic dissection and pneumothorax. Additional labs or imaging may be necessary depending on the most likely differential diagnosis. The main differential diagnoses (DDx) include ACS, musculoskeletal pain, pleuritic chest pain, pulmonary embolism (PE), gastroesophageal reflux disease (GERD), peptic ulcer disease (PUD), gastritis, gallstones, pancreatitis, aortic dissection, pericarditis, anxiety-induced precordial catch syndrome, and pneumothorax. Provide analgesia based on the most likely diagnosis. If the diagnosis remains unclear, continue with serial examinations, EKGs, and troponin measurements every 1–6 h until you are confident the pain is not cardiac in origin and the symptoms have resolved.

Pearl

Precordial catch syndrome is a benign condition characterized by a sharp, stabbing pain on the left side of the chest, typically just below the nipple. It most commonly affects young adults but can occur at any age. The pain normally lasts from a few seconds to a few minutes and may be triggered by certain movements or deep breaths. It is not associated with serious underlying health issues; the symptoms resolve independently. Although it can cause anxiety for those experiencing it, treatment is usually unnecessary. To help relieve the pain, the patient can try standing or sitting up straight and taking slow, shallow breaths while trying to relax.

Hospitalist Tip

Chest tenderness in patients with chest pain has limited diagnostic value if there is a history of coronary artery disease (CAD), as it does not rule out the possibility of ischemic chest pain. However, it can decrease the probability of acute coronary syndrome (ACS). Similarly, if chest pain is relieved by a GI cocktail, it may suggest a gastrointestinal cause rather than ischemic pain, but it should not be used to rule out ACS [15] definitively. Careful consideration of the overall clinical picture, including risk factors, history, and additional diagnostic tests, is necessary to diagnose accurately.

5.6 STEMI

5.6.1 Clinical Approach

- ST-segment elevation with elevated troponin is a hallmark of acute myocardial infarction, often resulting from sudden thrombotic ischemia due to plaque rupture. The diagnosis is primarily clinical, relying on a combination of patient history, electrocardiography (ECG), and troponin levels. A thorough assessment of historical data, particularly regarding anginal pain and dyspnea, is essential. For chest pain evaluation, the SOCRATES mnemonic should be utilized. Additionally, an examination should focus on pertinent findings associated with heart failure and its underlying causes. However, no single clinical sign is considered diagnostic, and neither the Levine sign nor the palm sign significantly increases the probability of acute coronary syndrome (ACS) [16].
- An ECG should be performed immediately upon presentation to assess for ST-segment elevation. However, approximately 30% of patients may present with a normal ECG. If the initial ECG is unremarkable but the patient remains symptomatic, it should be repeated within 15–30 min, and lead positioning should be adjusted to evaluate for posterior or inferior STEMI. Nonspecific ECG findings are generally not useful in diagnosis.
- High-sensitivity troponin testing is recommended for all patients. Repeat testing should be conducted within 1–6 h if the initial result is negative. A rising trend in troponin levels is highly suggestive of acute ischemia. However, in patients with chronic cardiac stress, congestive heart failure (CHF), or end-stage renal disease (ESRD), chronically elevated troponin levels may be observed without a significant delta change upon presentation.
- Transthoracic echocardiography (TTE) benefits all patients at initial evaluation, upon clinical deterioration, or near discharge to assess left ventricular function. TTE may reveal regional wall motion abnormalities or complications related to ACS. Additionally, inpatient telemetry monitoring is recommended for all patients to detect potential cardiac events or arrhythmias [17].

Pearl

Conditions that mimic STEMI on EKG include hypercalcemia, acute pericarditis, left ventricular aneurysm, and occasionally SAH.

Pearl

Patients presenting with ST-segment elevation myocardial infarction (STEMI) and elevated troponin but without significant obstructive coronary artery disease (CAD) (defined as <50% stenosis on angiography) do not benefit from perfusion therapy. This condition, known as cardiac syndrome X, is more prevalent in women. Management focuses on supportive care and addressing underlying atherosclerotic risk factors when present.

5.6.2 Treatment Approach in Acute Settings [34]:

1. Reperfusion is the main goal, either:
   I. **PCI with DES for the culprit vessel [31]**
   - Optimal reperfusion should be achieved within 90 min of first medical contact or 120 min if the patient is at a PCI-equipped center. If successful, repeating PCI before discharge is considered the standard of care to ensure the culprit lesion is fully treated. Current guidelines recommend radial access over femoral access for PCI.
   - Management of non-culprit vessel lesions with significant stenosis following STEMI may be considered, with evidence suggesting benefits of revascularization within 4 to 6 weeks post-STEMI [7]. If PCI is not available in-house, the patient should be stabilized and, if appropriate, receive thrombolytic therapy before being transferred to a facility equipped for PCI.
   - Following PCI or thrombolytic therapy, an ECG should be repeated within 60–90 min to assess for reperfusion. A reduction in ST-segment elevation by at least 50% indicates successful reperfusion. However, up to 30% of patients may not respond adequately to initial treatment. In such cases, repeat PCI should be considered in consultation with cardiology. Routine angiography post-PCI is not recommended unless clinically indicated.

- Urgent coronary artery bypass grafting (CABG) should be considered when PCI is unsuccessful or technically challenging or when a large myocardial territory is at risk.

II. Thrombolytics

- If PCI is unavailable within 120 min, thrombolytic therapy should be administered within 12 h of symptom onset, with the greatest efficacy observed within 3–6 h. Regardless of the thrombolytic treatment outcome, transferring the patient to a PCI-capable center is crucial for further evaluation and management.
- The preferred thrombolytic agent is tissue plasminogen activator (tPA) due to its superior patency rates and lower risk of allergic reactions. Before administering thrombolytics, clinicians must carefully assess absolute and relative contraindications, as outlined in clinical decision tools such as MedCalc. Thrombolytics can be life-saving, particularly in rural or resource-limited settings; thus, familiarity with available thrombolytic options and institutional protocols is essential. However, the most recent guidelines do not recommend routine aspiration thrombectomy [17, 18].

Pearl

Common complications of coronary angiograms include vascular complications (hematoma, pseudoaneurysm, AV fistula), contrast allergy, and contrast nephropathy. If the patient has severe contrast allergy, proceeding with urgent PCI may require premedication with steroids and antihistamines per hospital policy.

Hospitalist Tip

A post-ROSC patient suspected of ACS should have a cardiac cath to rule out STEMI [17].

2. **Antiplatelets**. Patients should receive an aspirin loading dose of 325 mg and a daily maintenance dose of 81 mg. In addition, a P2Y12 inhibitor should be administered if angiography will likely be delayed, with ticagrelor as the preferred first-line agent due to its faster onset of action and lack of known genetic polymorphisms. Clopidogrel is considered second-line, except in cases where thrombolytics are used. So, Administration of clopidogrel or ticagrelor may be considered in patients scheduled for coronary angiography beyond 24 hours. However, in those undergoing early invasive angiography (within 24 hours), the

routine pre-procedural use of a P2Y12 inhibitor alongside aspirin has an uncertain benefit. Post-acute coronary syndrome (ACS) treatment with dual antiplatelet therapy (DAPT) is recommended for at least 12 months. Among P2Y12 inhibitors, prasugrel has been shown to lower the incidence of myocardial infarction and stroke compared to ticagrelor when PCI is planned [19]. However, prasugrel is generally not recommended for patients over 75 years old or those with a history of transient ischemic attack (TIA) or stroke due to an increased risk of bleeding. For patients with ACS who require anticoagulation and undergo PCI with stenting, a P2Y12 inhibitor (preferably clopidogrel) should be used instead of triple therapy to minimize bleeding risk [20]. If triple treatment is necessary, it should be limited to 1–4 weeks, based on cardiology guidance [20]. In patients at high risk of bleeding, proton pump inhibitors (PPIs) should be initiated to reduce gastrointestinal complications.

Pearl

For patients with high bleeding risk who cannot continue on DAPT, a shorter duration of around 3 months of combination is reasonable, followed by clopidogrel or Ticagrelol alone. More evidence is building up for the safety of this approach of P2Y12 inhibitor monotherapy after PCI in ACS [34].

3. **Anticoagulation**. According to institutional protocol, all STEMI patients must receive anticoagulation therapy, preferably unfractionated heparin (UFH) as an infusion, which should be continued until PCI or coronary artery bypass grafting (CABG) is completed. For patients with unstable angina (UA) or non-ST elevation myocardial infarction (NSTEMI) managed medically, anticoagulation is typically maintained until discharge or for at least 48 h. Low molecular weight heparin (LMWH) may be considered in cases where an invasive approach is unlikely, as it carries a higher risk of thrombosis during intervention [17]. However, LMWH dosing must be carefully adjusted in patients with renal impairment to prevent accumulation and bleeding complications.

Pearl

Glycoprotein IIb/IIIa inhibitors should not be administered routinely in patients with ACS due to their lack of ischemic benefit and increased risk of bleeding [17]. If needed, the cardiologist, not the hospitalist, should decide on the cath site.

4. **Oral B-blockers**. All patients with acute coronary syndrome (ACS) should be started on beta-blockers within 24 h, as they help reduce myocardial oxygen demand and control tachycardia in acute settings. However, beta-blockers are contraindicated in patients with acute decompensated heart failure (ADHF) and should be used with extreme caution in cases of inferior myocardial infarction (MI) with a high risk of cardiogenic shock or atrioventricular (AV) blocks. Despite these considerations, beta-blockers have been shown to reduce the risk of reinfarction and arrhythmias [17].
5. **Oral ACE/ARBS**. Within 24 h, especially for ADHF and DM patients.
6. **Nitrates**. Oral nitrates are preferred as the initial treatment for angina relief. However, in cases of persistent angina, hypertensive emergencies associated with ACS, or acute decompensated heart failure (ADHF), intravenous (IV) nitrate infusion may be required. Nitrates should be avoided in patients with inferior myocardial infarction (MI) involving right ventricular infarction, as well as those who have recently used phosphodiesterase-5 inhibitors (within the past 48 h) due to the risk of severe hypotension. Additional contraindications include systolic blood pressure (SBP) <90 mmHg or a drop in SBP >30 mmHg from baseline [17]. It is important to note that tachyphylaxis may develop after approximately 24 h of continuous nitrate use, necessitating periodic nitrate-free intervals to maintain efficacy.
7. **Aldosterone antagonist agents**. Should be initiated within 1 week in patients with an ejection fraction (EF) of 40% or less, particularly those with diabetes mellitus (DM). Potassium levels should be closely monitored to prevent hyperkalemia, and these medications should be avoided in patients with significant acute kidney injury (AKI) or chronic kidney disease (CKD) with a glomerular filtration rate (GFR) below 30 mL/min to reduce the risk of further renal impairment.
8. **Anemia**. Aim for target Hb of ≥10 g/dL [17, 32].
9. **Statin**. ASAP, preferably before PCI, as it lowers the risk of interim ischemic events due to its pleiotropic effects.
10. **Pain control**. For persistent chest pain, you may use morphine or fentanyl (both can delay the effects of oral P2Y12 therapy), but avoid NSAIDs as they increase cardiac events [21].
11. **Oxygen**. All patients should have oxygen if their oxygen saturation is less than 90% [17]. It does not need to be 100% (actually, it could be harmful). Also, keep in mind that subjective Shortness of breath with normal oxygenation, rather than chest pain, is a side effect of ticagrelor and would be an indication to switch to clopidogrel.

Pearl

Intravenous (IV) antihypertensives are generally avoided in patients with acute coronary syndrome (ACS) due to the risk of hypotension, except in cases of hypertensive emergency.

5.6.3 Summary of Treatment Approach in Post-acute Settings for ACS

Medication or treatment class	Indications
DAPT	All patients for 1 year, followed by antiplatelets preferably aspirin

Comments

Aspirin combined with ticagrelor is the preferred regimen for dual antiplatelet therapy (DAPT) [22]. In patients who have tolerated DAPT with ticagrelor, transitioning to ticagrelor monotherapy at least 1 month post-PCI is beneficial to reduce the risk of bleeding [17].
For patients allergic to aspirin or those taking direct oral anticoagulants (DOACs) for another indication, clopidogrel should be used in those with a high bleeding risk, while ticagrelor is appropriate for patients with a low bleeding risk.
Prasugrel is contraindicated in patients over 75 years of age or those with a history of stroke, transient ischemic attack (TIA), or brain hemorrhage.

Medication or treatment class	Indications
Oral β-blockers	Continued mostly indefinitely in all patients with ACS

Comments
In patients with a low ejection fraction (EF) of <50% or systolic dysfunction, only metoprolol succinate, carvedilol, or bisoprolol should be used as beta-blockers. Metoprolol is preferred in patients with significant obstructive lung diseases such as chronic obstructive pulmonary disease (COPD), as it is more selective for beta-1 receptors, minimizing the risk of bronchoconstriction compared to non-selective beta-blockers.

Medication or treatment class	Comments
Oral ACE/ARBS	Used in patients with LV systolic dysfunction (HefreF <40%), DM, CKD, HTN Do not combine ACE with ARBS

Medication or treatment class	Indications
Aldosterone antagonist agents	LVEF ≤40% and either clinical heart failure or diabetes

Comments
When using ACE inhibitors or ARBs in patients with chronic kidney disease (CKD), it is essential to monitor potassium levels closely and avoid significant acute kidney injury (AKI) or further renal deterioration in patients with a glomerular filtration rate (GFR) less than 30 mL/min. These medications should not be used in patients with CKD if the serum creatinine (Cr) is greater than 2.5 mg/dL in men or greater than 2.0 mg/dL in women, or if the serum potassium exceeds 5 mEq/L, as these conditions increase the risk of severe adverse effects such as hyperkalemia and worsening renal function.

Medication or treatment class	Indications
Statin high dose	Continue indefinitely

Comments
High dose includes atorvastatin 40–80 mg/day and rosuvastatin 20–40 mg/day. If intolerant, use a lower dose.

Medication or treatment class	Indications
Nitrates or nondihydropyridine calcium channel blockers (diltiazem, verapamil)	For intermittent angina, or IV infusion for continues angina, HTN emergency, and ADHF

Comments
Phosphodiesterase-5 inhibitors should not be used with nitrates due to the risk of significant hypotension, which can be life-threatening. This contraindication applies if the phosphodiesterase-5 inhibitor was used within the past 24–48 h. Additionally, caution should be exercised when nitrates are used in patients with severe aortic stenosis (AS), as this condition also carries a high risk of hypotension and poor cardiac output. If nitrates are ineffective for angina relief, calcium channel blockers can be used as an alternative. However, continuous use of nitrates for 24–48 h may lead to tachyphylaxis (a reduced response overtime). Cardiac selective calcium channel blockers should be avoided in patients with systolic dysfunction (e.g., Hefref), as their use is contraindicated in this population and may worsen mortality. Overall, calcium channel blockers provide symptomatic relief for angina but do not offer a mortality benefit.

Medication or treatment class	Indications	Comments
Cardiac rehab	All patients	Does improve mortality

Medication or treatment class	Indications	Comments
Colchicine	Selected patients per the cardiologist discretion	In patients after ACS, low-dose colchicine (0.5 mg daily) may be reasonable to reduce risk of MACE [17]

Pearl

Current guidelines recommend that high-risk patients, such as those with acute coronary syndrome (ACS), initiate high-intensity statin therapy to achieve at least a 50% reduction in LDL cholesterol levels, with the ideal target being an LDL cholesterol level of <70 mg/dL. If this target is not achieved despite maximal statin therapy or the patient cannot tolerate high-dose statins, ezetimibe (up to 10 mg daily) can be added to lower LDL cholesterol levels. If LDL cholesterol remains >70 mg/dL within 2 months post-discharge despite the use of both statins and ezetimibe, consider initiating a proprotein convertase subtilisin–kexin type 9 (PCSK9) inhibitor [23].

5.6.4 Complications of STEMI and Their Treatment

Time zone and evaluation	Medication	Treatment	Comments
Within 48 h Post 48 h	Arrhythmias	If ventricular tachycardia (VT) occurs within 48 h and the patient is stable, no ICD is typically indicated. After 48 h, management depends on the clinical situation. An implantable cardioverter-defibrillator (ICD) is reasonable if the patient experiences sustained VT or VF. For symptomatic low-grade heart block, temporary transvenous pacing may be required. Permanent pacemaker placement should be reserved for those with sinus node dysfunction or high-degree AV block that persists for greater than 72 hours after MI.	Accelerated idioventricular rhythm (AIVR) is a common and typically benign arrhythmia. It resembles ventricular tachycardia (VT) but is distinguished by a rate of less than 100 beats per minute. AIVR often occurs in the setting of reperfusion after acute myocardial infarction or other transient ischemic events. Since AIVR is generally self-limiting and asymptomatic, no specific treatment is typically required. Nonsustained ventricular tachycardia (NSVT) is a common finding within the first 24 hours after myocardial infarction (MI). Premature ventricular complexes (PVCs) without hemodynamic compromise and accelerated idioventricular rhythms following reperfusion do not warrant specific antiarrhythmic therapy beyond standard post-MI management. Consequently, the use of amiodarone or referral for electrophysiologic evaluation and ablation is not indicated. The former practice of prophylactically suppressing ventricular ectopy with antiarrhythmic agents is now discouraged due to an increased risk of fatal bradyarrhythmias and asystole. Implantable cardioverter-defibrillator (ICD) placement is reserved for sustained ventricular arrhythmias occurring more than 48 hours after MI; thus, ICD therapy is mostly inappropriate in cases of early NSVT.
	Cardiogenic shock	Will need cardiac ICU, with pressors, and likely mechanical support if all fails	Common postanterior MI It has a high mortality rate, especially if followed by ventricular wall rupture.

Time zone and evaluation	Medication	Treatment	Comments
	LV thrombus	Need to be treated with anticoagulation for at least 3 months, followed by imaging to document resolution [24]	
	LV aneurysm	No treatment indicated	May trigger arrhythmias. In patients with a prior anterior STEMI without symptoms of ischemia, the most likely etiology of the persistent ST-segment elevations is an LV aneurysm. Warfarin anticoagulation may be considered (Class IIb) in patients with a large anterior myocardial infarction accompanied by apical aneurysm or akinesis.
Within 48 h Post 48 h	RV shock	In cases of severe hypotension or cardiogenic shock, patients may require fluid resuscitation along with pressor support (e.g., norepinephrine or dopamine) to maintain blood pressure. Inotropic agents (such as dobutamine or milrinone) may also be necessary to improve cardiac contractility and support the heart's pumping function. In cases where medical management is insufficient, mechanical circulatory support (e.g., intra-aortic balloon pump [IABP] or ventricular assist devices [VAD]) may be required to provide additional cardiac support and improve tissue perfusion. However, keep in mind, the use of a left ventricular assist device or intraaortic balloon pump is not recommended in patients with right ventricular myocardial infarction in the absence of left ventricular dysfunction, as these interventions provide limited benefit and may be detrimental in isolated right ventricular failure.	The triad of hypotension, high jugular venous distension (JVD), and clear lungs is commonly seen in patients after a right coronary artery (RCA) or inferior myocardial infarction (MI). This combination is indicative of right ventricular (RV) failure, which is often preload-dependent. In these patients, fluids are essential to improve preload and cardiac output, as they are dependent on adequate filling to maintain circulation. Vasodilators, such as nitroglycerin, are contraindicated in this scenario, as they can further decrease preload, exacerbating hypotension and worsening right ventricular function. The primary focus should be on maintaining adequate volume status and supporting right ventricular function.

5

Time zone and evaluation	Medication	Treatment	Comments
Within 5 days	VSD	In ventricular septal defect (VSD), afterload reduction with nitroprusside is used to decrease systemic vascular resistance and improve hemodynamics. Mechanical support (e.g., IABP or VAD) may be required in severe cases, and surgery is typically indicated for large or symptomatic VSDs, especially with heart failure or significant shunting. Surgical repair is essential to prevent complications like pulmonary hypertension and long-term heart failure.	Triad of sudden pulmonary edema with pansystolic murmur, and shock
	MR	After load reduction and IABP placement, followed by emergent surgery.	Due to papillary muscle rupture. It could present as VSD. Presents with acute pulmonary edema, mobile mass in the left atrium (papillary muscle) Sometimes, it could be functional dysfunction due to ischemia, so that will need PCI treatment.

5.6.5 Mimics to STEMI Presentation

Condition	Description	Treatment	Comments
Coronary vasospasm	Sudden coronary artery constriction caused either spontaneously, by medications, or illicit drug use such as cocaine	Treated with nitrates, benzodiazepines, or calcium channel blockers. If possible, avoid B-blockers in the acute stage unless highly indicated (may lead to theoretical risk of unopposed alpha vascular stimulation with uncontrolled HTN and spasm)	It mainly affects women at night. They could present atypically with new dyspepsia and fatigue.

Condition	Description	Treatment	Comments
Cardiac syndrome X (MINOCA)	CAD with no significant stenosis on angiography (less than 50%)	Treatment includes β-blockers, calcium channel blockers, nitrates, and ranolazine. Novel therapies include potassium channel openers, metabolic modulators, rho-kinase inhibitors, angiotensin-converting enzyme inhibitors, late sodium channel blockers, ivabradine, phosphodiesterase-5 inhibitors, and statins.	It is more common in women and should be treated with supportive care and treatment of underlying atherosclerotic risk factors if present. It could present as STEMI, with limited cath findings.
Takotsubo cardiomyopathy	ADHF/Transient LV systolic dysfunction with reduced LVEF, elevated troponin, and ischemic changes on ECG with negative LHC	Supportive	Usually triggered due to stressors Echo is diagnostic with apical ballooning, sparing the base of the heart. If coronary disease is found, the diagnosis of stress cardiomyopathy can still be made if the wall motion abnormalities are not in the distribution of the coronary disease.
Spontaneous coronary artery dissection (SCAD)	Enlarging hematoma in the false lumen compresses the coronary artery leading to ischemia and possible STEMI	Needs PCI with stent placement by a cardiologist if significant ischemia is present	Highly suspected if young, or pregnant lady presents with STEMI

5.6.6 Post Discharge Plan

- All patients will benefit from close discharge follow-up with a cardiac rehab program. A clear verbal and written plan for discharge, medication reconciliation, and follow-up is vital [17].
- In patients undergoing PCI, de-escalating DAPT to single antiplatelet therapy and switching from ticagrelor or prasugrel to clopidogrel after 1 month may be reasonable to reduce bleeding risk in high-risk patients [17]. Most high-bleeding-risk patients encountered as a hospitalist include ESRD, platelets $<100 \times 10^9$/L, liver cirrhosis with portal hypertension, previous ICH, long-term use of oral NSAIDs or steroids, and recent major surgery.

- All patients must be up to date with their vaccinations, especially the influenza vaccine, which would be optimum if given before discharge.
- A few questions that may come up:
  - (i) When can the patient resume sex? Usually, it is okay after 1–4 weeks if there is no significant ACS; otherwise, it should be once at baseline, cardiology cleared, and at least 6–8 weeks after any intervention [25]. Sexual activity should be deferred for patients with unstable or refractory angina until their condition is stabilized and optimally managed [25]. The general advice is that the patient should be able to climb one flight of stairs before considering intercourse.
  - (ii) Is the life vest (temporary wearable cardioverter-defibrillator) indicated after STEMI? Generally, no. It may be of benefit only in patients with a high risk of death, like those with sudden death, sustained VT, or ADHF with EF of ≤35% and present with symptoms [17]. Overall, ICD for primary prevention should not be placed after MI with low ejection fraction of ≤40% for at least 40 days, hoping the heart muscle will recover, and after 3 months for PCI intervention.
  - (iii) What should I screen for after STEMI to improve my well-being? Screening for depression is important.

5.7 NSTEMI

5.7.1 Clinical Approach

- An incomplete obstruction to blood flow in acute coronary syndrome (ACS) can progress to a complete obstruction, leading to STEMI if left untreated.
- In addition to a thorough history and physical examination (H&P), diagnostic tests such as EKG, echocardiogram (Echo), CBC, CMP, and serial troponin measurements should be conducted to monitor the patient's progress.
- Risk stratification is essential, and tools like the TIMI and GRACE scores (available on MDcalc) are useful for predicting the severity of ACS. These scoring systems help guide treatment decisions by assessing the risk of adverse outcomes, allowing clinicians to determine the most appropriate treatment approach based on the patient's risk profile.

5.7.2 Treatment Approach in Post-acute Settings for ACS [26]

- Cardiologists always need to be involved.
- For medical management, follow the same approach as in STEMI, except thrombolytics, which is not indicated in US/NSTEMI due to the high risk of hemorrhagic stroke and major noncerebral bleeding.

- Suppose the patient is unstable (hypotensive, AMS, significant ventricular arrhythmias, ADHF, persistent chest pain despite initial medical treatment). In that case, they should go for urgent PCI for the culprit lesion only within 2 h, ASAP [17]. Otherwise, for stable patients, the following approaches could be followed for treatment:
  A. **Invasive strategy (PCI/CABG)**
     (i) **TIMI score of 3–4/GRACE 109–140**. Recommended delayed invasive strategy within 72 h
     (ii) **TIMI score above 5/GRACE above 140**. Early strategy within 24 h

Hospitalist Tip

If the patient has a limited life expectancy of less than 2 years or advanced dementia, it is preferable to proceed with medical management alone without an invasive approach after discussing the options with the family or patient [17].

  B. **Ischemia-guided treatment/conservative approach**. A noninvasive approach is often reasonable for patients with a TIMI score of less than 2 or a GRACE score of less than 109, as evidence supports this strategy for low-risk patients. A recent study showed that, in older adults (aged 75 years) with NSTEMI, an invasive strategy did not significantly lower the risk of cardiovascular death or nonfatal myocardial infarction [26, 27]. As previously discussed, medical treatment should follow the same approach as STEMI management. For patients managed with an ischemia-guided strategy, the initial antiplatelet regimen includes aspirin combined with either clopidogrel or ticagrelor (Class I). Ticagrelor is preferred over clopidogrel, which carries a Class IIa recommendation. Noninvasive stress testing is recommended in low- and intermediate-risk patients who have been free of ischemia at rest or with low-level activity for a minimum of 12-24 hours. If results are normal or the patient is deemed low-risk, follow-up with a cardiologist on an outpatient basis within 1–2 weeks is appropriate [17]. However, suppose the patient's condition deteriorates or chest pain persists. In that case, the cardiologist should be notified for urgent angiography while the patient is an inpatient, followed by an invasive strategy and potential PCI.

Pearl

UFH will continue for at least 48 h or near discharge in NSTEMI/US. LMWH or fondaparinux could be used in low- risk patients (TIMI less than 2) [28].

Pearl

Hold clopidogrel or ticagrelor for at least 5 days if the patient will go for CABG due to the increased risk of bleeding. Hold for at least 24 h if the procedure is urgent. Therefore, in most of my ACS patients, I defer initiating additional antiplatelet therapy beyond aspirin until after cardiology evaluation, given the potential need for urgent coronary artery bypass grafting (CABG).

5.8 Acute Myocardial Injury

5.8.1 What Is Acute Myocardial Injury [29]

- Acute myocardial injury refers to a nonischemic form of heart injury, typically caused by factors such as acute illness (e.g., postoperative state), severe stress (e.g., sepsis), or trauma. Unlike myocardial infarction, where the underlying cause is ischemic, acute myocardial injury occurs without the blockage of coronary arteries.
- This condition is associated with higher mortality, primarily due to non-cardiovascular causes, which suggests that the underlying illness (such as infection, surgery, or trauma) is the primary factor, rather than complications arising from ischemia or necrosis of the heart muscle.
- Other terms used to describe this condition include acute nonischemic myocardial injury, troponin leak, or stress cardiomyopathy.

Pearl

MI is divided into five categories according to its underlying cause of ischemia. It is most important for a hospitalist to know type 1, which is attributable to acute atherothrombosis, or supply/demand mismatch without acute atherothrombosis (type 2 MI). Myocardial infarction is characterized by a dynamic change in cardiac troponin levels, specifically, a rise and/or fall with at least one value above the 99th percentile upper reference limit ,accompanied by evidence of Myocardial ischemia. This evidence may include acute ischemic symptoms, new ischemic changes on the electrocardiogram, the emergence of pathological Q waves, or imaging findings demonstrating new loss of viable myocardium or regional wall motion abnormalities consistent with an ischemic etiology. If there is no evidence of myocardial ischemia, the patient is more likely experiencing acute or chronic non-ischemic myocardial injury rather than a Type 2 myocardial infarction, which by definition requires documented evidence of ischemia in addition to elevated troponin.

Pearl

When an acute myocardial injury occurs in the context of another acute illness or surgical procedure, type 2 MI and nonischemic myocardial injury are more likely than type 1 MI, although it should be recognized that plaque rupture events can be triggered by acute infectious illness or precipitated by perioperative stressors [29].

5.8.2 Myocardial Injury Taxonomy [29]

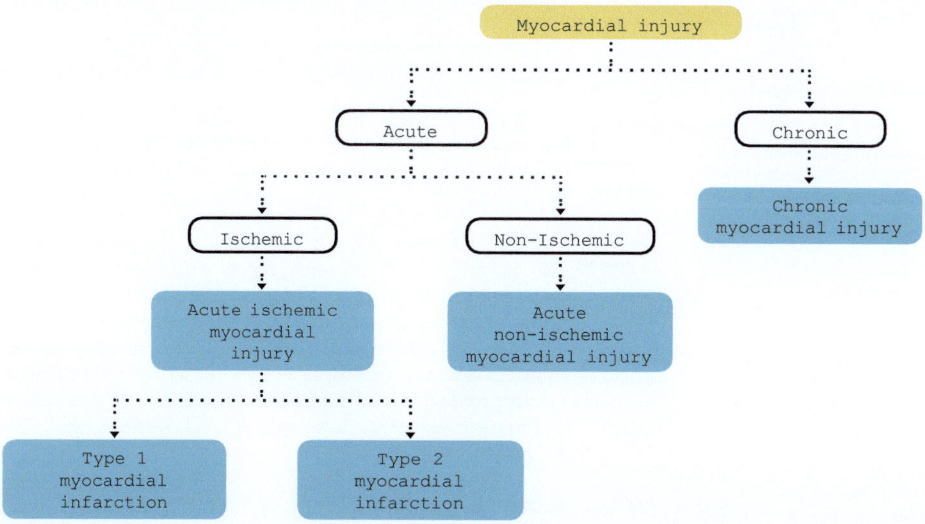

5.8.3 Myocardial Injury Description

Type 1 MI

MI caused by atherothrombotic CAD and usually precipitated by atherosclerotic plaque disruption.

Type 2 MI

MI is caused by a mismatch between oxygen supply and demand by a pathophysiological mechanism (no plaque disruption) other than coronary atherothrombosis type 1 MI. Common triggers include significant anemia, Hypotension, uncontrolled HTN, significant tachycardia, and severe hypoxia. Other primary causes include spasms, dissection, and embolization.

Acute nonischemic myocardial injury

Acute myocardial injury with elevated Troponin without in the absence of a primary ischemic cause. A classic example is takotsubo) cardiomyopathy.

Chronic myocardial injury

Chronic myocardial injury with elevated stable Troponin without an acute EKG change. It could be seen in ESRD or chronic CHF.

Pearl

Although cardiac troponin is highly specific for myocardial injury, it does not differentiate between the etiologically diverse types of MI or non-MI causes of myocardial injury. However, the higher the troponin, the more likely the injury is ischemic.

5.8.4 Clinical Approach

- Acute nonischemic myocardial injury is commonly observed in hospital settings, particularly in patients with significant illnesses such as sepsis. The condition is often asymptomatic, although some patients may experience chest pain (27%) or shortness of breath (33%). Troponin levels are typically elevated, and the EKG may show nonspecific findings.
- This condition is largely a diagnosis of exclusion, made by ruling out acute coronary syndrome (ACS), which is not always straightforward. Dynamic ST changes on the EKG may prompt further ischemic evaluation, such as a stress test or invasive angiography, once the patient's condition stabilizes.
- Echocardiography can provide useful insights: regional wall motion abnormalities in specific coronary territories support an ischemic cause. In contrast, diffuse myocardial abnormalities or a normal echo are more indicative of nonischemic myocardial injury. This pattern is also true for myocardial perfusion testing.
- Coronary or cardiac computed tomography angiography (CTA) can be a valuable tool when type 1 MI is suspected, as the absence of atherosclerotic disease on CTA can effectively rule out type 1 MI.
- A cardiac MRI may also be helpful. Ischemia-related myocardial injury typically affects the subendocardium to the epicardium, while nonischemic myocardial injury tends to be localized to the epicardium or mid-wall. Cardiac MRI is especially useful for identifying conditions like acute myocarditis or cardiomyopathy that are not related to MI.

Hospitalist Tip

As a hospitalist approaches a patient with elevated troponin, your chain of thoughts should rule out the possibility of ischemia based on how probable it is according to clinical assessment, EKG findings, TTE, and, if needed, cardiac CTA. When the probability is borderline and inconclusive, you should consult your cardiologist and proceed with further testing, such as nuclear stress testing, Coronary angiogram, or cardiac MRI.

Hospitalist Tip

Keep in mind in the absence of clear evidence for type 1 MI, it is more likely to follow the diagnosis of acute nonischemic myocardial injury for patients presenting with evidence of elevated cardiac troponin with ADHF, sepsis, or postoperative state, and to reserve the diagnosis of type 2 MI for those patients with acute myocardial injury and clear evidence of ischemia or notable extracardiac supply/demand mismatch (e.g., significant tachycardia, hypertension, hypotension, hypoxemia, or anemia) or acute non-atherothrombotic coronary obstruction (e.g., dissection and embolization).

5.8.5 Treatment Approach

- If the likelihood of type 1 MI is high (e.g., known coronary artery disease (CAD), no specific triggers, typical symptoms, dynamic ECG changes, or very high troponin levels), treat the patient as ACS (either STEMI or NSTEMI) until proven otherwise.
- For type 2 MI or acute cardiac injury, the focus should be on treating the underlying stressor (such as sepsis, hypotension, or surgery). A beta-blocker may be useful in high-demand states (e.g., tachycardia or hypertension) to reduce myocardial workload and oxygen demand [30].
- Once the patient's clinical condition is more stable, assessing the presence or absence of CAD and structural cardiac disease is recommended if this has not already been done. This can be accomplished with functional or anatomic studies (such as stress tests, coronary angiography, or cardiac imaging), provided this aligns with the patient's overall goals of care [29]. These studies can be done either non-urgently during the inpatient stay or on an outpatient basis, with input from a cardiologist.

Hospitalist Tip

Suppose there is a dilemma about distinguishing between type 1 and type 2 MI/acute myocardial injury. In that case, it may be reasonable to manage the patient conservatively until more conclusive evidence arises or the patient's clinical status is more appropriate for the angiography or antithrombotic approach. Consult your cardiologist for further advice.

References

1. Swap CJ, Nagurney JT. Value and limitations of chest pain history in the evaluation of patients with suspected acute coronary syndromes. JAMA. 2005;294(20):2623–9. https://doi.org/10.1001/jama.294.20.2623. Erratum in: JAMA. 2006 May 17;295(19):2250. PMID: 16304077
2. Cullen L, Greenslade JH, Than M, Brown AF, Hammett CJ, Lamanna A, Flaws DF, Chu K, Fowles LF, Parsonage WA. The new Vancouver Chest Pain Rule using troponin as the only biomarker: an external validation study. Am J Emerg Med. 2014;32(2):129–34. https://doi.org/10.1016/j.ajem.2013.10.021. Epub 2013 Oct 14. PMID: 24238485
3. Steffel J, Eikelboom JW, Anand SS, Shestakovska O, Yusuf S, Fox KAA. The COMPASS Trial: net clinical benefit of low-dose rivaroxaban plus aspirin as compared with aspirin in patients with chronic vascular disease. Circulation. 2020;142(1):40–8. https://doi.org/10.1161/CIRCULATIONAHA.120.046048. Epub 2020 May 21. Erratum in: Circulation. 2020 Jul 7;142(1):e23. doi: 10.1161/CIR.0000000000000880. PMID: 32436455
4. Chun AA, McGee SR. Bedside diagnosis of coronary artery disease: a systematic review. Am J Med. 2004;117(5):334–43. https://doi.org/10.1016/j.amjmed.2004.03.021. PMID: 15336583
5. Solomon CG, Lee TH, Cook EF, Weisberg MC, Brand DA, Rouan GW, Goldman L. Comparison of clinical presentation of acute myocardial infarction in patients older than 65 to younger patients: the Multicenter Chest Pain Study experience. Am J Cardiol. 1989;63(12):772–6. https://doi.org/10.1016/0002-9149(89)90040-4. PMID: 2648786

6. Thompson A, Fleischmann KE, Smilowitz NR, de Las FL, Mukherjee D, Aggarwal NR, Ahmad FS, Allen RB, Altin SE, Auerbach A, Berger JS, Chow B, Dakik HA, Eisenstein EL, Gerhard-Herman M, Ghadimi K, Kachulis B, Leclerc J, Lee CS, Macaulay TE, Mates G, Merli GJ, Parwani P, Poole JE, Rich MW, Ruetzler K, Stain SC, Sweitzer B, Talbot AW, Vallabhajosyula S, Whittle J, Williams KA Sr, Peer Review Committee Members. 2024 AHA/ACC/ACS/ASNC/HRS/SCA/SCCT/SCMR/SVM Guideline for Perioperative Cardiovascular Management for Non-cardiac Surgery: a report of the American College of Cardiology/American Heart Association Joint Committee on Clinical Practice Guidelines. Circulation. 2024;150(19):e351–442. https://doi.org/10.1161/CIR.0000000000001285. Epub 2024 Sep 24. Erratum in: Circulation. 2024 Nov 19;150(21):e466. doi: 10.1161/CIR.0000000000001298. PMID: 39316661.
7. Mehta SR, Wood DA, Storey RF, Mehran R, Bainey KR, Nguyen H, Meeks B, Di Pasquale G, López-Sendón J, Faxon DP, Mauri L, Rao SV, Feldman L, Steg PG, Avezum Á, Sheth T, Pinilla-Echeverri N, Moreno R, Campo G, Wrigley B, Kedev S, Sutton A, Oliver R, Rodés-Cabau J, Stanković G, Welsh R, Lavi S, Cantor WJ, Wang J, Nakamya J, Bangdiwala SI, Cairns JA. COMPLETE Trial Steering Committee and Investigators. Complete revascularization with multivessel PCI for myocardial infarction. N Engl J Med. 2019;381(15):1411–21. https://doi.org/10.1056/NEJMoa1907775. Epub 2019 Sep 1. PMID: 31475795
8. De Vita A, Covino M, Pontecorvo S, Buonamassa G, Marino AG, Marano R, Natale L, Liuzzo G, Burzotta F, Franceschi F. Coronary CT angiography in the emergency department: state of the art and future perspectives. J Cardiovasc Dev Dis. 2025;12(2):48. https://doi.org/10.3390/jcdd12020048. PMID: 39997482; PMCID: PMC11856466
9. Thuijs DJFM, Kappetein AP, Serruys PW, Mohr FW, Morice MC, Mack MJ, Holmes DR Jr, Curzen N, Davierwala P, Noack T, Milojevic M, Dawkins KD, da Costa BR, Jüni P, Head SJ. SYNTAX Extended Survival Investigators. Percutaneous coronary intervention versus coronary artery bypass grafting in patients with three-vessel or left main coronary artery disease: 10-year multicentre randomized controlled SYNTAX trial follow-up. Lancet. 2019;394(10206):1325–34. https://doi.org/10.1016/S0140-6736(19)31997-X. Epub 2019 Sep 2. Erratum in: Lancet. 2020 Mar 14;395(10227):870. doi: 10.1016/S0140-6736(20)30249-X. PMID: 31488373
10. Fihn SD, Gardin JM, Abrams J, Berra K, Blankenship JC, Dallas AP, Douglas PS, Foody JM, Gerber TC, Hinderliter AL, King SB 3rd, Kligfield PD, Krumholz HM, Kwong RY, Lim MJ, Linderbaum JA, Mack MJ, Munger MA, Prager RL, Sabik JF, Shaw LJ, Sikkema JD, Smith CR Jr, Smith SC Jr, Spertus JA, Williams SV, Anderson JL, American College of Cardiology Foundation/American Heart Association Task Force. 2012 ACCF/AHA/ACP/AATS/PCNA/SCAI/STS guideline for the diagnosis and management of patients with stable ischemic heart disease: a report of the American College of Cardiology Foundation/American Heart Association task force on practice guidelines, and the American College of Physicians, American Association for Thoracic Surgery, Preventive Cardiovascular Nurses Association, Society for Cardiovascular Angiography and Interventions, and Society of Thoracic Surgeons. Circulation. 2012;126(25):e354–471. https://doi.org/10.1161/CIR.0b013e318277d6a0. Epub 2012 Nov 19. Erratum in: Circulation. 2014 Apr 22;129(16):e463. PMID: 23166211
11. Boden WE, O'Rourke RA, Teo KK, Hartigan PM, Maron DJ, Kostuk WJ, Knudtson M, Dada M, Casperson P, Harris CL, Chaitman BR, Shaw L, Gosselin G, Nawaz S, Title LM, Gau G, Blaustein AS, Booth DC, Bates ER, Spertus JA, Berman DS, Mancini GB, Weintraub WS, COURAGE Tri- al Research Group. Optimal medical therapy with or without PCI for stable coronary disease. N Engl J Med. 2007;356(15):1503–16. https://doi.org/10.1056/NEJMoa070829. Epub 2007 Mar 26. PMID: 17387127
12. Cho MS, Kang DY, Ahn JM, Yun SC, Oh YS, Lee CH, Choi EK, Lee JH, Kwon CH, Park GM, Choi HO, Park KH, Park KM, Hwang J, Yoo KD, Cho YR, Kim JH, Hwang KW, Jin ES, Kwon O, Kim KH, Park SJ, Park DW, Nam GB. EPIC-CAD Investigators. Edoxaban antithrombotic therapy for atrial fibrillation and stable coronary artery disease. N Engl J Med. 2024; https://doi.org/10.1056/NEJMoa2407362. Epub ahead of print. PMID: 39225258

13. Yasuda S, Kaikita K, Akao M, Ako J, Matoba T, Nakamura M, Miyauchi K, Hagiwara N, Kimura K, Hirayama A, Matsui K, Ogawa H. AFIRE Investigators. Antithrombotic therapy for atrial fibrillation with stable coronary disease. N Engl J Med. 2019;381(12):1103–13. https://doi.org/10.1056/NEJMoa1904143. Epub 2019 Sep 2. Erratum in: N Engl J Med. 2021 Oct 21;385(17):1632. doi: 10.1056/NEJMx210010. PMID: 31475793
14. Brown KN, Hussain K, Richards JR. Radiation-induced coronary artery disease. [Updated 2023 Jun 12]. In: StatPearls [Internet]. Treasure Island (FL): StatPearls Publishing. p. 2025. Available from: https://www.ncbi.nlm.nih.gov/books/NBK536948/.
15. Virani SS, Newby LK, Arnold SV, Bittner V, Brewer LC, Demeter SH, Dixon DL, Fearon WF, Hess B, Johnson HM, Kazi DS, Kolte D, Kumbhani DJ, LoFaso J, Mahtta D, Mark DB, Minissian M, Navar AM, Patel AR, Piano MR, Rodriguez F, Talbot AW, Taqueti VR, Thomas RJ, van Diepen S, Wiggins B, Williams MS, Peer Review Committee Members. 2023 AHA/ACC/ACCP/ASPC/NLA/PCNA Guideline for the Management of Patients With Chronic Coronary Disease: a report of the American Heart Association/American College of Cardiology Joint Committee on Clinical Practice Guidelines. Circulation. 2023;148(9):e9–e119. https://doi.org/10.1161/CIR.0000000000001168. Epub 2023 Jul 20. Erratum in: Circulation. 2023 Sep 26;148(13):e148. doi: 10.1161/CIR.0000000000001183. Erratum in: Circulation. 2023 Dec 5;148(23):e186. doi: 10.1161/CIR.0000000000001195. PMID: 37471501
16. Marcus GM, Cohen J, Varosy PD, Vessey J, Rose E, Massie BM, Chatterjee K, Waters D. The utility of gestures in patients with chest discomfort. Am J Med. 2007;120(1):83–9. https://doi.org/10.1016/j.amjmed.2006.05.045. PMID: 17208083
17. Rao SV, O'Donoghue ML, Ruel M, Rab T, Tamis-Holland JE, Alexander JH, Baber U, Baker H, Cohen MG, Cruz-Ruiz M, Davis LL, de Lemos JA, DeWald TA, Elgendy IY, Feldman DN, Goyal A, Isiadinso I, Menon V, Morrow DA, Mukherjee D, Platz E, Promes SB, Sandner S, Sandoval Y, Schunder R, Shah B, Stopyra JP, Talbot AW, Taub PR, Williams MS. ACC/AHA/ACEP/NAEMSP/SCAI guideline for the management of patients with acute coronary syndromes: a report of the American College of Cardiology/American Heart Association Joint Committee on Clinical Practice Guidelines. Circulation. 2025;2025 https://doi.org/10.1161/CIR.0000000000001309. Epub ahead of print. PMID: 40014670
18. Ibanez B, James S, Agewall S, Antunes MJ, Bucciarelli-Ducci C, Bueno H, Caforio ALP, Crea F, Goudevenos JA, Halvorsen S, Hindricks G, Kastrati A, Lenzen MJ, Prescott E, Roffi M, Valgimigli M, Varenhorst C, Vranckx P, Widimský P, ESC Scientific Document Group. 2017 ESC Guidelines for the management of acute myocardial infarction in patients presenting with ST-segment elevation: The Task Force for the management of acute myocardial infarction in patients presenting with ST-segment elevation of the European Society of Cardiology (ESC). Eur Heart J. 2018;39(2):119–77. https://doi.org/10.1093/eurheartj/ehx393. PMID: 28886621
19. Schüpke S, Neumann FJ, Menichelli M, Mayer K, Bernlochner I, Wöhrle J, Richardt G, Liebetrau C, Witzenbichler B, Antoniucci D, Akin I, Bott-Flügel L, Fischer M, Landmesser U, Katus HA, Sibbing D, Seyfarth M, Janisch M, Boncompagni D, Hilz R, Rottbauer W, Okrojek R, Möllmann H, Hochholzer W, Migliorini A, Cassese S, Mollo P, Xhepa E, Kufner S, Strehle A, Leggewie S, Allali A, Ndrepepa G, Schühlen H, Angiolillo DJ, Hamm CW, Hapfelmeier A, Tölg R, Trenk D, Schunkert H, Laugwitz KL, Kastrati A. ISAR-REACT 5 Trial Investigators. Ticagrelor or prasugrel in patients with acute coronary syndromes. N Engl J Med. 2019;381(16):1524–34. https://doi.org/10.1056/NEJMoa1908973. Epub 2019 Sep 1. PMID: 31475799
20. Angiolillo DJ, Bhatt DL, Cannon CP, Eikelboom JW, Gibson CM, Goodman SG, Granger CB, Holmes DR, Lopes RD, Mehran R, Moliterno DJ, Price MJ, Saw J, Tanguay JF, Faxon DP. Antithrombotic therapy in patients with atrial fibrillation treated with oral anticoagulation undergoing percutaneous coronary intervention: A North American perspective: 2021 update. Circulation. 2021;143(6):583–96. https://doi.org/10.1161/CIRCULATIONAHA.120.050438. Epub 2021 Feb 8. PMID: 33555916
21. Bally M, Dendukuri N, Rich B, Nadeau L, Helin-Salmivaara A, Garbe E, Brophy JM. Risk of acute myocardial infarction with NSAIDs in real world use: Bayesian meta-analysis of individual patient data. BMJ. 2017;357:j1909. https://doi.org/10.1136/bmj.j1909. PMID: 28487435; PMCID: PMC5423546

22. James SK, Roe MT, Cannon CP, Cornel JH, Horrow J, Husted S, Katus H, Morais J, Steg PG, Storey RF, Stevens S, Wallentin L, Harrington RA, PLATO Study Group. Ticagrelor versus clopidogrel in patients with acute coronary syndromes intended for non-invasive management: sub-study from prospective randomised PLATelet inhibition and patient Outcomes (PLATO) trial. BMJ. 2011;342:d3527. https://doi.org/10.1136/bmj.d3527. PMID: 21685437; PMCID: PMC3117310
23. Grundy SM, Stone NJ, Bailey AL, Beam C, Birtcher KK, Blumenthal RS, Braun LT, de Ferranti S, Faiella-Tommasino J, Forman DE, Goldberg R, Heidenreich PA, Hlatky MA, Jones DW, Lloyd-Jones D, Lopez-Pajares N, Ndumele CE, Orringer CE, Peralta CA, Saseen JJ, Smith SC Jr, Sperling L, Virani SS, Yeboah J. 2018 AHA/ACC/AACVPR/AAPA/ABC/ACPM/ADA/AGS/APhA/ASPC/NLA/PCNA guideline on the management of blood cholesterol: executive summary: a report of the American College of Cardiology/American Heart Association Task Force on Clinical Practice Guidelines. J Am Coll Cardiol. 2019;73(24):3168–209. https://doi.org/10.1016/j.jacc.2018.11.002. Epub 2018 Nov 10. Erratum in: J Am Coll Cardiol. 2019 Jun 25;73(24):3234–7. doi: 10.1016/j.jacc.2019.05.012. PMID: 30423391
24. Goh FQ, Sia CH, Chan MY, Yeo LL, Tan BY. What's the optimal duration of anticoagulation in patients with left ventricular thrombus? Expert Rev Cardiovasc Ther. 2023;21(12):947–61. https://doi.org/10.1080/14779072.2023.2270906. Epub 2023 Dec 13. PMID: 37830297
25. Levine GN, Steinke EE, Bakaeen FG, Bozkurt B, Cheitlin MD, Conti JB, Foster E, Jaarsma T, Kloner RA, Lange RA, Lindau ST, Maron BJ, Moser DK, Ohman EM, Seftel AD, Stewart WJ, American Heart Association Council on Clinical Cardiology; Council on Cardiovascular Nursing; Council on Cardiovascular Surgery and Anesthesia; Council on Quality of Care and Outcomes Research. Sexual activity and cardiovascular disease: a scientific statement from the American Heart Association. Circulation. 2012;125(8):1058–72. https://doi.org/10.1161/CIR.0b013e3182447787. Epub 2012 Jan 19. PMID: 22267844
26. Amsterdam EA, Wenger NK, Brindis RG, Casey DE Jr, Ganiats TG, Holmes DR Jr, Jaffe AS, Jneid H, Kelly RF, Kontos MC, Levine GN, Liebson PR, Mukherjee D, Peterson ED, Sabatine MS, Smalling RW, Zieman SJ. 2014 AHA/ACC guideline for the management of patients with Non-ST-elevation acute coronary syndromes: a report of the American College of Cardiology/American Heart Association Task Force on Practice Guidelines. J Am Coll Cardiol. 2014;64(24):e139–228. https://doi.org/10.1016/j.jacc.2014.09.017. Epub 2014 Sep 23. Erratum in: J Am Coll Cardiol. 2014 Dec 23;64(24):2713-4. Dosage error in article text. PMID: 25260718
27. Kunadian V, Mossop H, Shields C, Bardgett M, Watts P, Teare MD, Pritchard J, Adams-Hall J, Runnett C, Ripley DP, Carter J, Quigley J, Cooke J, Austin D, Murphy J, Kelly D, McGowan J, Veerasamy M, Felmeden D, Contractor H, Mutgi S, Irving J, Lindsay S, Galasko G, Lee K, Sultan A, Dastidar AG, Hussain S, Haq IU, de Belder M, Denvir M, Flather M, Storey RF, Newby DE, Pocock SJ, Fox KAA. British Heart Foundation SENIOR-RITA Trial Team and Investigators. Invasive treatment strategy for older patients with myocardial infarction. N Engl J Med. 2024; https://doi.org/10.1056/NEJMoa2407791. Epub ahead of print. PMID: 39225274
28. Onwordi EN, Gamal A, Zaman A. Anticoagulant therapy for acute coronary syndromes. Interv Cardiol. 2018;13(2):87–92. https://doi.org/10.15420/icr.2017:26:1. PMID: 29928314; PMCID: PMC5980649
29. DeFilippis AP, Chapman AR, Mills NL, de Lemos JA, Arbab-Zadeh A, Newby LK, Morrow DA. Assessment and treatment of patients with Type 2 myocardial infarction and acute non-ischemic myocardial injury. Circulation. 2019;140(20):1661–78. https://doi.org/10.1161/CIRCULATIONAHA.119.040631. Epub 2019 Aug 16. PMID: 31416350; PMCID: PMC6855329
30. Sandoval Y, Smith SW, Sexter A, Thordsen SE, Bruen CA, Carlson MD, Dodd KW, Driver BE, Hu Y, Jacoby K, Johnson BK, Love SA, Moore JC, Schulz K, Scott NL, Apple FS. Type 1 and 2 myocardial infarction and myocardial injury: clinical transition to high-sensitivity cardiac Troponin I. Am J Med. 2017;130(12):1431–1439.e4. https://doi.org/10.1016/j.amjmed.2017.05.049. Epub 2017 Jul 21. PMID: 28739197

31. Roiron C, Sanchez P, Bouzamondo A, Lechat P, Montalescot G. Drug eluting stents: an updated meta-analysis of randomised controlled trials. Heart. 2006;92(5):641–9. https://doi.org/10.1136/hrt.2005.061622. Epub 2005 Oct 10. PMID: 16216853; PMCID: PMC1860942
32. Portela GT, Carson JL, Swanson SA, Alexander JH, Hébert PC, Goodman SG, Steg PG, Bertolet M, Strom JB, Fergusson DA, Simon T, White HD, Cooper HA, Abbott JD, Rao SV, Chaitman BR, Fordyce CB, Lopes RD, Daneault B. MINT Investigators. Effect of four hemoglobin transfusion threshold strategies in patients with acute myocardial infarction and anemia: a target trial emulation using MINT trial data. Ann Intern Med. 2024;177(11):1489–98. https://doi.org/10.7326/M24-0571. Epub 2024 Oct 1. PMID: 39348705
33. Raphael CE, Sandoval Y, Beachey JD, Roger V, Singh M, Johnson MP, Tweet MS, Bell MR, Lerman A, Hayes SN, Holmes DR, Gersh BJ, Jaffe AS, Gulati R. Causes of Myocardial Infarction in Younger Patients: Troponin-Elevation in Persons ≤65 Years Old in Olmsted County. J Am Coll Cardiol. 2025 Sep 23;86(12):877–888. https://doi.org/10.1016/j.jacc.2025.07.012. Epub 2025 Aug 27. PMID: 40864006; PMCID: PMC12445014
34. Guimarães PO, Franken M, Tavares CAM, Antunes MO, Silveira FS, Andrade PB, Bergo RR, Joaquim RM, Tinoco de Paula JE, Nascimento BR, Pitta FG, Arruda JA, Serpa RG, Ohe LN, Mangione FM, Furtado RHM, Ferreira E, Sampaio FBA, T do Nascimento C, Genelhu LOO, Bezerra CG, Sarmento-Leite R, Maia LN, Oliveira FRA, Wainstein MV, Dall'Orto FTC, Monfardini F, Assis SRL, Nicolau JC, Sposito AC, Lopes RD, Onuma Y, Valgimigli M, Angiolillo DJ, Serruys PWJC, Berwanger O, Bacal F, Lemos PA; NEO-MINDSET Trial Investigators. Early Withdrawal of Aspirin after PCI in Acute Coronary Syndromes. N Engl J Med. 2025 Aug 31. https://doi.org/10.1056/NEJMoa2507980. Epub ahead of print. PMID: 40888723

Valvular Heart Disease (VHD)

Contents

M. Salih, *Practical Hospitalist Guide to Inpatient Cardiology*, https://doi.org/10.1007/978-3-032-03240-9_6

This chapter offers a comprehensive overview of valvular heart disease, focusing on the diagnosis, clinical presentation, and management of the most common native and prosthetic valve disorders encountered by adult care providers. It details the pathophysiology and hallmark findings of **aortic stenosis (AS)** and **aortic regurgitation (AR)** including systolic outflow obstruction and diastolic volume overload, respectively, as well as **mitral stenosis (MS)** and **mitral regurgitation (MR)**, emphasizing their etiologies, murmur characteristics, and implications for left atrial and pulmonary pressures. The evaluation of **prosthetic valve dysfunction**, whether mechanical or bioprosthetic, includes recognizing complications such as thrombosis, pannus formation, endocarditis, and structural deterioration.

6.1 Aortic Regurgitation

6.1.1 When to Suspect and Major Etiology

- Unexplained shortness of breath (SOB) accompanied by significant dilation of the left ventricle and evidence of aortic regurgitation (AR) on objective assessment. It is less common than aortic stenosis (AS) or mitral regurgitation (MR). AR can arise from either valve pathology or root pathology.
- The most prevalent causes of chronic AR in developed countries include [1]:
  1. Dilation of the aortic root: Connective tissue disorders such as Marfan syndrome and Ehlers-Danlos syndrome (EDS) can lead to aortic dilation and aneurysms. Other rarer causes include large vessel vasculitis, syphilis, and ankylosing spondylitis, which should be considered in the appropriate clinical context.
  2. Primary valve pathology: Congenital bicuspid aortic valves.
  3. Loss of support for the aortic valve cusp: Conditions such as radiation exposure, rheumatic fever, ventricular septal defect (VSD), or degenerative diseases can cause calcification or fibrosis of the aortic valves. A rare cause is rheumatoid arthritis, which can result in rheumatoid nodules on the valves, preventing adequate closure.

Pearl

Long-standing HTN leads to aortic root dilation, which could lead to AR [3]. Treat the HTN.

6.1.2 Clinical Approach

- Patients with chronic aortic regurgitation (AR) may present with nonspecific symptoms such as shortness of breath (SOB), exertional angina, and extreme fatigue. Unique early findings can include palpitations, especially when lying on the left side, likely due to premature ventricular contractions (PVCs). In advanced stages, symptoms may progress to congestive heart failure with pulmonary hypertension and volume overload. Physical examination findings in chronic AR include bounding, large-volume peripheral pulses with wide pulse pressure, a laterally displaced apex beat, and a diastolic murmur auscultated at the third left (valvular pathology) or right (aortic pathologies such as Marfan syndrome, dissection, or syphilis) intercostal space. In acute AR, these signs may be subtle due to a sudden increase in volume causing diastolic pressure equilibrium between the aorta and ventricle, leading to shock with under-compensating contractility. In chronic AR, this mechanism fails over the years, gradually leading to symptom onset.
- The basic workup includes a transthoracic echocardiogram (TTE) to assess AR severity and cardiac function. An electrocardiogram (EKG) may reveal arrhythmias and signs of left atrial dilation (LAD) or left ventricular hypertrophy (LVH). At the same time, a chest X-ray may show cardiomegaly due to eccentric hypertrophy and aortic dilation.

Hospitalist Tip

If you suspect acute AR with dissection, the investigation of choice is CTA with contrast.

Pearl

Most signs for chronic AR are not sensitive, specific enough, or suitable to assess severity [2].

6.1.3 Major DD

- All other VHDs may present similarly.

6.1.4 Treatment Approach [1]

- Aortic valve replacement(AVR) or surgical correction is preferred for patients with symptomatic aortic regurgitation (AR) when symptoms are attributed to AR rather than other conditions. Surgery is also considered for asymptomatic patients with a left ventricular ejection fraction (LVEF) below 55% or significant left ventricular dilation (end-systolic diameter greater than 50 mm), regardless of the ejection fraction. The timing of surgery is crucial to prevent irreversible myocardial dysfunction.
- Medical therapy with afterload reduction in hypertensive patients using vasodilators and diuretics is reasonable for patients with uncontrolled hypertension, acute decompensated heart failure (ADHF), and chronic AR. Vasodilators include dihydropyridine calcium channel blockers, ACE inhibitors, ARBs, hydralazine, and isosorbide mononitrate. If the patient has congestive heart failure (CHF), it should be managed similarly to other heart failure patients with guideline-directed medical therapy (GDMT), but mainly start with Entresto@, ACE, and ARB for HFrEF patients (for afterload reduction). That's especially true if the patient is not a good surgical candidate.
- In acute settings, surgery is the appropriate choice, with aggressive blood pressure control needed in cases of aortic dissection. If the patient is hypertensive, do not use B-blockers (Lopressor@/or labetalol), as they will lower the already physiologically increased heart rate to compensate for lower cardiac output. In cardiogenic shock, inotropes like dobutamine may be required. Intra-aortic balloon pump (IABP) and norepinephrine are contraindicated, as they can increase regurgitation pressure and left ventricular diastolic pressure, thereby worsening cardiac output.

Pearl

To simplify indications for aortic valve replacement (AVR) or surgical intervention, consider surgery if the patient is symptomatic, has left ventricular dysfunction, or exhibits left ventricular dilation.

6.2 Aortic Stenosis

6.2.1 When to Suspect and Major Etiology

- In elderly populations, particularly those aged 70 to 80, it is important to suspect aortic stenosis when patients present with exertional angina, exertional dyspnea, and syncopal episodes. In hospital settings, these symptoms may manifest as acute decompensated heart failure (ADHF) or unexplained exertional syncope, and it is crucial to rule out acute coronary syndrome (ACS) due to its similar presentation. The symptoms of aortic stenosis are caused by increased pressure on the left ventricle, leading to left ventricular hypertrophy (LVH) and diastolic dysfunction, particularly during events that elevate cardiac output. The prognosis becomes poor once the patient develops congestive heart failure (CHF). Cardiac implantable electronic device (CIED) infections are categorized as pocket infections or bacteremia, with a cardiac device and imaging revealing lead or valve vegetation.
- The most common cause of aortic stenosis:
    1. Calcification due to degenerative changes [4]. This process begins with sclerosis, which is clinically silent and progresses gradually to aortic stenosis over the years. It is associated with atherosclerotic risk factors such as ischemic heart disease (IHD).
    2. Another cause is the congenital bicuspid aortic valve, which leads to aortic stenosis due to abnormal mechanical stress and shear tension. This condition typically affects patients younger than 70 years and is linked to coarctation of the aorta, dilated aortic root, Turner syndrome, and other congenital heart diseases.

Pearl

The most common cause for AS is senile degenerative calcification. Most VHDs (60%) in developed countries are caused mainly by degenerative pathology [5].

Pearl

Additional, less common causes of aortic stenosis include rheumatic heart disease, which is not prevalent in developed countries but may be considered in patients from developing regions. Other rare causes encompass exposure to radiation, connective tissue disorders, cardiac amyloidosis, and end-stage renal disease (ESRD), which can lead to abnormal calcification over time, primarily affecting the aorta.

6.2.2 Clinical Approach

- Patients with aortic stenosis may present with a triad of symptoms: angina, dyspnea on exertion (more than usual), and exertional syncope, which indicate a poor prognosis and severe aortic stenosis. Acute decompensated heart failure (ADHF) and, rarely, bleeding events may also occur. A physical examination typically reveals a systolic murmur at the second right intercostal space that radiates to the carotids, along with diminished carotid pulse volume. As the stenosis becomes more severe, the A2 heart sound becomes softer, and the murmur may occasionally become louder [4, 6]. However, based on physical examination findings alone, physical examination findings demonstrated poor sensitivity and specificity in diagnosing significant AS [6]. Coexisting coronary artery disease (CAD) is common, necessitating an ischemic heart disease (IHD) workup with left heart catheterization (LHC) in many patients. Differential diagnoses for a systolic flow murmur include anemia, pregnancy, fever, and hyperdynamic states. Treatment is primarily indicated for severe aortic stenosis.

Pearl

Syncope could be due to low flow to the brain or arrhythmias.

Pearl

The Gallavardin phenomenon occurs when the murmur of aortic stenosis is heard at the apex of the heart due to the transmission of sound waves through the aortic descending wall. This phenomenon can sometimes be misleading, as it may be mistaken for a mitral regurgitation (MR) murmur. However, unlike MR, the Gallavardin phenomenon does not cause the murmur to radiate to the axilla. In aortic stenosis, the murmur intensity is loudest at the right sternal border, not at the apex.

Hospitalist Tip

A useful clinical tip but not diagnostic for differentiating aortic stenosis from non-clinically significant aortic sclerosis involves assessing distal pulses, such as the brachial or radial artery, with a preference for the carotid pulse [4, 6]. In cases of severe aortic stenosis, the pulse is typically faint and difficult to palpate, in contrast to aortic sclerosis, where the pulse is more palpable. Additionally, the murmur is mild in aortic sclerosis, and the A2 heart sound is normal, with echocardiography not showing a significant pressure gradient.

Pearl

Patients with aortic stenosis (AS) have an increased risk of lower gastrointestinal bleeding (LGIB) due to an association with angiodysplasia or arteriovenous malformations (AVM). It is hypothesized that the turbulent flow across the valve in severe AS can damage large multimers of von Willebrand factor, leading to acquired von Willebrand disease (VWD) and an increased risk of mucosal bleeding, known as Heyde syndrome.

- The basic diagnostic workup for aortic stenosis (AS) includes an electrocardiogram (EKG) to check for left ventricular hypertrophy (LVH) criteria, with possible conduction blocks due to the proximity of the atrioventricular (A-V) conduction pathway. A chest X-ray is performed to identify pulmonary edema in cases of acute decompensated heart failure (ADHF). Troponin and B-type natriuretic peptide (BNP) tests rule out acute coronary syndrome (ACS) or ADHF. An echocardiogram (Echo/TTE) determines AS severity based on the pressure gradient and valve area. Additional, less common tests include:
  - (i) Dobutamine stress echocardiography is useful in patients with significantly reduced ejection fraction (advanced heart failure with reduced ejection fraction, HFrEF) to differentiate between true severe AS and pseudo-stenosis, particularly when there is discordance between the calculated aortic valve area and the mean transvalvular gradient. In pseudo-stenosis, dobutamine increases cardiac output and opening forces on the aortic valve, causing the valve area to expand and ruling out severe AS if the area improves to more than 1 cm^2. This prevents unnecessary surgery. Another option is CT aortic valve calcium scoring which can quantify valve calcification and AS severity. An aortic valve calcium score >1300 Agatston units in women and >2000 Agatston units in men correlates with hemodynamically severe stenosis [7].
  - (ii) Exercise stress testing can be performed on asymptomatic patients with AS to determine if surgery is needed if symptoms develop or to assess functional capacity [30]. However, due to significant hemodynamic compromis [4], this test should not be conducted in acutely hospitalized symptomatic patients. The development of symptoms during exercise testing constitutes a Class 1 indication for aortic valve replacement (AVR).
  - (iii) Left heart catheterization (LHC) is used for precise valve area measurement and stroke volume assessment in patients with suspected low-flow, low-gradient AS with preserved left ventricular function. It may also be necessary before surgery to assess for concomitant coronary artery disease (CAD) and potential interventions in severe AS cases. In summary, if noninvasive testing does not provide a definitive diagnosis or if there is discordance between clinical assessment and echocardiographic results, cardiac catheterization should be performed to determine the severity of aortic stenosis.

Pearl

Severe AS is defined as maximum aortic velocity ≥ 4 m/s or mean pressure gradient ≥ 40 mmHg, and valve area typically ≤ 1.0 cm^2. However, the gradient is influenced by stroke volume.

Pearl

Stress testing is generally contraindicated in patients with severe, symptomatic AS. Determining the severity of the AS via an Echo would be indicated before performing stress testing, which could be considered, if possible, with cardiology consult advice.

Pearl

Always evaluate for the aorta in patients with bicuspid aortic valve disease to rule out aortic diseases.

6.2.3 Major DD

- The most typical differential diagnosis for aortic stenosis (AS) is coronary artery disease (CAD) or acute coronary syndrome (ACS). Left heart catheterization (LHC) can reveal abnormalities that help attribute symptoms to CAD rather than AS. An electrocardiogram (EKG) may show ischemic findings, and regional wall motion abnormalities can be detected through echocardiography. It is important to note that both conditions may coexist. Other pathological causes of systolic murmurs include mitral regurgitation (MR), hypertrophic obstructive cardiomyopathy (HOCM), ventricular septal defect (VSD), and pulmonary stenosis. Innocent systolic murmurs can also arise from conditions such as pregnancy, fever, anemia, and thyrotoxicosis.

6.2.4 Treatment Approach [8]

- Medical management of aortic stenosis (AS) should focus on controlling atherosclerotic risk factors. While ACE inhibitors or ARBs may reduce mortality in patients undergoing transcatheter aortic valve replacement (TAVR), they must be used cautiously in patients with low blood pressure. It is important to note that medical treatment alone is insufficient for AS.

Pearl

Notable complications for TAVR include paravalvular regurgitation, heart blocks, AKI, aortic rupture, strokes, and coronary occlusion.

- All symptomatic patients with severe AS, including younger patients with bicuspid AS, should undergo aortic valve replacement (AVR). Surgical AVR (SAVR) is generally recommended for patients younger than 65 years, those undergoing other cardiac surgeries, or those with a life expectancy greater than 20 years. TAVR is preferred for high-risk patients older than 80 years or those with a life expectancy of less than 10 years, but a minimum of 1 year.
- Patients with mechanical AVR devices should be on warfarin anticoagulation therapy. Anticoagulation depends on other risk factors for those with a biological valve, but generally, all patients should be on aspirin.

Hospitalist Tip

In individuals with AS and ADHF, afterload reduction may be useful in stabilizing patients before considering AVR/TAVR. However, being cautious with close hemodynamic monitoring is vital to avoid compromising cardiac output. Vasodilators should be avoided in patients with borderline low blood pressure/soft BP, as they can further compromise cardiac output and lead to hypotension.

Pearl

Aortic valve correction (with SAVR/TAVR) for AS is indicated for patients:

A. Symptomatic severe AS

B. Asymptomatic severe AS who are either:

(i) *Undergoing other cardiac surgeries.* Patients with severe AS may also qualify for upfront PCI in severe CAD stenosis (angiographic stenosis ≥90%) [9]. So, all patients with severe AS will need a cardiology evaluation for the double procedure.

(ii) *Those who have a left ventricular ejection fraction <50%*

(iii) *In unclear conditions (asymptomatic severe AS, but no above indications), it is reasonable to perform stress testing to confirm the presence of symptoms. However, more recent evidence does support TAVR in severe asymptomatic AS* [8].

Hospitalist Tip

When treatment would be futile (in cases of terminal illness, advanced dementia, short life expectancy, multiorgan failure, or extreme frailty/deconditioning), you should consider palliative care/hospice instead of valvular replacement.

6.3 Mitral Regurgitation

6.3.1 When to Suspect and Major Etiology

- Mitral regurgitation (MR) presents similarly to other valvular heart diseases (VHDs) with predominant volume overload, leading to congestive heart failure (CHF), and in acute phases, it may manifest as cardiogenic shock. If untreated, MR can lead to CHF, strokes, and arrhythmias. The causes of MR are classified as either primary (affecting the valve itself) or secondary which is the most common of all causes (due to a dilated left ventricle) and as either acute or chronic. The most common direct cause of chronic primary MR is mitral valve prolapse (MVP), followed by Ischemia and IE.
  1. Primary causes (valve problems) of MR can be acute or chronic. Acute conditions include acute coronary syndrome (ACS) with papillary muscle dysfunction or rupture and infective endocarditis (IE). Chronic causes include MVP, HOCM, post-radiation effects, and rheumatic fever.

2. Secondary causes/functional (ventricular problems) involve left ventricular dilation, which leads to leaflet tethering. Ventricular dysfunction can lead to secondary MR by dilating the mitral annulus and tethered chordae. It is more common than primary pathology. Any cardiomyopathy can lead to this.

Pearl

Dopaminergic drugs such as cabergoline could lead to valve MR.

Pearl

Mitral valve prolapse (MVP) is the most common cause of primary mitral regurgitation (MR) in developed countries. Patients may experience unique symptoms such as panic attacks, atypical chest pain, and occasional palpitations. On physical examination, (MVP) is most commonly characterized by a midsystolic click, produced by abrupt tensing of the mitral leaflet or chordae tendineae as they prolapse into the left atrium, followed by a late systolic murmur audible at the apex. A reduced left ventricular cavity size causes earlier leaflet prolapse, resulting in an earlier click and murmur. For symptomatic patients without heart failure, beta-blockers are the treatment of choice. In cases of advanced MR or heart failure symptoms, surgical repair or replacement of the mitral valve may be necessary.

6.3.2 Clinical Approach

- Mitral regurgitation (MR) presents with symptoms of congestive heart failure (CHF), fatigue with shortness of breath (SOB), and abdominal or chest pain. A physical examination may reveal a systolic murmur at the apex and a heaving apex beat, indicating volume overload. The S1 heart sound might be soft, and a palpable or loud P2 could indicate pulmonary hypertension. Acute MR can lead to acute decompensated heart failure (ADHF) with acute pulmonary edema and possible cardiogenic shock due to the sudden reduced compliance of the left atrium, which struggles to accommodate a significant increase in volume and pressure. In such cases, a murmur may be absent due to the equalization of pressure between the left atrium and ventricle. This condition should be considered when a patient presents with severe acute pulmonary edema and normal left ventricular function on transthoracic echocardiography (TTE).
- The basic workup includes TTE or transesophageal echocardiography (TEE) if TTE is inconclusive or the severity of MR is in question to assess MR severity

and possible underlying causes. An electrocardiogram (EKG) may show arrhythmias and signs of left atrial dilation (LAD) or left ventricular hypertrophy (LVH). At the same time, a chest X-ray may reveal cardiomegaly due to eccentric hypertrophy, similar to aortic regurgitation (AR). A stress test is indicated when MR is asymptomatic or cannot explain the patient's presentation. The same indications go for left heart catheterization and cardiac MRI. B-type natriuretic peptide (BNP) correlates with the severity of symptoms and prognostic information [1].

Hospitalist Tip

In acute mitral regurgitation (MR), the patient often presents with pulmonary edema, cardiogenic shock, and a mild or absent murmur due to the rapid equalization of pressures. In chronic MR, pulmonary edema and elevated right-sided pressures are rare in the early stages. Atrial fibrillation (AF) is common in chronic MR/AR due to a dilated atrium [10].

Pearl

Patients scheduled for elective valve surgery should undergo preoperative cardiac catheterization with coronary angiography to evaluate for the presence and severity of obstructive coronary artery disease (CAD). If significant CAD is identified, the patient may undergo coronary artery bypass grafting (CABG) at the time of valve surgery. This approach is particularly important for patients with prior symptoms of CAD or a high suspicion of its presence. This guideline applies to nearly all cases of elective valve surgery.

6.3.3 Major DD

- All other valvular heart diseases (VHDs) may present with similar symptoms. However, conditions such as aortic regurgitation (AR) and other hyperdynamic states, including severe hyperthyroidism, advanced heart failure, and severe anemia, can also present similarly.

6.3.4 Treatment Approach

- Surgical repair, which is preferred due to its association with lower mortality rates, or replacement is considered for primary mitral regurgitation (MR) if the patient meets the following criteria:
  (i) They are symptomatic, regardless of left ventricular (LV) systolic function.

(ii) They are asymptomatic with an ejection fraction (EF) less than or equal to 60%.
(iii) They are asymptomatic with an LV end-systolic dimension of 40 mm or more.

- For secondary moderate to severe MR, the treatment focuses on the underlying congestive heart failure (CHF) using guideline-directed medical therapy (GDMT) and addressing any underlying ischemia. If these measures are ineffective, referral for transcatheter edge-to-edge repair (TEER) should be considered, as this procedure enhances valve closure mechanics and has been shown in studies to improve mortality [11, 12]. TEER is also indicated in patients with severe, symptomatic, primary mitral regurgitation (MR) who are considered to be at high risk for cardiac surgery, as assessed by a cardiac surgeon. If any type of surgery is prohibited, then Vasodilator therapy is generally indicated in patients with severe MR and hypertension.
- In cases of acute MR, surgical repair is typically needed as soon as possible, necessitating consultation with a cardiothoracic surgeon. Consult immediately with your cardiologist and cardiothoracic surgeon. In the interim, the patient should be managed with afterload reduction or vasodilators (if blood pressure is stable; otherwise, use with inotropes/Dobutamine) and possibly an intra-aortic balloon pump (IABP), which aids in pushing blood forward and improving stroke volume.

Pearl

When the ejection fraction (EF) falls below normal in mitral regurgitation (MR), it signifies the left ventricle's inability to handle the increased stroke volume due to chronic wall tension. This indicates ventricular failure, and surgery should be considered before irreversible damage occurs.

6.4 Mitral Stenosis

6.4.1 When to Suspect and Major Etiology

- Presents predominantly at later ages, usually above 60, with symptoms of low cardiac output, such as generalized weakness and fatigue, along with right-sided heart failure due to backflow pressure. It should be suspected in immigrant patients with a history of rheumatic fever or childhood cardiac conditions. In developed countries, it may be considered in patients with a history of chest radiation, mitral valve pathology, or intervention [13]. Symptoms arise from poor forward flow or high back-pressure flow. Most patients die either due to advanced HF or thromboembolic events with strokes. The most common causes include:

1. Rheumatic fever, which occurs in developing countries or among migrants, is caused by shared M antigen with the endocardium or direct deposition on the valve structure. This triggers an inflammatory response, leading to valve retraction and initial regurgitation. Eventually, this progresses to valve commissure healing with fibrosis and fusion, resulting in mitral stenosis (MS).
2. Mitral annular calcification due to aging results in calcium deposits obstructing the mitral valve orifice.
3. Infiltrative or fibrosis-induced conditions include infective endocarditis (IE), carcinoid syndrome (especially bronchial), systemic lupus erythematosus (SLE), and other rare diseases.

Hospitalist Tip

MS usually presents as CHF, Afib, or systemic emboli, mainly strokes. However, MS is not as common as MR.

Pearl

Mitral valve calcification is common in patients with CKD/ESRD and PVD. This could lead to MS.

Pearl

Valvular heart diseases (VHDs) are predominantly degenerative. The second most common etiology is rheumatic valve disease, particularly in stenotic lesions, followed by infective endocarditis [1].

6.4.2 Clinical Approach

- Mitral stenosis (MS) progresses slowly over decades, primarily manifesting as symptoms of congestive heart failure (CHF), pulmonary hypertension (PHT), and right-sided heart failure. These symptoms can include generalized anasarca, gastrointestinal dyspepsia or discomfort, abdominal pain, congestive hepatopathy, and facial flushing due to vasodilation with hypoxemia and CO_2 retention. In rare instances, hemoptysis or hoarseness may occur due to rupture of bronchial vessels or damage to the recurrent laryngeal nerve around the left main bronchus due to a dilated left atrium.
- Physical examination reveals findings consistent with CHF and PHT. The diastolic murmur is more pronounced when the patient is in the left lateral decubitus position at the apex, though it is usually faint. The S1 heart sound becomes soft in advanced stages, and an opening snap closer to S2 indicates severe disease. Atrial fibrillation (AF) is common, and a diagnosis of severe MS is unlikely in its absence.
- The most crucial diagnostic tool is transthoracic echocardiography (TTE), which assesses the severity of MS [15]. Doppler echocardiography, considered the gold standard, or transesophageal echocardiography (TEE), is the next step to determine severity and confirm the presence of a thrombus. EKG is necessary for diagnosing AF [19]. Per current guidelines, in patients with rheumatic mitral stenosis (MS) who exhibit a discrepancy between resting echocardiographic findings and clinical symptoms, exercise testing with Doppler or invasive hemodynamic assessment is recommended to evaluate symptomatic response, exercise capacity, and changes in the mean mitral gradient. Other tests are similar to those used for valvular heart diseases [1].

Hospitalist Tip

Patients with mitral stenosis (MS) are highly sensitive to intravenous fluids due to elevated atrial pressures, which can lead to pulmonary edema. This is similar to the effects of uncontrolled tachycardia. A clue to this sensitivity may be significant shortness of breath postoperatively with pulmonary edema, even if the patient did not receive excessive fluids preoperatively.

6.4.3 Major DD

- All valvular heart diseases (VHD) can present with similar symptoms. Still, a particular case is atrial myxoma, which can mimic mitral stenosis (MS) due to the tumor blocking the mitral orifice. Echocardiography is diagnostic for identifying the mass.

6.4.4 Treatment Approach [16]

- Mitral valve surgery with mitral balloon commissurotomy or replacement (for significantly stiff, calcified valves, severe MR, or atrial thrombus) is recommended for severe MS (gradient >5 mmHg, valve area <1.5 cm^2). Indications:
  - (i) Symptomatic patient
  - (ii) Asymptomatic with pulmonary artery systolic pressure greater than 50 mm Hg
  - (iii) Going for another heart surgery
- If the patient is unsuitable for surgery or is pending evaluation treatment with diuretics + vasodilators like Imdur, it is reasonable to lower preload and afterload, respectively. B-blockers or rate control agents should be used if Afib is present; ivabradine may be considered if the patient is in sinus rhythm [17, 31].

- Anticoagulation with warfarin with a target INR of 2.0 to 3.0 is necessary for a patient [18]:
  - (i) With AF, irrespective of their "CHA2DS2-VASc score. Target INR of 2.5 to 3.5.
  - (ii) A history of LA thrombus.
  - (iii) Systemic embolization, such as stroke, even if there is no AF.

Pearl

Never use DOAC for MS, as it increases the risk for the composite endpoint of cardiovascular events. Use warfarin instead [19].

Pearl

For pregnant patients, try to maintain sinus rhythm or control the rate with B-blockers. Warfarin/or LMWH is used for AF, and diuretics are used for pulmonary edema.

6.5 Tricuspid Regurgitation

6.5.1 When to Suspect and Major Etiology

- Usually asymptomatic. When it is symptomatic, it is likely due to advanced severe TR. It presents usually as right-sided heart failure, with ascites and liver dysfunction. Most are commonly due to long-standing right ventricular failure with pulmonary hypertension.
- Tricuspid regurgitation was once considered less significant than mitral valve issues but is now acknowledged for its serious impact on patient outcomes. Severe cases have high mortality rates, and even mild regurgitation is linked to an increased risk of long-term mortality [14].
- It is either due to:
  A. Primary valve pathology, most commonly congenital myxomatous degeneration, rheumatic fever, carcinoid syndrome, trauma, tumors, infective endocarditis with IV drug users (suspect when acute and h/o drug use, unexplained leukocytosis, fever), and pacemaker disruption.
  B. Secondary valve pathology (leaflets are normal) is mainly due to pulmonary HTN (the most common cause). Another common secondary cause is atrial arrhythmias, particularly atrial fibrillation, which are prevalent and contribute to tricuspid regurgitation by causing atrial annulus dilatation [20].
  C. Tricuspid regurgitation associated with an implantable electronic device. Around 25–29% of patients with pacemakers experience tricuspid regurgitation, with devices implicated in 7–45% of cases [21].

Pearl

Heart failure with preserved ejection fraction shows high tricuspid regurgitation rates due to annular and atrial dilatation [22].

Pearl

Tricuspid stenosis is almost due to rheumatic etiology and usually accompanies mitral stenosis. In industrialized nations, the most prevalent etiology of tricuspid stenosis is prosthetic valve dysfunction.

Pearl

Valvular heart diseases (VHDs) are predominantly degenerative. The second most common etiology is rheumatic valve disease, particularly in stenotic lesions, followed by infective endocarditis [1].

6.5.2 Clinical Approach

- It is usually discovered incidentally for another reason on TTE. The patients may feel a neck pulsation sensation. Other common symptoms include fatigue, weight loss, and syncope when advanced. In advanced cases, right ventricle failure symptoms may develop. The physical exam is consistent with large neck systolic pulsation/V wave, lower limb edema, ascites, and hepatomegaly in later stages. A typical murmur is pansystolic in the left lower sternal border, worse on inspiration (more preload to the right heart).
- The EKG is consistent with right axis deviation, a large P wave in lead II, and right ventricular hypertrophy criteria. TTE is diagnostic and prognostic at the same time.
- Cardiac MRI is the reference standard for evaluating right ventricular size and volumes, and it can identify patients at high risk. Cardiac MRI is useful when echocardiographic results are inconclusive or do not align with clinical findings [23].

6.5.3 Major DD

- Significant pulmonary HTN due to other causes and left ventricular failure

6.5.4 Treatment Approach [1]

- Treat the underlying cause. GDMT for tricuspid regurgitation is primarily limited to diuretics and addressing underlying causes. Managing secondary tricuspid regurgitation involves assessing pulmonary hypertension severity, left ventricular function, and rhythm control for atrial fibrillation. If the cardiac device is thought to be the cause, timely lead removal can prevent severe right ventricular issues, though it may worsen regurgitation in some cases [24].
- Guidelines recommend surgical treatment for severe cases during left heart surgery, but management of secondary tricuspid regurgitation is complex due to

late diagnosis and diverse patient profiles. Isolated tricuspid valve surgery is advised for symptomatic, severe cases without pulmonary hypertension or left heart disease when medical treatment fails. In summary, if the patient is symptomatic, is not responsive to diuretics, and has severe TR during left heart surgery, consult your cardiac team/surgeon for possible intervention [1].

Pearl

Surgery for TR is indicated in:

(i) Severe cases during left heart surgery

(ii) Severe symptomatic TR, not responding to diuretics

6.6 Prosthetic Valves [25]

6.6.1 What Valves Do You Expect in Your Patients

- Two types of heart valves are used in valve replacement surgeries: mechanical and bioprosthetic valves. Younger patients, typically under 50–65 years old, are often given mechanical valves due to their durability and longevity despite the higher thrombotic risk, as these patients generally do not have major contraindications to taking warfarin. Conversely, older patients, usually over 65 years old, are more suitable candidates for bioprosthetic valves because these valves have a shorter lifespan of 10–20 years, and there are concerns about polypharmacy and potential drug interactions with warfarin in the elderly population or expected future pregnancy.
  1. Rheumatic fever, which occurs in developing countries or among migrants, is caused by shared M antigen with the endocardium or direct deposition on the valve structure. This triggers an inflammatory response, leading to valve retraction and initial regurgitation. Eventually, this progresses to valve commissure healing with fibrosis and fusion, resulting in mitral stenosis (MS).
  2. Mitral annular calcification due to aging results in calcium deposits obstructing the mitral valve orifice.
  3. Infiltrative or fibrosis-induced conditions include infective endocarditis (IE), carcinoid syndrome (especially bronchial), systemic lupus erythematosus (SLE), and other rare diseases.

Pearl

Valve replacement or TAVR is not indicated in patients with a life expectancy of less than 1 year.

6.6.2 Clinically Approaching Patients with Prosthetic Valves

- Occasionally, you will encounter patients with prosthetic heart valves presenting with cardiac-related issues. Workups and investigations should focus on detecting prosthetic valve dysfunction, systemic clots, or cardiac complaints. Clues suggesting prosthetic valve dysfunction include a new regurgitation murmur on examination, new acute decompensated heart failure (ADHF), evidence of hemolysis (such as lab findings of new jaundice), and unexplained thromboembolic phenomena. All patients with suspected valve dysfunction should undergo at least a transthoracic echocardiogram (TTE) to assess the prosthetic valve [25]. A basic hemolytic workup is reasonable and includes a complete blood count (CBC), reticulocyte index, lactate dehydrogenase (LDH), haptoglobin, unconjugated bilirubin levels, and urine bilirubin as part of urinalysis. The workup for ADHF, clots, or strokes should follow standard approaches based on the clinical setting.
- All patients with prosthetic valves should receive prophylactic antibiotic therapy before dental procedures to minimize the risk of endocarditis.

6.6.3 Managing Patients with Prosthetic Valves

A. **Mechanical heart valves (MHV)**
   - Mechanical heart valves carry a high risk of thrombosis. Consequently, all patients with mechanical valves require lifelong anticoagulation with warfarin. Direct oral anticoagulants (DOACs) should never be used for mechanical valves. The international normalized ratio (INR) goal is 3. A specific INR target is preferable, as it minimizes the risk of values consistently approaching the upper or lower limits of the therapeutic range. Still, it is crucial to verify the specific INR target for each patient from previous records or by consulting the patient's cardiologist, as it may vary. The IMPROVE Bleeding Risk Score is useful for assessing bleeding risk in inpatient settings. Unless there are other indications for low-dose aspirin, it should not be added routinely.

- If a patient with a mechanical heart valve has additional high-risk factors for thromboembolism, a higher INR target is typically recommended [26]. High-risk thrombotic factors include atrial fibrillation (AF), a history of transient ischemic attacks (TIA) or strokes, previous valve thrombosis, rheumatic valve disease, congestive heart failure (CHF), hypertension (HTN), diabetes mellitus (DM), and age over 75. Patients are usually considered high risk when multiple factors are present.

Hospitalist Tip

If anticoagulation must be stopped for a procedure, all patients with mechanical heart valves generally require bridging, except those with bileaflet aortic valve replacements who have low thrombotic risk factors. However, patients with bileaflet aortic valve replacements and multiple high thrombotic risk factors might benefit from bridging, though this decision is not always clear-cut. Consulting a cardiologist in ambiguous situations is crucial. More details are in ► Chap. 10.

Pearl

Therapeutic warfarin is key when managing pregnant patients with MHV. UFH is the preferred regimen near delivery. Always consult your patient, cardiologist, and obstetrician before adjusting any medications.

B. **Bioprosthetic valves**
- Aspirin 75–100 mg daily is indicated in all patients with bioprosthetic valves. Some patients may need short-term (3–6 months) anticoagulation after placing the valve [27].
- One of two options is available for patients with TAVR and low bleeding risk for the first 3–6 months [1].
  (a) VKA with a target INR of 2.5
  (b) Clopidogrel 75 mg added to aspirin (75–100 mg)

Pearl

Aspirin does decrease the risk of stroke and death in patients with prosthetic valves [28].

6.6.4 Common Complications of Prosthetic Valves

(i) Bioprosthesis calcification with stenosis
(ii) Perivalvular leak and regurgitation
(iii) Valve thrombosis acutely or pannus formation chronically
(iv) Infective endocarditis (IE)
(v) Hemolysis

- Most of the complications mentioned above can lead to heart failure symptoms and systemic clots. A valve regurgitation murmur may be detected on examination, indicating valve failure to close, along with possible jaundice and anemia findings suggestive of hemolysis. Diagnosis is usually confirmed with a doppler transthoracic echocardiogram (TTE), which may reveal an increased gradient, abnormal motion, thrombus, or severe valve regurgitation. However, mild regurgitation on TTE is mostly physiological. Transesophageal echocardiography (TEE) or cardiac computed tomography (CCT) may be needed for complex valve issues or concerns for IE. If hemolysis is suspected, a hemolytic workup should be conducted. Based on the underlying complication, consultation with a cardiac specialist is essential to explore options such as repeat surgery, thrombolytics (unstable), or anticoagulation (stable) with warfarin for valve thrombosis. The duration of anticoagulation usually depends on the specific thrombus but is generally around 30 days [29]. Pannus formation may require surgical intervention.

Hospitalist Tip

Acute valve thrombosis is likely if the patient has recently stopped anticoagulation, has acute cardiological symptoms, and has a short interval between implantation and presentation. The lack of crisp mechanical valve sounds is suspicious for valve thrombosis in acute settings.

Pearl

Any patient with a prosthetic valve that presents with new ADHF will need evaluation of prosthetic valve complications.

References

1. Otto CM, Nishimura RA, Bonow RO, Carabello BA, Erwin JP 3rd, Gentile F, Jneid H, Krieger EV, Mack M, McLeod C, O'Gara PT, Rigolin VH, Sundt TM 3rd, Thompson A, Toly C. 2020 ACC/AHA guideline for the management of patients with valvular heart disease: executive summary: a report of the American College of Cardiology/American Heart Association Joint Committee on Clinical Practice Guidelines. Circulation. 2021;143(5):e35–71. https://doi.org/10.1161/CIR.0000000000000932. Epub 2020 Dec 17. Erratum in: Circulation. 2021 Feb 2;143(5):e228. Erratum in: Circulation. 2021 Mar 9;143(10):e784. PMID: 33332149
2. Babu AN, Kymes SM, Carpenter Fryer SM. Eponyms and the diagnosis of aortic regurgitation: what says the evidence? Ann Intern Med. 2003;138(9):736–42. https://doi.org/10.7326/0003--4819-138-9-200305060-00010. PMID: 12729428.
3. Nazarzadeh M, Pinho-Gomes AC, Smith Byrne K, Canoy D, Raimondi F, Ayala Solares JR, Otto CM, Rahimi K. Systolic blood pressure and risk of valvular heart disease: a Mendelian Randomization Study. JAMA Cardiol. 2019;4(8):788–95. https://doi.org/10.1001/jamacardio.2019.2202. PMID: 31290937; PMCID: PMC6624812
4. Hoagland PM, Cook EF, Wynne J, Goldman L. Value of noninvasive testing in adults with suspected aortic stenosis. Am J Med. 1986;80(6):1041–50. https://doi.org/10.1016/0002--9343(86)90663-7. PMID: 3728503
5. Santangelo G, Bursi F, Faggiano A, Moscardelli S, Simeoli PS, Guazzi M, Lorusso R, Carugo S, Faggiano P. The global burden of valvular heart disease: from clinical epidemiology to management. J Clin Med. 2023;12(6):2178. https://doi.org/10.3390/jcm12062178. PMID: 36983180; PMCID: PMC10054046
6. Forssell G, Jonasson R, Orinius E. Identifying severe aortic valvular stenosis by bedside examination. Acta Med Scand. 1985;218(4):397–400. https://doi.org/10.1111/j.0954-6820.1985.tb08864.x. PMID: 4083081
7. Pawade T, Sheth T, Guzzetti E, Dweck MR, Clavel MA. Why and how to measure aortic valve calcification in patients with aortic stenosis. JACC Cardiovasc Imaging. 2019;12(9):1835–48. https://doi.org/10.1016/j.jcmg.2019.01.045. PMID: 31488252
8. Généreux P, Schwartz A, Oldemeyer JB, Pibarot P, Cohen DJ, Blanke P, Lindman BR, Babaliaros V, Fearon WF, Daniels DV, Chhatriwalla AK, Kavinsky C, Gada H, Shah P, Szerlip M, Dahle T, Goel K, O'Neill W, Sheth T, Davidson CJ, Makkar RR, Prince H, Zhao Y, Hahn RT, Leipsic J, Redfors B, Pocock SJ, Mack M, Leon MB. EARLY TAVR Trial Investigators. Transcatheter aortic-valve replacement for asymptomatic severe aortic stenosis. N Engl J Med. 2025;392(3):217–27. https://doi.org/10.1056/NEJMoa2405880. Epub 2024 Oct 28. PMID: 39466903
9. Stone GW, Kappetein AP, Sabik JF, Pocock SJ, Morice MC, Puskas J, Kandzari DE, Karmpaliotis D, Brown WM 3rd, Lembo NJ, Banning A, Merkely B, Horkay F, Boonstra PW, van Boven AJ, Ungi I, Bogáts G, Mansour S, Noiseux N, Sabaté M, Pomar J, Hickey M,

Gershlick A, Buszman PE, Bochenek A, Schampaert E, Pagé P, Modolo R, Gregson J, Simonton CA, Mehran R, Kosmidou I, Généreux P, Crowley A, Dressler O, Serruys PW. EXCEL Trial Investigators. Five-year outcomes after PCI or CABG for left main coronary disease. N Engl J Med. 2019;381(19):1820–30. https://doi.org/10.1056/NEJMoa1909406. Epub 2019 Sep 28. Erratum in: N Engl J Med. 2020 Mar 12;382(11):1078. doi: 10.1056/NEJMx200004. PMID: 31562798

10. DePace NL, Nestico PF, Morganroth J. Acute severe mitral regurgitation. Pathophysiology, clinical recognition, and management. Am J Med. 1985;78(2):293–306. https://doi.org/10.1016/0002-9343(85)90440-1. PMID: 3881945
11. Anker SD, Friede T, von Bardeleben RS, Butler J, Khan MS, Diek M, Heinrich J, Geyer M, Placzek M, Ferrari R, Abraham WT, Alfieri O, Auricchio A, Bayes-Genis A, Cleland JGF, Filippatos G, Gustafsson F, Haverkamp W, Kelm M, Kuck KH, Landmesser U, Maggioni AP, Metra M, Ninios V, Petrie MC, Rassaf T, Ruschitzka F, Schäfer U, Schulze PC, Spargias K, Vahanian A, Zamorano JL, Zeiher A, Karakas M, Koehler F, Lainscak M, Öner A, Mezilis N, Theofilogiannakos EK, Ninios I, Chrissoheris M, Kourkoveli P, Papadopoulos K, Smolka G, Wojakowski W, Reczuch K, Pinto FJ, Wiewiórka Ł, Kalarus Z, Adamo M, Santiago-Vacas E, Ruf TF, Gross M, Tongers J, Hasenfuss G, Schillinger W, Ponikowski P. RE-SHAPE-HF2 Investigators. Transcatheter valve repair in heart failure with moderate to severe mitral regurgitation. N Engl J Med. 2024;391(19):1799–809. https://doi.org/10.1056/NEJMoa2314328. Epub 2024 Aug 31. PMID: 39216092
12. Baldus S, Doenst T, Pfister R, Gummert J, Kessler M, Boekstegers P, Lubos E, Schröder J, Thiele H, Walther T, Kelm M, Hausleiter J, Eitel I, Fischer-Rasokat U, Bufe A, Schmeisser A, Ince H, Lurz P, von Bardeleben RS, Hagl C, Noack T, Reith S, Beucher H, Reichenspurner H, Rottbauer W, Schulze PC, Müller W, Frank J, Hellmich M, Wahlers T, Rudolph V. MATTERHORN Investigators. Transcatheter repair versus mitral-valve surgery for secondary mitral regurgitation. N Engl J Med. 2024;391(19):1787–98. https://doi.org/10.1056/NEJMoa2408739. Epub 2024 Aug 31. PMID: 39216093
13. Maganti K, Rigolin VH, Sarano ME, Bonow RO. Valvular heart disease: diagnosis and management. Mayo Clin Proc. 2010;85(5):483–500. https://doi.org/10.4065/mcp.2009.0706. PMID: 20435842; PMCID: PMC2861980
14. Hahn RT. Tricuspid regurgitation. N Engl J Med. 2023;388(20):1876–91. https://doi.org/10.1056/NEJMra2216709. PMID: 37195943
15. Pearlman AS, Scoblionko DP, Saal AK. Assessment of valvular heart disease by Doppler echocardiography. Clin Cardiol. 1983;6(12):573–87. https://doi.org/10.1002/clc.4960061202. PMID: 6362941
16. Iung B, Baron G, Butchart EG, Delahaye F, Gohlke-Bärwolf C, Levang OW, Tornos P, Vanoverschelde JL, Vermeer F, Boersma E, Ravaud P, Vahanian A. A prospective survey of patients with valvular heart disease in Europe: The Euro Heart Survey on Valvular Heart Disease. Eur Heart J. 2003;24(13):1231–43. https://doi.org/10.1016/s0195-668x(03)00201-x. PMID: 12831818
17. Patel S, Singh R, Preuss CV, et al. Warfarin. [Updated 2024 Oct 5]. In: StatPearls [Internet]. Treasure Island (FL): StatPearls Publishing; 2025. Available from: https://www.ncbi.nlm.nih.gov/books/NBK470313/.
18. Carnicelli AP, Hong H, Connolly SJ, Eikelboom J, Giugliano RP, Morrow DA, Patel MR, Wallentin L, Alexander JH, Cecilia Bahit M, Benz AP, Bohula EA, Chao TF, Dyal L, Ezekowitz MAA, Fox K, Gencer B, Halperin JL, Hijazi Z, Hohnloser SH, Hua K, Hylek E, Toda Kato E, Kuder J, Lopes RD, Mahaffey KW, Oldgren J, Piccini JP, Ruff CT, Steffel J, Wojdyla D, Granger CB. COMBINE AF (A Collaboration Between Multiple Institutions to Better Investigate Non-Vitamin K Antagonist Oral Anticoagulant Use in Atrial Fibrillation) Investigators. Direct oral anticoagulants versus Warfarin in patients with atrial fibrillation: patient-level network meta-analyses of Randomized Clinical Trials with interaction testing by age and sex. Circulation.

2022;145(4):242–55. https://doi.org/10.1161/CIRCULATIONAHA.121.056355. Epub 2022 Jan 5. Erratum in: Circulation. 2022 Feb 22;145(8):e640. doi: 10.1161/CIR.0000000000001058. PMID: 34985309; PMCID: PMC8800560

19. Omran AS, Arifi AA, Mohamed AA. Echocardiography in mitral stenosis. J Saudi Heart Assoc. 2011;23(1):51–8. https://doi.org/10.1016/j.jsha.2010.07.007. Epub 2010 Sep 7. PMID: 23960637; PMCID: PMC3727554
20. Itakura K, Hidaka T, Nakano Y, Utsunomiya H, Kinoshita M, Susawa H, Harada Y, Izumi K, Kihara Y. Successful catheter ablation of persistent atrial fibrillation is associated with improvement in functional tricuspid regurgitation and right heart reverse remodeling. Heart Vessels. 2020;35(6):842–51. https://doi.org/10.1007/s00380-019-01546-3. Epub 2020 Jan 2. PMID: 31897639
21. Addetia K, Harb SC, Hahn RT, Kapadia S, Lang RM. Cardiac implantable electronic device lead-induced tricuspid regurgitation. JACC Cardiovasc Imaging. 2019;12(4):622–36. https://doi.org/10.1016/j.jcmg.2018.09.028. PMID: 30947905
22. Harada T, Obokata M, Omote K, Iwano H, Ikoma T, Okada K, Yoshida K, Kato T, Kurosawa K, Nagai T, Anzai T, Borlaug BA, Kurabayashi M. Functional tricuspid regurgitation and right atrial remodeling in heart failure with preserved ejection fraction. Am J Cardiol. 2022;162:129–35. https://doi.org/10.1016/j.amjcard.2021.09.021. Epub 2021 Oct 24. PMID: 34702555
23. Zhan Y, Debs D, Khan MA, Nguyen DT, Graviss EA, Khalaf S, Little SH, Reardon MJ, Nagueh S, Quiñones MA, Kleiman N, Zoghbi WA, Shah DJ. Natural history of functional tricuspid regurgitation quantified by cardiovascular magnetic resonance. J Am Coll Cardiol. 2020;76(11):1291–301. https://doi.org/10.1016/j.jacc.2020.07.036. PMID: 32912443
24. Polewczyk A, Jacheć W, Nowosielecka D, Tomaszewski A, Brzozowski W, Szczęśniak-Stańczyk D, Duda K, Kutarski A. Tricuspid valve damage related to transvenous lead extraction. Int J Environ Res Public Health. 2022;19(19):12279. https://doi.org/10.3390/ijerph191912279. PMID: 36231579; PMCID: PMC9566121
25. Zoghbi WA, Jone PN, Chamsi-Pasha MA, Chen T, Collins KA, Desai MY, Grayburn P, Groves DW, Hahn RT, Little SH, Kruse E, Sanborn D, Shah SB, Sugeng L, Swaminathan M, Thaden J, Thavendiranathan P, Tsang W, Weir-McCall JR, Gill E. Guidelines for the Evaluation of prosthetic valve function with cardiovascular imaging: a report from the American Society of Echocardiography Developed in Collaboration With the Society for Cardiovascular Magnetic Resonance and the Society of Cardiovascular Computed Tomography. J Am Soc Echocardiogr. 2024;37(1):2–63. https://doi.org/10.1016/j.echo.2023.10.004.
26. Mohamed H. Antithrombotic therapy in patients with prosthetic heart valves. Libyan J Med. 2009;4(1):54–6. https://doi.org/10.4176/090115. PMID: 21483507; PMCID: PMC3066703
27. Papak JN, Chiovaro JC, Noelck N, Healy LD, Freeman M, Quin JA, Paynter R, Low A, Kondo K, McCarty OJT, Kansagara D. Antithrombotic strategies after bioprosthetic aortic valve replacement: a systematic review. Ann Thorac Surg. 2019;107(5):1571–81. https://doi.org/10.1016/j.athoracsur.2018.10.016. Epub 2018 Nov 17. PMID: 30458159; PMCID: PMC6743973
28. Leiria TL, Lopes RD, Williams JB, Katz JN, Kalil RA, Alexander JH. Anti-thrombotic therapies in patients with prosthetic heart valves: guidelines translated for the clinician. J Thromb Thrombolysis. 2011;31(4):514–22. https://doi.org/10.1007/s11239-011-0574-9. PMID: 21327503; PMCID: PMC3699194
29. Otto CM, Nishimura RA, Bonow RO, Carabello BA, Erwin JP 3rd, Gentile F, Jneid H, Krieger EV, Mack M, McLeod C, O'Gara PT, Rigolin VH, Sundt TM 3rd, Thompson A, Toly C. 2020 ACC/AHA guideline for the management of patients with valvular heart disease: executive summary: a report of the American College of Cardiology/American Heart Association Joint Committee on Clinical Practice Guidelines. J Am Coll Cardiol. 2021;77(4):450–500. https://doi.org/10.1016/j.jacc.2020.11.035. Epub 2020 Dec 17. Erratum in: J Am Coll Cardiol. 2021 Mar 9;77(9):1276. doi: 10.1016/j.jacc.2021.02.008. PMID: 33342587

30. Das P, Rimington H, Chambers J. Exercise testing to stratify risk in aortic stenosis. Eur Heart J. 2005;26(13):1309–13. https://doi.org/10.1093/eurheartj/ehi250. Epub 2005 Apr 8. PMID: 15820999
31. Agrawal V, Kumar N, Lohiya B, Sihag BK, Prajapati R, Singh TB, Subramanian G. Metoprolol vs ivabradine in patients with mitral stenosis in sinus rhythm. Int J Cardiol. 2016;221:562–6. https://doi.org/10.1016/j.ijcard.2016.07.022. Epub 2016 Jul 9. PMID: 27420578

Selected Cardiac Infection

Contents

M. Salih, *Practical Hospitalist Guide to Inpatient Cardiology*, https://doi.org/10.1007/978-3-032-03240-9_7

This chapter focuses on the recognition, diagnosis, and *management of cardiac implantable electronic device (CIED) infections and infective endocarditis, as well as* conditions associated with significant morbidity and mortality, particularly in hospitalized patients. It outlines the clinical presentations ranging from localized pocket infections to systemic bacteremia and device-related endocarditis, emphasizing the importance of high clinical suspicion in patients with fever, positive blood cultures, and CIEDs. This chapter guides hospitalists through diagnostic pathways, including the use of *transesophageal echocardiography (TEE), blood culture timing*, and key laboratory findings. It distinguishes between *simple device-site infections and invasive CIED endocarditis*, which necessitates complete device removal and prolonged antibiotic therapy. For *infective endocarditis*, the modified Duke criteria are reviewed alongside common causative organisms (e.g., *Staphylococcus aureus*, streptococci, and enterococci), and the implications of prosthetic valves or prior endocarditis. Management principles cover empiric and pathogen-directed antibiotic selection, surgical indications, and coordination with infectious disease and cardiology teams. Special considerations are given to patients with *prosthetic valves*, *immunosuppression*, or recent healthcare exposures. This chapter equips hospitalists with the tools to initiate timely diagnosis, reduce complications, and facilitate multidisciplinary care in these high-risk cardiac infections.

7.1 Infective Endocarditis

7.1.1 When to Suspect and Major Etiology [1]

- When a patient presents with an unexplained fever, positive blood cultures indicative of typical pathogens, septic emboli, new-onset valvular regurgitation, and underlying risk factors, further evaluation for infectious endocarditis should be considered.

Pearl

The major risk factors for infective endocarditis (IE) include intravenous drug use (IVDU), diabetes mellitus (DM), immunosuppression, indwelling intravenous catheters, congenital heart disease, cardiac transplantation with valvulopathy, and the presence of an implanted cardiac device.

7.1.2 Clinical Approach [1]

- The hospitalist should maintain a high index of suspicion for infective endocarditis (IE), as its symptoms are often nonspecific and subtle. While fever is the most common symptom, it is not always present, and not all patients appear acutely ill. Cardiac symptoms may or may not be evident. In subacute or chronic cases, often caused by less virulent organisms, patients may present with weight loss, fatigue, and generalized malaise. In elderly patients, confusion may be the only presenting symptom.
- Characteristic physical examination findings to assess include splinter hemorrhages, conjunctival hemorrhages, Osler nodes, Janeway lesions, and Roth spots. However, due to the widespread early use of antibiotics, these findings are now infrequent and should not be solely relied upon for diagnosis.
- Diagnosis is often established using Duke's criteria. A definitive diagnosis requires either two major criteria (one major and three minor criteria) or five minor criteria.

7.1.3 Modified Duke Criteria [1]

Major criteria
Blood culture positive for IE Typical microorganisms consistent with IE from 2 separate blood cultures*: Viridans streptococci, *Streptococcus bovis*, HACEK group (*Haemophilus* spp., *Actinobacillus actinomycetemcomitans*, *Cardiobacterium hominis*, *Eikenella* spp., and *Kingella kingae*), *S. aureus*; or community-acquired enterococci, in the absence of a primary focus; or Microorganisms consistent with IE from persistently positive blood Culture results, defined as follows: At least 2 positive culture results of blood samples drawn 12 h apart; or All of 3 or most of ≥4 separate culture samples of blood (with first and last samples drawn at least 1 h apart) Single positive blood culture result for *Coxiella burnetii* or antiphase I IgG antibody titer >1:800
Evidence of endocardial involvement Echocardiogram positive for IE defined as follows: Oscillating intracardiac mass on valve or supporting structures, in the path or regurgitant jets, or on implanted material in the absence of an alternative anatomic explanation Abscess; or New partial dehiscence of prosthetic valve New valvular regurgitation (worsening or changing of preexisting Murmur not sufficient)
Minor criteria
Predisposition: predisposing heart condition, or injection drug use
Fever: temperature >38° (100.4 °F)

Vascular phenomena: major arterial emboli, septic pulmonary infarcts, mycotic aneurysm, intracanial hemorrhage, conjunctival hemorrhages, and Janeway lesions
Immunological phenomena: glomerulonephritis, Osler's nodes, Roth's spots, and rheumatoid factor
Microbiological evidence: positive blood culture but does not meet a major criterion as noted above* or serological evidence of active infection with organism consistent with IE

Pearl

Streptococcus bovis IE is linked to gastrointestinal diseases and cancer [2]. Do Colonoscopy when able.

7.1.4 IE Diagnosis [1]

Definite IE
Pathological criteria
Microorganisms demonstrated by culture or histological examination of vegetation, a vegetation that has embolized, or an intracardiac abscess specimen; or
Pathologic lesions: vegetation or intracardiac abscess confirmed by histological examination showing active endocarditis
Clinical criteria
2 major criteria; or
1 major criterion and 3 minor criteria; or
5 minor criteria
Possible IE
1 major criterion and 1 minor criterion; or
3 minor criteria
Rejected
Firm alternative diagnosis explaining evidence of IE; or
Resolution of IR syndrome with antibiotic therapy for <4 days; or
No pathological evidence of IE at surgery or autopsy, with antibiotic therapy for <4 days; or
Does not meet criteria for possible IE as listed above

7.1.5 Workup Inclusion

(i) *Blood cultures* are essential for all patients with suspected infective endocarditis (IE), with a sensitivity of approximately 90%. They should be obtained as soon as possible before initiating antibiotic therapy, as antibiotic administration significantly reduces their sensitivity. The standard practice involves collecting two to three blood cultures from different sites, spaced approximately 1 h apart, to maximize diagnostic yield.

Pearl

In patients with early prosthetic valve endocarditis (PVE), occurring within 60 days of surgery, *Staphylococcus aureus* and gram-negative bacteria are the most commonly identified pathogens. For intermediate PVE (60 days and 1 year post-surgery), *coagulase-negative staphylococci* (e.g., *Staphylococcus epidermidis*) are frequently detected. While these organisms are normal skin commensals and often considered contaminants in asymptomatic patients, persistent bacteremia or multiple positive blood culture sets in a patient with prosthetic material should raise strong suspicion for true infection rather than contamination. Late PVE (occurring more than 1 year after surgery) typically mirrors the microbiological profile of native valve endocarditis, as outlined in the table above.

Hospitalist Tip

Additional biochemical abnormalities commonly observed in hospitalized patients with infective endocarditis (IE) include acute kidney injury (AKI), elevated liver function tests (LFTs), and increased inflammatory markers such as C-reactive protein (CRP), erythrocyte sedimentation rate (ESR), and procalcitonin. Polyclonal hypergammaglobulinemia, reduced complement levels (C3/C4), proteinuria, and red blood cell casts suggestive of glomerulonephritis may also be noted. Furthermore, a positive rheumatoid factor test is frequently seen. While none of these findings are specific to IE, their presence can support the clinical suspicion of the disease.

(ii) *TTE* [4]. Transthoracic echocardiography (TTE) is a prerequisite for all suspected infective endocarditis (IE) patients. However, if TTE results are negative but clinical suspicion remains high, transesophageal echocardiography (TEE) should be performed for further evaluation. TEE is particularly indicated in the following scenarios:

1. *Non-diagnostic* TTE with persistent clinical suspicion of IE.
2. *Suspected complications*, such as abscess formation, perforation, or valve dehiscence.

3. *Presence of prosthetic heart material* in a patient with persistent, unexplained fever.
4. *Bacteremia is caused by highly virulent organisms*, including *Staphylococcus aureus*, *Enterococcus*, or fungal pathogens.

Hospitalist Tip

Normal TTE does not exclude IE

Hospitalist Tip

Given the high risk associated with this pathogen [3], all patients with *Staphylococcus aureus* bacteremia should be thoroughly evaluated for infective endocarditis (IE). This is particularly crucial in patients with underlying risk factors such as diabetes mellitus, end-stage renal disease (ESRD) requiring hemodialysis, or persistent bacteremia despite appropriate antibiotic therapy.

(iii) *Cardiac CT/FDG PET/CT* is typically indicated when there is suspicion of valvular complications, particularly abscess formation, or in cases of possible prosthetic valve infection. These modalities are especially useful when transthoracic echocardiography (TTE) or transesophageal echocardiography (TEE) is nondiagnostic or not feasible.

Hospitalist Tip

The presence of multiple septic lung emboli or small abscesses is strongly suggestive of right-sided infective endocarditis (IE), which is commonly seen in intravenous drug users. In such cases, a urine drug screen should be performed to help identify potential substance abuse. If transthoracic echocardiography (TTE) results are negative but clinical suspicion for IE remains high, transesophageal echocardiography (TEE) should be performed for further evaluation. Other differential diagnoses for right-sided valve masses or lesions include metastatic carcinoid tumors, which can present with symptoms such as flushing and bronchospasm, and myxomas, which typically affect the left side of the heart, especially the left atrium.

7.1.6 Treatment Approach [1]

- All patients should begin intravenous (IV) antibiotic therapy immediately, preferably after obtaining blood cultures. Consultation with infectious disease (ID) specialists is recommended to determine the most appropriate antibiotic regimen and treatment duration, typically 4–6 weeks of IV antibiotics, starting from the first day of negative blood cultures. For community-acquired native valve endocarditis with a low risk of resistant organisms, initial treatment should consist of vancomycin and ceftriaxone. In cases of early prosthetic valve endocarditis (within 1 year of surgery) or healthcare-associated endocarditis, a regimen of vancomycin and cefepime is recommended, with the addition of gentamicin or rifampin as per ID recommendations. Blood cultures should be repeated every 1–4 days to monitor for clearance. Antibiotic therapy should be adjusted based on the results of these cultures.
- Early surgery is indicated for the following reasons after consulting your cardiothoracic surgeon. It is preferred to operate during initial hospitalization before completion of the antibiotics course [4]:
    1. Symptomatic heart failure due to severe valvular dysfunction (commonly missed).
    2. High-risk resistant organisms (like fungal infections, *Staphylococcus aureus*, ESBL, KPC, VRE) with persistent bacteremia (usually more than 5 days) despite IV antibiotics.
    3. Destructive valvular lesions such as abscesses, fistulating disease, and lesions near the AV node lead to heart blocks.
    4. Recurrent septic emboli/septic stroke not responding to IV antibiotics.
    5. More than 1 cm of left-sided vegetation (high risk of embolization).
    6. Cardiac device infection is cured by removing the entire system.

Pearl

Occasionally, despite successful antimicrobial therapy, some sterile vegetations may persist indefinitely. It is also important to note that not all vegetations indicate infective endocarditis (IE). Differential diagnoses should include benign masses, Libman-Sacks endocarditis, tumors, and Marantic vegetations, which are malignant masses associated with other cancers.

Pearl

Prosthetic valve endocarditis (PVE) follows the same surgical indications for native valves stated above.

Hospitalist Tip

Patients with known VHD should not receive antibiotics before blood cultures are obtained for unexplained fever [1].

Pearl

Anticoagulation should be temporarily withheld in patients with atrial fibrillation (AF), pulmonary embolism (PE), and acute infective endocarditis who also present with an embolic stroke, regardless of other indications for anticoagulation. Additionally, aspirin and other antiplatelet agents are not indicated in cases of infected embolic stroke [4].

7.1.7 Major Complication

I. CHF. The condition is typically due to significant valve dysfunction, primarily aortic regurgitation (AR). Without surgical intervention, the mortality rate is high [4]. This situation represents a class I indication for surgical intervention; therefore, it is essential to involve a cardiothoracic surgeon promptly for a comprehensive risk assessment.

II. Perivalvular abscess. This condition is typically associated with staphylococcal infections and should be suspected when fever and elevated inflammatory markers fail to resolve with medical management. Surgical intervention is generally indicated in these cases.

III. AKI. This condition is not uncommon and may result from immune-mediated glomerulonephritis (GN), sepsis with prerenal failure, embolic infarction, or medication-induced interstitial nephritis. If symptoms do not resolve with supportive care, it is advisable to consult a nephrologist for further evaluation and management.

IV. Embolic events. The incidence is lower if antibiotics are initiated early. The most commonly affected organs include the brain (the most frequent site), kidneys, lungs (particularly in intravenous drug users), bones, and spleen. This condition can lead to the formation of a mycotic aneurysm in the brain, which is often fatal if it ruptures.

7.1.8 Prophylaxis [1]

- Antibiotic prophylaxis is only indicated for patients undergoing selected procedures with specific underlying predisposing risk factors. Always ask these two questions to determine which patients and procedures require prophylaxis.

Selected procedures	*Specific underlying predisposing risk factors (Mostly any prosthetic material in the heart)*

- Manipulation of the gingival tissue, the periapical region of the teeth, or the oral mucosa's perforation
  – Placement or adjustment of orthodontic appliances and bleeding from trauma to oral mucosa is not considered
- Incision into active skin or soft tissue infection
- Incision or biopsy in the respiratory tract
  – Prevention is unnecessary if there is no biopsy or incision diagnostic scope
	- Prosthetic material used for cardiac valve repair
	- LVAD
	- Unrepaired congenital heart disease
	- Repaired congenital heart disease with residual defects
	- A defect that has been repaired with prosthetic material within the previous 6 months
	- Surgical or transcatheter pulmonary artery valve
	- History of endocarditis
	- Cardiac transplantation with residual valve regurgitation
	- Prosthetic valve

- If indicated, antibiotics should be given 30–60 min before the procedure. Preferably, oral amoxicillin 2 g or IM/IV ampicillin, cefazolin, or ceftriaxone should be used. If allergic, azithromycin 500 mg or doxycycline 100 mg should be used.

7.2 CIED Infections

7.2.1 When to Suspect and Major Etiology [5]

- In patients presenting with unexplained bacteremia or localized inflammation alongside a cardiac device, one should consider the possibility of a cardiac implantable electronic device (CIED) infection.

Fig. 7.1 CIED infections

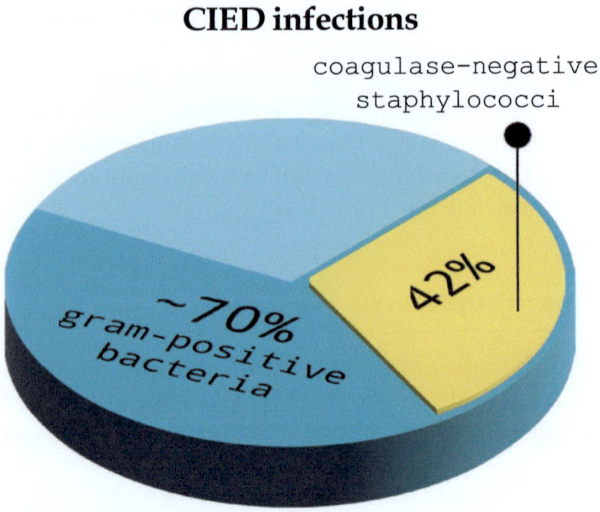

- CIED infections are categorized as pocket infections or bacteremia, with a cardiac device and imaging revealing lead or valve vegetation.
- Over 70% of these infections are attributed to gram-positive bacteria, predominantly staphylococci, with coagulase-negative staphylococci accounting for about 42% of cases. Nonetheless, infections involving gram-negative organisms such as *Pseudomonas aeruginosa* and *Candida* species, although less frequent, remain possible (Fig. 7.1).

Hospitalist Tip

Hospitalists must exercise caution before dismissing it as a contaminant when confronting persistent coagulase-negative staphylococcus bacteremia, such as *Staphylococcus epidermidis*. This bacteremia may sometimes be the sole indication of a cardiac implantable electronic device (CIED) infection in patients with a cardiac device. In cases where bacteremia remains unexplained and does not resolve spontaneously, it is advisable to conduct a thorough evaluation for CIED infection.

Pearl

Other notable complications include lead thrombosis, perforation, and pericardial effusion.

7.2.2 Clinical Approach [5]

- The most frequent clinical manifestation of a cardiac implantable electronic device (CIED) infection is inflammation at the pocket site. This pocket infection is characterized by device erosion through the skin, purulent drainage, fluctuance, and the formation of a sinus tract, which may occur with or without positive blood cultures or PET/CT scans indicating increased uptake activity at the site. Obtaining blood cultures for all patients is crucial, ideally at least two sets from different sites. In cases where blood cultures are positive for typical infections associated with CIED and other conditions do not explain the bacteremia, a transthoracic echocardiogram (TTE) should be performed, followed by a transesophageal echocardiogram (TEE) if the TTE results are negative, due to the high likelihood of CIED infection. Echocardiography may reveal a dense mass on the lead or new valve vegetation suggestive of infective endocarditis in the presence of a cardiac device. If TEE remains inconclusive, PET/CT is the preferred imaging modality, as it may detect increased uptake activity within the leads or valves. While the utility of inflammatory markers like ESR and CRP is limited, an elevated procalcitonin level could indicate a systemic infection in the context of a CIED.

Hospitalist Tip

The diagnostic algorithm for a suspected cardiac implantable electronic device (CIED) infection involves the following steps: assessing the clinical context, obtaining blood cultures, conducting a transthoracic echocardiogram (TTE) or transesophageal echocardiogram (TEE), and proceeding to PET/CT imaging. In cases where more advanced diagnostic options are available, such as 16S rRNA gene polymerase chain reaction/sequencing of sonicate fluid or metagenomic next-generation sequencing, it is essential to consult a specialist before ordering these tests.

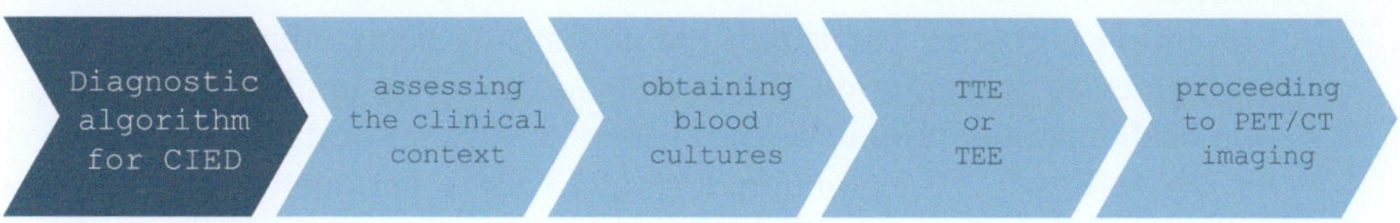

Hospitalist Tip

If there are alternative clinical explanations for bacteremia, it is advisable not to diagnose a cardiac implantable electronic device (CIED) infection. For instance, if a patient presents with pneumonia and positive blood cultures for *Streptococcus pneumoniae*, which resolves with antibiotic treatment, it is highly unlikely that the cardiac device is infected. Moreover, suppose cardiac imaging with transesophageal echocardiography (TEE) is performed for conditions such as congestive heart failure (CHF) or as part of a stroke workup, and it reveals echo density within the leads. In that case, this should not be immediately diagnosed as a CIED infection. This is particularly true in the absence of symptoms or signs of disease. It is important to note that TEE cannot differentiate between infectious and noninfectious lead echo densities nor exclude lead infection without an echo density.

Hospitalist Tip

Superficial cellulitis, retained suture inflammation, or allergic contact dermatitis do not constitute a pocket infection. These conditions are common in the initial period following the implantation of a new device and are typically resolved with a short 5–10-day course of antistaphylococcal antibiotics. In contrast, changes at the generator pocket, such as fluctuance, purulent drainage, device erosion through the skin, or sinus tract formation, indicate a definite pocket infection.

Differentiating between a pocket and superficial infection can be challenging; PET/CT scans are useful in uncertain cases. Percutaneous aspiration of the pocket site should be avoided in patients with indeterminate changes at the pocket site due to the risk of introducing an infection through needle insertion.

7.2.3 Treatment and Prevention Approach [5]

I. *Prevention*

- Prevention is crucial, particularly in minimizing hematoma formation following device implantation. This can be achieved by limiting anticoagulation bridging, maintaining warfarin therapy without bridging while aiming for an INR of 2–3.5, and managing DOACs perioperatively, as both approaches have demonstrated a low risk of bleeding.
- Cefazolin is the standard antibiotic prophylaxis for patients receiving new implantable cardiac devices. Vancomycin is an acceptable alternative for patients who are allergic to penicillin or have a history of MRSA.

Pearl

Patients experiencing persistent, unexplained *Staphylococcus aureus* or coagulase-negative staphylococcal bacteremia face a heightened risk of cardiac implantable electronic device infection (CIEDI) and should promptly undergo device removal in conjunction with antimicrobial therapy. It is essential to involve an experienced cardiologist in the management process.

II. *Treatment*

- Early removal of a cardiac implantable electronic device (CIED) has been linked to enhanced patient outcomes, with prompt action being beneficial in pocket and bloodstream infections. However, removing the device is complex, particularly when extracting attached leads, posing significant risks and complications.
- For pocket infections requiring device removal, a treatment duration of approximately 7–10 days with antibiotics is typical. In cases involving bacteremia, potential infective endocarditis (IE), or complicated cardiac implantable electronic device (CIED) infections, alongside device removal, an extended course of parenteral antibiotics for 4–6 weeks is advisable. Once the pathogen's sensitivity is determined, transitioning to oral antibiotics after the clearance of bacteremia may be considered, though consultation with an infectious disease specialist is essential.
- Reimplantation of a cardiac device should only be undertaken once local and systemic infection signs and symptoms have resoved, assuming the original indication for device placement remains essential. In cases of delayed reimplantation, utilizing a wearable defibrillator (Life Vest) and a temporary pacemaker (externalized pacemaker) is a reasonable interim solution. It is advisable to wait until at least 3 days of negative blood cultures are achieved before placing a new permanent device, extending up to 14 days in patients with valvular infective endocarditis (IE). The new device should preferably be implanted on the contralateral side, iliac vein, or in an epicardial position, with leadless pacemakers (LPM) and subcutaneous implantable cardioverter-defibrillators (S-ICD) being favored due to their reduced risk of reinfection.
- For patients not eligible for device removal due to a high risk of surgery or comorbidities, the following could be considered:
  (i) Percutaneous mechanical aspiration [6].
  (ii) Chronic oral antimicrobial suppression, transitioning from an IV once clinically stable, and blood cultures are negative. As long as the device is there, it will most often be a lifelong treatment. An ID input is vital with cardiologist feedback [7].

Pearl

If you suspect residual infection at the leads or pocket, PET/CT is the imaging of choice.

References

1. Writing Committee Members, Otto CM, Nishimura RA, Bonow RO, Carabello BA, Erwin JP 3rd, Gentile F, Jneid H, Krieger EV, Mack M, McLeod C, O'Gara PT, Rigolin VH, Sundt TM 3rd, Thompson A, Toly C. 2020 ACC/AHA guideline for the management of patients with valvular heart disease: executive summary: a report of the American College of Cardiology/American Heart Association Joint Committee on Clinical Practice Guidelines. J Am Coll Cardiol. 2021;77(4):450–500. https://doi.org/10.1016/j.jacc.2020.11.035. Epub 2020 Dec 17. Erratum in: J Am Coll Cardiol. 2021;77(9):1276. https://doi.org/10.1016/j.jacc.2021.02.008. PMID: 33342587.
2. Murray HW, Roberts RB. Streptococcus bovis bacteremia and underlying gastrointestinal disease. Arch Intern Med. 1978;138(7):1097–9. PMID: 666468.
3. Rasmussen RV, Høst U, Arpi M, Hassager C, Johansen HK, Korup E, Schønheyder HC, Berning J, Gill S, Rosenvinge FS, Fowler VG Jr, Møller JE, Skov RL, Larsen CT, Hansen TF, Mard S, Smit J, Andersen PS, Bruun NE. Prevalence of infective endocarditis in patients with Staphylococcus aureus bacteraemia: the value of screening with echocardiography. Eur J Echocardiogr. 2011;12(6):414–20. https://doi.org/10.1093/ejechocard/jer023. PMID: 21685200; PMCID: PMC3117467.
4. Otto CM, Nishimura RA, Bonow RO, Carabello BA, Erwin JP 3rd, Gentile F, Jneid H, Krieger EV, Mack M, McLeod C, O'Gara PT, Rigolin VH, Sundt TM 3rd, Thompson A, Toly C. 2020 ACC/AHA guideline for the management of patients with valvular heart disease: executive summary: a report of the American College of Cardiology/American Heart Association Joint Committee on Clinical Practice Guidelines. Circulation. 2021;143(5):e35–71. https://doi.org/10.1161/CIR.0000000000000932. Epub 2020 Dec 17. Erratum in: Circulation. 2021;143(5):e228. https://doi.org/10.1161/CIR.0000000000000960. Erratum in: Circulation. 2021;143(10):e784. https://doi.org/10.1161/CIR.0000000000000966. PMID: 33332149.
5. Baddour LM, Esquer Garrigos Z, Rizwan Sohail M, Havers-Borgersen E, Krahn AD, Chu VH, Radke CS, Avari-Silva J, El-Chami MF, Miro JM, De-Simone DC, American Heart Association Council on Lifelong Congenital Heart Disease and Heart Health in the Young (Young Hearts) and Council on Clinical Cardiology. Update on cardiovascular implantable electronic device infections and their prevention, diagnosis, and management: a scientific statement from the American Heart Association: endorsed by the International Society for Cardiovascular Infectious Diseases. Circulation. 2024;149(2):e201–16. https://doi.org/10.1161/CIR.0000000000001187. Epub2023Dec4. PMID: 38047353.

6. Starck CT, Schaerf RHM, Breitenstein A, Najibi S, Conrad J, Berendt J, Esmailian F, Eulert-Grehn J, Dreizler T, Falk V. Transcatheteraspiration of large pacemaker and implantable cardioverter-defibrillator lead vegetations facilitating safe transvenous lead extraction. Europace. 2020;22:133–8. https://doi.org/10.1093/europace/euz283.
7. Baddour LM, Epstein AE, Erickson CC, Knight BP, Levison ME, Lock-hart PB, Masoudi FA, Okum EJ, Wilson WR, Beerman LB, et al. On behalf of the American Heart Association Rheumatic Fever, Endocarditis, and Kawasaki Disease Committee of the Council on Cardiovascular Disease in the Young; Council on Cardiovascular Surgery and Anesthesia; Council on Cardiovascular Nursing; Council on Clinical Cardiology; and the Interdisciplinary Council on Quality of Care and Outcomes Research. Update on cardiovascular implantable electronic device infections and their management: a scientific statement from the American Heart Association. Circulation. 2010;121:458–77. https://doi.org/10.1161/CIRCULATIONAHA.109.192665.

Pericardial Disease

Contents

M. Salih, *Practical Hospitalist Guide to Inpatient Cardiology*, https://doi.org/10.1007/978-3-032-03240-9_8

This chapter provides a focused overview of *acute pericarditis* and *constrictive pericarditis*, emphasizing clinical features, diagnostic criteria, and management strategies relevant to hospitalists. Acute pericarditis is characterized by chest pain, pericardial friction rub, and ECG changes such as diffuse ST elevation, typically managed with anti-inflammatory therapy. Constrictive pericarditis involves chronic pericardial thickening and fibrosis, leading to impaired diastolic filling and signs of right heart failure. This chapter highlights key diagnostic tools, including echocardiography, cardiac MRI, and invasive hemodynamics, to distinguish constrictive pericarditis from *restrictive cardiomyopathy*, which presents with similar symptoms but involves myocardial stiffness rather than pericardial restriction. Differentiating features such as respiratory variation in ventricular filling pressures, septal bounce, and pericardial thickness guide diagnosis and management. Treatment options range from medical therapy for acute inflammation to pericardiectomy for chronic constriction. This chapter equips hospitalists with practical approaches to diagnosis and tailored treatment, ensuring optimal care for patients with pericardial and restrictive cardiac diseases.

8.1 Acute Pericarditis

8.1.1 When to Suspect and Major Etiology

- You will need two out of the four criteria for confirmation, Typical chest pain is necessary for the diagnosis to be made [1, 27]:
  1. Typical pleuritic severe chest pain (the pericardium is highly innervated, that is why it is so painful; also may irritate nearby structures like the sternum or diaphragm)
  2. Pericardial effusion or inflammation on imaging
  3. Pericardial friction rub
  4. EKG findings consistent with the diagnosis or Elevated inflammatory markers

Pearl

Other supportive findings include elevated inflammatory markers, C-reactive protein, ESR, and white blood cell count elevation.

- Most common causes
  (i) Viral infections (the most common). It is expected that the condition is preceded by viral nonspecific symptoms or gastrointestinal complaints [2].

(ii) Post-cardiac injury. Including all types of procedures, even LHC. It is a growing cause in developed countries due to more frequent cardiac surgeries or interventions. It may occur weeks after the procedure.
(iii) Others (▫ Table 8.1).

▫ Table 8.1 Selected common examples of acute pericarditis causes

Etiology	Comments
Infections	The etiology of infections is predominantly viral, although atypical infections, including bacterial and fungal, should also be considered as potential causes. It is critical to suspect an infectious etiology in the presence of a high-grade fever.
	Bacterial infections are relatively rare and should be considered when the patient exhibits signs of sepsis, confirmed by positive blood cultures, or if the patient has recently undergone cardiothoracic surgery or interventions.
Metabolic	Uremia and hypothyroidism are significant clinical conditions. Uremia commonly arises from inadequately managed renal failure, whether it is acute or chronic in nature.
Cancer	This phenomenon is predominantly observed in metastatic cancers of various types, including leukemia and lymphoma.
Drug-induced	Medications such as hydralazine necessitate careful monitoring of potential side effects. It is imperative to consistently review the side effects experienced by patients as a result of their medications.
Autoimmune	These conditions primarily encompass systemic lupus erythematosus (SLE), Sjögren's syndrome, rheumatoid arthritis (RA), systemic sclerosis, mixed connective tissue disease, and sarcoidosis.
Radiation therapy	May occur up to weeks after radiation therapy.
Post ACS/MI	Dressler Syndrome is a post–myocardial infarction inflammatory condition that generally manifests 1 to 8 weeks after the event. Clinically, it is characterized by malaise, fever, pericardial discomfort, leukocytosis, elevated erythrocyte sedimentation rate, and the presence of a pericardial effusion. First-line management consists of high-dose aspirin, commonly administered at 750 mg three times daily. Typically, it is a benign condition that responds favorably to treatment.

Hospitalist Tip

No cause is usually found around 50% of the time [3]. It is unnecessary to determine the etiology of all patients with the presentation if they improved with supportive care alone.

Pearl

TB is considered the most typical cause in developing countries. Consider the diagnosis when a patient is a traveler or an immigrant from an endemic area [4].

8.1.2 Clinical Approach

- Most patients present with sharp, central, pleuritic chest pain, characterized by its exacerbation when lying flat and alleviation when leaning forward. This pain is neither aggravated by physical exertion nor relieved by rest or nitroglycerin. Notably, it may radiate to the trapezius muscle, sharing the same phrenic nerve supply as the heart. Such pain could be accompanied by low-grade fever, fatigue, and myalgia. When gathering additional history, it is crucial to consider potential underlying causes such as end-stage renal disease (ESRD), hypothyroidism, recent cardiac surgery, prior chest radiation, and malignancy. A pericardial friction rub at the left lower sternal border is a significant clinical finding, though it may be intermittent and lacks high sensitivity, with prevalence estimates ranging from 35% to 85% [5].
- A comprehensive admission workup for this condition should include tests such as a complete blood count (CBC), comprehensive metabolic panel (CMP), erythrocyte sedimentation rate (ESR), C-reactive protein (CRP), electrocardiogram (EKG), serum troponin, chest X-ray, and transthoracic echocardiogram (TTE). If the patient shows signs of sepsis, blood cultures are warranted. Should the initial diagnosis remain elusive and the patient's condition not improve, further testing may be necessary. This could involve ordering an antinuclear antibody (ANA) complete profile with a vasculitis-targeted panel,

thyroid-stimulating hormone (TSH) test, and respiratory pathogen viral panel, focusing on common viruses such as echovirus, coxsackievirus, parvovirus B19, and human herpesvirus 6. Additionally, pericardial fluid analysis and computed tomography (CT) of the chest, abdomen, and pelvis may be employed to identify complications, atypical infections, malignancies, or lymphomas.
- It could be recurrent in around 30% of patients [20].

8.1.3 Test for Acute Pericarditis and Their Significance

Test	Clinical significance	Comments
CBC	Leukocytosis	Mainly left shift

Test	Clinical significance	Comments
CMP	Elevated BUN	Typically above 100 mg/dL [6]

Test	Clinical significance	Comments
ESR/CRP	Elevated	Monitoring disease activity and recovery can be beneficial in assessing the progression and response to treatment.

Test	Clinical significance	Comments
EKG	Upwardly concave ST-segment elevations with PR segment depressions in most leads, except lead aVR where it is elevated.	These changes are not consistently present across all cases. The stages of electrocardiographic (ECG) changes typically progress as follows: Stage 1 involves diffuse ST elevation and PR depression. Stage 2 is the normalization of ST and PR segments. Stage 3 features diffuse T-wave inversions with isoelectric ST segments. Stage 4 is characterized by the normalization of the ECG [7].

Test	Clinical significance	Comments
Troponin	Could be elevated in 35–50% of patients with pericarditis [7].	Concomitant myocarditis is observed in approximately 15% of cases, yet it lacks prognostic significance [8]. It cannot be utilized to distinguish from acute coronary syndrome (ACS), as its levels can occasionally be substantially elevated.

Test	Clinical significance	Comments
Chest X-ray/CT chest/MRI chest	May show an enlarged heart with sizable pericardial effusion (bottle-shaped heart).	Imaging plays a crucial role in identifying underlying etiologies, such as tuberculosis (TB) in the chest, mediastinal masses in lymphoma, or lytic lesions indicative of cancer. It is also essential for ruling out other potential causes. Computed tomography (CT) can diagnose constrictive pericarditis and is useful for differentiating causes based on contrast enhancement. Magnetic resonance imaging (MRI) can reveal pericardial inflammation, indicated by pericardial thickening and late gadolinium enhancement, but it should be routinely requested only for surgical planning or monitoring persistent inflammation.

Test	Clinical significance	Comments
TTE	May show effusion, but not always; normal in 40% of cases [6].	Its significance lies in monitoring for complications such as cardiac tamponade and excluding underlying regional wall motion abnormalities associated with acute coronary syndrome (ACS).

Test	Clinical significance	Comments
Pericardial fluid analysis and possible biopsy by a cardiologist or cardiothoracic surgeon.	Diagnostic procedures may reveal the underlying etiology. It is advisable to conduct a cell count and cultures for bacteria, acid-fast bacilli (AFB), and fungi and to test for adenosine deaminase to screen for tuberculosis (TB). Biopsy is primarily utilized in the context of suspected TB.	Interpretation is challenging and should be considered when the etiology remains unclear despite persistent symptoms, when the patient exhibits a lack of response to treatment in the context of sepsis and bacteremia, or when the patient is critically ill with cardiac tamponade.

Pearl

CT attenuation values below 10 Hounsfield units (HU) indicate transudative fluids, whereas values exceeding 10 HU indicate exudative fluids. Attenuation values ranging from 20 to 60 HU may indicate a purulent, malignant, or myxedematous origin, while values above 60 HU suggest the presence of hemorrhagic fluid [9].

8.1.4 Common DD

Condition	How to differentiate
ACS/MI	Chest pain characterized by a pressure-like sensation is typically exacerbated by physical exertion and alleviated by rest or administration of nitroglycerin. Electrocardiogram (EKG) findings of ST elevation are localized rather than diffuse. Echocardiography may reveal regional wall motion abnormalities.
PE	Dyspnea is commonly observed in conjunction with hypoxemia. Although the chest pain may appear similar, it is not positional. Most patients present with tachypnea and tachycardia. Electrocardiogram (EKG) findings typically do not show diffuse ST elevations but are more localized. A CT scan of the chest with contrast is diagnostic.

Condition	How to differentiate
Myocarditis	It may coexist with other conditions and is often associated with symptoms such as dyspnea, as well as worsening ventricular function or the occurrence of arrhythmias. If it solely presents with nonspecific ST segment changes on an electrocardiogram (EKG), TTE may show global systolic dysfunction or regional. Left heart catheterization (LHC) is essential for excluding acute coronary syndrome (ACS) when there is uncertainty. Routine endomyocardial biopsy is generally not necessary. However, if there is suspicion of autoimmune myocarditis, sarcoidosis, or eosinophilic myocarditis, conducting a biopsy is a reasonable course of action. Viral blood serology results often do not align with findings from biopsies; thus, it is not recommended to order them routinely. Most common virus infections includes parvoviruses (PV B19) and human herpesvirus 6 (HHV 6).
Aortic dissection	Patients commonly present with acute, sharp tearing pain that radiates towards the back. A significant number of these patients exhibit hypertension upon presentation. A computed tomography angiography (CTA) is the definitive diagnostic tool for this condition. In cases where there is a low probability of dissection, a D-dimer test, known for its high sensitivity, can be utilized to effectively rule out the possibility of dissection.
Cardiac contusion	Following trauma, there may be an elevation in troponin levels accompanied by nonspecific electrocardiogram (EKG) findings. Additionally, there can be indications of possible pericardial effusion and abnormal wall motion in the heart.
Pneumonia with Pleurisy	The pain experienced may have a pleuritic characteristic, although it is infrequently positional. It is often accompanied by a cough and fever, with either localized or diffuse findings present on a chest X-ray.
Pneumothorax	While the pain may initially appear similar to other conditions, specific examination findings such as diminished breath sounds, reduced vocal resonance, and decreased chest expansion on the affected side help distinguish it. A chest X-ray serves as a diagnostic tool in this scenario.
Musculoskeletal	Localized tenderness. CBC, ESR/CRP, EKG, troponin, and TTE are normal.
GERD	Heart burn, and other GI symptoms. Improved with GI cocktail in some patients.

8.1.5 Treatment Approach

- If symptoms are sufficiently severe, hospital admission is necessary to monitor for complications such as cardiac tamponade. The primary treatment strategy involves reducing the inflammatory process and addressing the underlying cause. B-Blockers are used for symptomatic tachycardia [16, 25]. Physical activity should be restricted until the pain resolves, as elevated heart rates can increase shear stress across the pericardial layers, exacerbating inflammation and potentially prolonging the disease course [10].

Hospitalist Tip

The following criteria indicate a worse prognosis and the need for admission [10]:

- High fever (i.e., >100.4 °F [38 °C])
- Subacute course (symptoms over a couple of days without clear onset day)
- Evidence of a large pericardial effusion on echo
- Cardiac tamponade
- Failure to respond within 1 week to NSAID
- Oral anticoagulation therapy
- Lack of response within 1 week of symptoms

I. NSAIDs and aspirin: The first-line treatment for symptomatic relief in all patients typically involves the use of anti-inflammatory medications, continuing for a period of 1–4 weeks until both pain subsides and inflammatory mediators return to normal levels. These medications are effective in reducing inflammation, thereby alleviating pain and systemic symptoms. The choice of medication may vary based on the side effect profile of the patient. While effective for immediate relief, these treatments do not prevent future complications such as constrictive pericarditis or cardiac tamponade [1]. Given the high doses of NSAIDs or aspirin often required, most patients will benefit from concurrent use of proton pump inhibitors (PPIs) or H2 blockers to mitigate the risk of gastrointestinal bleeding.

Pearl

Remember NSAIDs increase the risk of bleeding, HTN, and kidney injury.

Hospitalist Tip

Post ACS/MI, aspirin or colchicine is preferred in post-ACS pericarditis patients, probably due to its antithrombotic effect. Avoid glucocorticoids and NSAIDs as they may impair healing and increase the risk of myocardial rupture, bleeding risk, and ischemic events [11]. If pain is not controlled, consider adding acetaminophen or opioids.

II. Colchicine: All patients, except those with advanced renal or liver dysfunction, should be prescribed colchicine in addition to NSAIDs or aspirin. Colchicine is effective in limiting inflammation by reducing neutrophil activation, decreasing recurrence rates, and enhancing the response to NSAIDs [12]. The typical duration of colchicine therapy ranges from 1 to 6 months, most commonly around 3 months. Common side effects of colchicine include gastrointestinal symptoms. For patients with renal or liver impairment, dose adjustments are necessary or the drug should be avoided, as it can lead to neuromuscular toxicity and bone marrow suppression. It is important to monitor these patients by regularly checking kidney function and complete blood counts (CBC).

III. Corticosteroids: Not generally recommended as first-line due to side effect profile and concern for prolonged disease recovery and recurrence [13]. A low dose is safer with a low risk of recurrence and adverse events (prednisone 0.2–0.5 mg/kg) [14]. Taper slowly over weeks to months after symptoms improve and inflammatory markers normalize. They should be added to first-line treatments.

Hospitalist Tip

Steroids are mainly indicated for the following:

1. If it does not resolve with multiple trials of NSAIDS/colchicine
2. Contraindication to the above medicine (pregnancy, advanced CKD, use of anticoagulation)
3. Autoimmune/vasculitis-related pericarditis (should be used with colchicine)

Pearl

All patients expected to be on long tapering dose of steroids (more than 3 weeks) should be on calcium (1200–1500 mg/day) and vitamin D supplements (1000 IU/day). If it is expected to be of prolonged duration, most patients will also need to be on bisphosphonates.

8.1.6 Treatment for Acute and Recurrent Pericarditis and Their Complications [2]

	Drug	Dose	Duration
Acute pericarditis	Aspirin	750-1,000 mg every 8 h	1-2 weeks
	Ibuprofen	600-800 mg every 8 h	1-2 weeks
	Colchicine	0.5-1.2 mg in one or divided doses	3 months
Recurrent pericarditis	Aspirin	750-1,000 mg every 8 h	Weeks-months
	Ibuprofen	600-800 mg every 8 h	Weeks-months
	Indomethacin	25-50 mg every 8 h	Weeks-months
	Colchicine	0.5-1.2 mg in one or divided doses	At least 6 months
	Prednisone	0.2-0.5 mg/kg/daily	Months
	Anakinra	1-2 mg/kg/daily up to 100 mg/daily	Months
	Rilonacept	320 mg once, than 160 mg weekly	Months
	Azathioprine	1 mg/kg/daily up to 2-3 mg/kg/daily	Months
	Methotrexate	10-15 mg weekly	Months
	MMF	2,000 mg daily	Months
	IVIGs	400-500 mg/kg/day	5 days

Tamponade
- Pericadiocentesis
- Pericardial window

Constrictive pericarditis
- Active inflammation:
  - Yes → Anti-inflammatory therapy as first line, pericardiectomy for refractory cases
  - No → Pericardiectomy

Hospitalist Tip

In case of acute pericarditis, stop any oral anticoagulation because of the risk of intrapericardial hemorrhage leading to possible tamponade.

8.1.7 Treatment of Special Conditions [2]

Condition	Treatment approach	Comments
Tuberculous pericarditis	Antituberculosis (TB) treatment is generally administered for a duration of approximately 6 months. If there is no significant response to this treatment, it may be necessary to consider a pericardiectomy	Steroids are not typically indicated. Mainly used in TB meningitis
Autoimmune disorders	Steroid +/– immunosuppressive therapy	Steroids should not be used for nonspecific myocarditis. However, steroid should be used in: (i) Giant-cell arteritis myocarditis (ii) Cardiac sarcoidosis (iii) Eosinophilic myocarditis
Purulent pericarditis	Need urgent pericardiocentesis, drain with a cardiologist and broad-spectrum antibiotics	Do not forget to send cultures for bacteria, AFB, and fungus
Recurrent pericarditis	If patients do not show improvement with nonsteroidal anti-inflammatory drugs (NSAIDs) or colchicine, consider the addition of steroids to the initial treatment regimen, thereby implementing a triple therapy approach	For resistant cases, IL-1 blockade with Anakinra is beneficial [15]. Other options include immunosuppressives and pericardiectomy (last option)
Uremic pericarditis	Dialysis will be necessary for a few weeks until the condition resolves	

8.1.8 Complication and Special Conditions

Constrictive Pericarditis

- The diagnosis should be suspected in cases of unexplained right-sided heart failure (collapse more easily than the left heart), normal EF, particularly when echocardiographic findings are inconclusive and there is a history of recurrent pericarditis, chest irradiation, mediastinal malignancy such as lymphoma, or cardiac surgery like coronary artery bypass grafting (CABG). This condition is not typically explained by advanced lung conditions, valvular heart disease, or advanced left heart failure with reduced ejection fraction (HFrEF), and it is important not to hastily conclude this diagnosis due to its rarity.

- Primary symptoms include heart failure-related manifestations with right-sided systemic congestion, such as generalized anasarca, gastrointestinal symptoms like dyspepsia (bowel edema/poor perfusion), and elevated liver function tests (LFTs) due to congestion or ischemia.
- Physical examination may reveal signs of right-sided heart failure, including elevated jugular venous distension (JVD), hepatomegaly, ascites, pleural effusion, and significant lower limb edema. Lung crackles may be minimal or absent. Cardiac examination might show a pericardial knock, muffled heart sounds, Kussmaul's sign (a sudden rise in JVD during inspiration followed by a sudden collapse on expiration)/nonspecific, and pulsus paradoxus.
- Diagnostic approaches, alongside history and physical examination, include electrocardiogram (EKG) showing low voltage, inflammatory markers, Doppler echocardiography indicating elevated diastolic pressure in all chambers (because of impaired filling capacity) and respiratory cycle filling variation (septal bounce), plethoric inferior vena cava (IVC) without inspiratory compression (highly sensitive), and cardiac CT demonstrating pericardial thickening, which is specific but not highly sensitive [23]. Cardiologists may opt for cardiac MRI to detect active inflammation [24], suggesting the potential effectiveness of anti-inflammatory treatments, and right heart catheterization to measure high diastolic pressure due to the inability of the heart to relax, in cases where the diagnosis remains unclear.

- *The most common causes are as follows* [26]:
  1. Cardiac surgery, 37%
  2. Recurrent history of idiopathic/viral pericarditis, 49% of cases
  3. Chronic atypical infections (TB, viral), radiation
  4. Rheumatological conditions/collagen vascular disease
- Following consultation with a cardiologist and cardiothoracic surgeon, the treatment plan typically involves the surgical removal of the pericardial sac, in addition to addressing the underlying condition. In a hospital setting, careful administration of diuretics is recommended to manage volume overload while ensuring adequate cardiac output. Beta-blockers may be employed to manage symptomatic tachycardia, in inflammatory stage [25]. Acute effusive constrictive pericarditis (usually diagnosed by MRI showing edema and active inflammation, chest pain, and raised inflammatory markers) can be treated with aggressive anti-inflammatory medications, akin to the treatment strategies used for acute pericarditis.
- Most common DD: The most classical differential diagnosis to consider against constrictive pericarditis is restrictive cardiomyopathy, which can present similarly. Restrictive cardiomyopathy may be primary (genetic), metabolic (such as Gaucher's or Fabry's disease), or secondary to infiltrative conditions like cardiac amyloidosis, radiation exposure, hemochromatosis, sarcoidosis, or hypereosinophilic syndromes. Consequently, it is prudent to rule out these secondary causes based on clinical context by performing appropriate tests, including complete blood count (CBC), iron studies/ferritin, flow cytometry for leukemia/lymphoma, lymph node biopsy, serum protein electrophoresis (SPEP), urine protein electrophoresis (UPEP), free light chain serum analysis, cardiac MRI,

and 99m-technetium pyrophosphate scintigraphy. Metabolic pathway and genetic testing may also be indicated in specific scenarios. Typically, brain natriuretic peptide (BNP) levels are moderately elevated, reflecting significant myocardial disease and stiffness, along with biventricular failure, which is not commonly observed in constrictive pericarditis unless it is advanced and primarily involves right ventricular failure. The primary pathophysiological issue is impaired left ventricular (LV) compliance. Echocardiography shows that systolic and diastolic pressures are higher in restrictive cardiomyopathy than in constrictive pericarditis, owing to more severely restricted filling pressures throughout the cardiac cycle, whereas constrictive pericarditis results in more available space within the heart. Echocardiography will also typically reveal biatrial dilatation, attributable to diastolic filling defects, but normal ventricular size and function. In constrictive pericarditis, Doppler echocardiography, which is more accurate in assessing blood flow and velocity throughout the cardiac cycle, may demonstrate ventricular interdependence, where increased right ventricular filling reciprocally decreases left ventricular filling, a phenomenon not typical in restrictive cardiomyopathy. Treatment primarily involves loop diuretics, but as in constrictive pericarditis, assessing volume status and balancing between filling pressure and overload present a narrow therapeutic index, given the enclosed heart requires relatively high filling pressures to maintain cardiac output. Beta-blockers and aggressive arrhythmia management are crucial, as rapid heart rates further compromise the already limited filling time. Heart transplantation remains a last resort; thus, patients with deteriorating heart failure should be referred to a transplant center promptly. Most patients succumb to congestive heart failure (CHF) and arrhythmias.

Hospitalist Tip

In short, to differentiate, send a BNP and Doppler echo, followed by a cardiology consult for the right heart catheter if it is inconclusive. In restrictive cardiomyopathy, elevated BNP and significantly elevated LA size/volume are characteristic. On the other hand, think about constrictive pericarditis when there is right-sided heart failure out of the proportion of VHD, myocardial findings on echo, or CT chest/lung pathology.

Pearl

Other less common DDs include SVC syndrome with obstruction.

Pericardial Effusion

- This condition presents with exertional dyspnea, orthopnea, and a sensation of fullness. The diagnostic workup is similar to that of acute pericarditis. Echo is the most important test to request. If complex or loculated effusion is suspected, cardiac CT, MRI, or TEE is mostly recommended [23, 27].
- Trivial, mild effusions of less than 50 ml can be considered a normal variant, and pericardiocentesis is generally unnecessary in these cases.
- The "Light'scriteria" should not be applied to analyze pericardial fluid content, as it often misclassifies exudative effusions due to the naturally high levels of lactate dehydrogenase (LDH), protein, and cells within the pericardial sac. Unfortunately, there are no specific criteria dedicated to pericardial effusion analysis [17]. That is why Pericardiocentesis for pericardial effusion without tamponade is mostly not recommended [27].
- When the effusion is pathological, it is most commonly caused by idiopathic or presumed viral pericarditis, and in developing countries, tuberculosis accounts for over 70% of cases [18]. In cases where the effusion is significantly large, metastatic malignancy should be suspected. Other common etiologies for moderately large effusion includes hypothyroidism and uremia.
- Hold diuretics and vasodilators specifically in large effusion that may lead to tamponade.

Pearl

Pericardial effusion is common and mostly benign after cardiac intervention/surgery. It usually resolves within weeks. Pericardiocentesis for pericardial effusion without tamponade is mostly not recommended.

8.1.9 Management Approach by 2015 European Society of Cardiology [1]

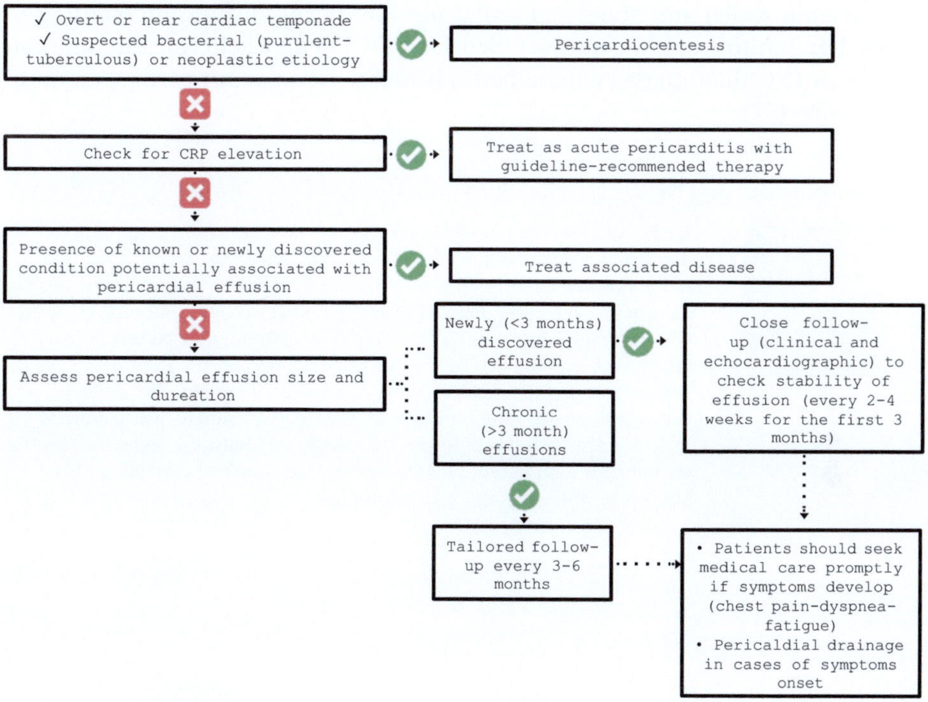

8.1.10 Cardiac Tamponade

- It is important to stress that a sizable pericardial effusion is not synonymous with cardiac tamponade, as large chronic effusions can be well tolerated by some patients. However, there is a higher risk associated with effusions due to *neoplastic causes, tuberculosis, and hypothyroidism* [2].
- Cardiac tamponade classically presents with Beck's triad, which includes hypotension, elevated jugular venous distension (JVD), and muffled heart sounds. Other symptoms in the early phase include SOB, chest fullness, and fatigue. These symptoms are related to low cardiac output. Tachycardia is considered the most sensitive sign, while pulsus paradoxus characterized by an absent pulse during inspiration is specific when observed in the appropriate clinical context [2]. Peripheral pulses will fade during inspiration (simple bedside technique, not accurate).

- An electrocardiogram (EKG) may reveal electrical alternans, resulting from the motion of the heart within the fluid-filled sac, or low voltage. A chest X-ray is typically not useful in this diagnosis. Echocardiography is essential, as it can demonstrate the collapse of right-sided heart chambers during diastole (thin walls) and abnormal septal motion during inspiration (shifting to the left, limiting cardiac output). Bedside POCUS may help rule out tamponade, as IVC dilation (>2 cm diameter) is highly sensitive for cardiac tamponade 92% [22].

Hospitalist Tip

Understanding the pulsus paradoxus sign can indeed be perplexing for many junior doctors. The key is to pay close attention while deflating the blood pressure cuff. Initially, as you deflate, the first Korotkoff sound you hear marks the upper limit of pulsus paradoxus, say at 140 mmHg. As you continue to listen, during inspiration, the sounds may become irregular or even muffled due to the pulsus paradoxus effect. Eventually, the sounds will become regular again, perhaps at 80 mmHg. The difference between these two values, 140 and 80 mmHg, is 60 mmHg, which exceeds the normal threshold of 10 mmHg, confirming pulsus paradoxus. This technique is essential for identifying conditions such as cardiac tamponade. I hope this explanation is helpful!

Pearl

The absence of a large effusion does not rule out tamponade. Early diastolic (RV) collapse on TTE has 85–100% specificity for tamponade [21]. In tamponade, the intrapericardial pressure transiently exceeds the RV filling pressure (normally low compared to left ventricle), leading to the collapse of the RV and hemodynamic compromise.

- Call your cardiologist ASAP. Treatment is by drainage with pericardiocentesis and drain placement/window by a cardiologist. To buy time, all patients need good fluid challenges, preferably isotonic fluids, 1 L at a time, to maintain preload and critical cardiac output. Most importantly, treat the patient, not the pericardial effusion volume; treat the patient, not the numbers. Avoid mechanical ventilation whenever possible (it increases intrathoracic pressure, limiting further compromised cardiac output).

8.1.11 Myopericarditis/Myocarditis [19]

- Myocarditis should be suspected when a patient presents with acute pericarditis accompanied by significant troponin elevation, acute decompensated heart failure (ADHF), or arrhythmias.
- The three classic presentations of myocarditis include chest pain, heart failure or shock, and symptoms related to arrhythmia, such as presyncope or syncope. This condition can mimic myocardial infarction due to the overlap in symptoms, making accurate diagnosis critical for appropriate management.

Hospitalist Tip

In young individuals, a history of a preceding viral infection or other risk factors, followed by cardiovascular symptoms, should raise the suspicion of myocarditis. The symptoms are often nonspecific, including gastrointestinal symptoms or signs of respiratory illness. Pure myocarditis may not commonly present with overt cardiac complaints, making diagnosis challenging. Clinicians should maintain a high index of suspicion, especially when typical cardiac symptoms are absent.

Hospitalist Tip

It is often challenging to rule out underlying acute coronary syndrome (ACS), so it is advisable to consult with cardiology when there is a significant elevation in troponin levels. This may include considering a left heart catheterization (LHC) or an ischemic evaluation with a stress test—if the patient is stable and under supervised monitoring due to concerns about acute arrhythmias. An echocardiogram and cardiac MRI can help identify global dysfunctions, as opposed to regional ones (ischemia), which are typical in myocarditis. If a patient presents with symptoms suggestive of ACS but has a negative LHC, myocarditis should be suspected.

- Troponin levels in myocarditis are often elevated, although not consistently. Electrocardiograms (EKG) may reveal nonspecific findings or arrhythmias. Inflammatory markers such as ESR and CRP might be elevated. Transthoracic echocardiography (TTE) can demonstrate new, otherwise unexplained, left or right ventricular structural and functional abnormalities. Cardiac MRI is considered the most crucial diagnostic tool; it can show myocardial inflammation, edema, tissue changes, or fibrosis. In severe cases, an endomyocardial biopsy remains the gold standard, under specific criteria [19].

- Myocarditis can lead to severe acute decompensated heart failure (ADHF), significant arrhythmias, and other nonspecific symptoms. Referral to an advanced heart failure center with a multidisciplinary myocarditis team is recommended for symptomatic patients. Patients with high-risk features, such as severely reduced ventricular function, symptomatic heart failure, or hemodynamic instability, should be transferred to a specialized center.
- Treatment focuses on removing the offending agent or medications, addressing underlying arrhythmias, applying immunosuppression in selected cases, and providing guideline-directed medical therapy (GDMT) for heart failure patients. Patients should abstain from competitive sports for at least 3–6 months, obtaining clearance from a specialist before resuming activities.
- Follow-up with a myocardial disease specialist on an outpatient basis is essential. Given the growing recognition of genetic contributions to myocarditis, genetic counseling and testing are advised for all consenting patients.

Pearl

Immunosuppression is indicated for specific types of myocarditis, including eosinophilic myocarditis, giant cell myocarditis, myocarditis related to immune checkpoint inhibitors, and autoimmune-associated conditions. In acute settings, a regimen of methylprednisolone at 7–14 mg/kg for 3 days is recommended, followed by prednisone at 1 mg/kg. This approach is tailored to mitigate the inflammatory response in these severe cases, aiming to preserve cardiac function and improve patient outcomes [19].

8.1.12 Risk Factors for Myocarditis [19]

Genetic variants	– Pathogenic gene variants linked to dilated and arrhythmogenic cardiomyopathy and neuromuscular disorders – Disease-causing variants in DSP and TTN are consistently associated with myocarditis
History of myocarditis	– Personal history of prior episode of myocarditis – Family history of myocarditis
Cardiotoxins	– Prescribed medications, including immune checkpoint inhibitors, doxorubicin, trastuzumab, and clozapine – Illicit substances: cocaine, methamphetamine
Thymoma	
Systemic immune-mediated/ connective tissue disease	Sarcoidosis, systemic lupus, rheumatoid arthritis, scleroderma, myositis, or vasculitis
Hypereosinophilia	

Infectious agents	Particularly viruses (e.g., adenovirus, enterovirus, parvovirus, human herpes virus 6, influenza, HIV, SARS-CoV-2) but also other organisms, including bacteria, fungi, and parasites
Vaccines	Including smallpox, mRNA COVID-19

COVID-19 coronavirus disease of 2019, *DSP* desmoplakin, *mRNA* messenger RNA, *TTN* titin

References

1. Y Adler, Charron P, Imazio M, Badano L, Barón-Esquivias G, Bogaert J, Brucato A, Gueret P, Klingel K, Lionis C, Maisch B, Mayosi B, Pavie A, Ristic AD, Sabaté Tenas M, Seferovic P, Swedberg K, Tomkowski W, ESC Scientific Document Group. 2015 ESC guidelines for the diagnosis and management of pericardial diseases: the task force for the diagnosis and management of pericardial diseases of the European Society of Cardiology (ESC) endorsed by: the European Association for Cardio-Thoracic Surgery (EACTS). Eur Heart J. 2015;36(42):2921–64. https://doi.org/10.1093/eurheartj/ehv318. Epub 2015 Aug 29. PMID: 26320112; PMCID: PMC7539677.
2. Chiabrando JG, Bonaventura A, Vecchié A, Wohlford GF, Mauro AG, Jordan JH, Grizzard JD, Montecucco F, Berrocal DH, Brucato A, Imazio M, Abbate A. Management of acute and recurrent pericarditis: JACC state-of-the-art review. J Am Coll Cardiol. 2020;75(1):76–92. https://doi.org/10.1016/j.jacc.2019.11.021. PMID: 31918837
3. Gouriet F, Levy P-Y, Casalta J-P, Zandotti C, Collart F, Lepidi H, Cautela J, Bonnet JL, Thuny F, Habib G, Raoult D. Etiology of pericarditis in a prospective cohort of 1162 cases. Am J Med. 2015;128(7):784.e1–8. ISSN 0002-9343.
4. Mayosi BM. Contemporary trends in the epidemiology and management of cardiomyopathy and pericarditis in sub-Saharan Africa. Heart. 2007;93:1176–83.
5. Chahine J, Siddiqui WJ. Pericardial friction rub. In: StatPearls [Internet]. Treasure Island: StatPearls Publishing; 2025.
6. Restrepo D, Vaduganathan M, Fenves AZ. Uremic pericarditis: distinguishing features in a now-uncommon clinical syndrome. South Med J. 2018;111(12):754–7. https://doi.org/10.14423/SMJ.0000000000000899. PMID: 30512129; PMCID: PMC6281170.
7. Masek KP, Levis JT. ECG diagnosis: acute pericarditis. Perm J. 2013;17(4):e146. https://doi.org/10.7812/TPP/13-044. PMID: 24361030; PMCID: PMC3854820
8. Imazio M, Gaita F. Acute and recurrent pericarditis. Cardiol Clin. 2017;35:505–13.
9. Lazaros G, et al. New approaches to management of pericardial effusions. Curr Cardiol Rep. 2021;23:106.
10. Sivalokanathan S, Chokshi N. Pericarditis in athletes: approach to exercise restriction. Published September 7, 2022.
11. Kang DO, An H, Park GU, Yum Y, Park EJ, Park Y, Jang WY, Kim W, Choi JY, Roh SY, Na JO. Cardiovascular and bleeding risks associated with nonsteroidal anti-inflammatory drugs after myocardial infarction. J Am Coll Cardiol. 2020;76:518–29.
12. Imazio M, et al. A randomized trial of colchicine for acute pericarditis. N Engl J Med. 2013. https://www.nejm.org/doi/full/10.1056/NEJMoa1208536.
13. Imazio M, Bobbio M, Cecchi E, et al. Colchicine as first-choice therapy for recurrent pericarditis: results of the CORE (COlchicine for REcurrent pericarditis) trial. Arch Intern Med. 2005;165:1987–91.
14. Imazio M, Brucato A, Cumetti D, et al. Corticosteroids for recurrent pericarditis: high versus low doses: a nonrandomized observation. Circulation. 2008;118:667–71.
15. Dagan A, Langevitz P, Shoenfeld Y, Shovman O. Anakinra in idiopathic recurrent pericarditis refractory to immunosuppressive therapy; a preliminary experience in seven patients. Autoimmun Rev. 2019;18:627–31.
16. Roubille F, Tournoux F, Roubille C, et al. Management of pericarditis and myocarditis: could heart-rate-reducing drugs hold a promise? Arch Cardiovasc Dis. 2013;106:672–9.

17. Buoro S, Tombetti E, Ceriotti F, Simon C, Cugola D, Seghezzi M, et al. What is the normal composition of pericardial fluid? Heart. 2020:heart-jnl-2020-317966. https://doi.org/10.1136/heartjnl-2020-317966.
18. Imazio M, Spodick DH, Brucato A, Trinchero R, Adler Y. Controversial issues in the management of pericardial diseases. Circulation. 2010;121(7):916–28.
19. Writing Committee, Drazner MH, Bozkurt B, Cooper LT, Aggarwal NR, Basso C, Bhave NM, Caforio ALP, Ferreira VM, Heidecker B, Kontorovich AR, Martín P, Roth GA, Van Eyk JE. 2024 ACC expert consensus decision pathway on strategies and criteria for the diagnosis and management of myocarditis: a report of the American College of Cardiology Solution Set Oversight Committee. J Am Coll Cardiol. 2024:S0735-1097(24)10040-X. https://doi.org/10.1016/j.jacc.2024.10.080. Epub ahead of print. PMID: 39665703.
20. Andreis A, Imazio M, Casula M, Avondo S, Brucato A. Recurrent pericarditis: an update on diagnosis and management. Intern Emerg Med. 2021;16(3):551–8. https://doi.org/10.1007/s11739-021-02639-6. Epub 2021 Feb 28. PMID: 33641044; PMCID: PMC7914388.
21. Refaat MM, Katz WE. Neoplastic pericardial effusion. Clin Cardiol. 2011;34(10):593–8. https://doi.org/10.1002/clc.20936. Epub 2011 Sep 16. PMID: 21928406; PMCID: PMC6652358.
22. Pérez-Casares A, Cesar S, Brunet-Garcia L, Sanchez-de-Toledo J. Echocardiographic evaluation of pericardial effusion and cardiac tamponade. Front Pediatr. 2017;5:79. https://doi.org/10.3389/fped.2017.00079. PMID: 28484689; PMCID: PMC5401877.
23. Khandaker MH, Espinosa RE, Nishimura RA, Sinak LJ, Hayes SN, Melduni RM, Oh JK. Pericardial disease: diagnosis and management. Mayo Clin Proc. 2010;85(6):572–93. https://doi.org/10.4065/mcp.2010.0046. PMID: 20511488; PMCID: PMC2878263.
24. Bolen MA, Rajiah P, Kusunose K, Collier P, Klein A, Popović ZB, Flamm SD. Cardiac MR imaging in constrictive pericarditis: multiparametric assessment in patients with surgically proven constriction. Int J Cardiovasc Imaging. 2015;31(4):859–66. https://doi.org/10.1007/s10554-015-0616-z. Epub 2015 Feb 12. PMID: 25672267.
25. Imazio M, Andreis A, Agosti A, Piroli F, Avondo S, Casula M, Paneva E, Squarotti GB, Giustetto C, De Ferrari GM. Usefulness of beta-blockers to control symptoms in patients with pericarditis. Am J Cardiol. 2021;146:115–9. https://doi.org/10.1016/j.amjcard.2021.01.032. Epub 2021 Feb 1. PMID: 33539856.
26. Yacoub M, Quintanilla Rodriguez BS, Mahajan K. Constrictive-effusive pericarditis. [Updated 2023 Jul 24]. In: StatPearls [Internet]. Treasure Island: StatPearls Publishing; 2025. Available from: https://www.ncbi.nlm.nih.gov/books/NBK519579/.
27. Wang TKM, Klein A, Cremer PC, Imazio M, Kohnstamm S, Luis SA, Mardigyan V, Mukherjee M, Ordovas K, Vakamudi S, Wohlford GF. 2025 Concise clinical guidance: an ACC expert consensus statement on the diagnosis and management of pericarditis. J Am Coll Cardiol. 2025;31. https://doi.org/10.1016/j.jacc.2025.05.023.

Cardiomyopathy

Contents

M. Salih, *Practical Hospitalist Guide to Inpatient Cardiology*, https://doi.org/10.1007/978-3-032-03240-9_9

This chapter reviews the clinical features, diagnostic challenges, and management principles of key cardiomyopathies encountered in hospitalized patients, focusing on *dilated cardiomyopathy (DCM)*, *hypertrophic obstructive cardiomyopathy (HOCM)*, and *cardiac amyloidosis*. DCM is characterized by ventricular dilation and systolic dysfunction, often presenting with heart failure symptoms. HOCM involves asymmetric septal hypertrophy causing dynamic outflow obstruction, frequently associated with exertional dyspnea, syncope, and arrhythmias. Cardiac amyloidosis results from extracellular amyloid protein deposition causing restrictive physiology, marked by diastolic dysfunction and signs of heart failure with preserved ejection fraction. This chapter emphasizes differentiating these entities through clinical clues, echocardiographic findings, cardiac MRI, and advanced imaging such as nuclear scintigraphy or biopsy in amyloidosis. Understanding these differences aids in tailoring treatment—ranging from medical therapy and device implantation in DCM and HOCM to targeted therapies in amyloidosis—and informs prognosis. Hospitalists are equipped with practical strategies for early recognition, appropriate diagnostic evaluation, and coordination with specialty care to optimize outcomes.

9.1 When to Suspect

- Infiltrative cardiac disease should be considered when cardiac dysfunction or symptomatology persists without a clear etiology after excluding common causative factors: ischemic heart disease (via left heart catheterization or stress testing), valvular heart disease (via echocardiographic findings), or significant hypertension (via clinical assessment). While often categorized as nonischemic cardiomyopathy by cardiologists, these conditions may present as acute decompensated heart failure in patients with preserved ejection fraction, necessitating careful diagnostic consideration before assuming primary HFpEF.
- Initial diagnostic evaluation should encompass electrocardiography, transthoracic echocardiography, ischemic assessment (stress testing or left heart catheterization based on coronary artery disease pretest probability), complete blood count (evaluating for significant anemia or eosinophilia), comprehensive metabolic panel (assessing hepatic function, uremia, and electrolyte disturbances), and thyroid function studies. Further targeted evaluation may be pursued based on clinical context.

Pearl

Patients presenting with new-onset unexplained cardiac dysfunction or heart failure with high pretest probability for coronary artery disease warrant direct left heart catheterization before classification as nonischemic cardiomyopathy.

Pearl

Endomyocardial biopsy should be selectively employed only when results alter the therapeutic approach, particularly in suspected giant cell myocarditis, hemochromatosis, amyloidosis, or sarcoidosis. This invasive diagnostic approach is typically reserved for cases of excluded ischemia presenting with new-onset ventricular arrhythmias or heart block.

9.2 Dilated Nonischemic Cardiomyopathy (DCM) [1]

- Nonischemic cardiomyopathytypically presents with new-onset systolic heart failure (HFrEF), cardiac conduction abnormalities (including bundle branch blocks and heart blocks), or sudden cardiac death. Ischemic evaluation typically reveals nonsignificant findings. While 50% of cases are idiopathic (potentially familial), secondary causes warrant thorough investigation. Dilated cardiomyopathy (DCM) often has a genetic basis, with autosomal dominant inheritance seen in about 25–40% of cases.

Pearl

Initial diagnostic uncertainty warrants expanded evaluation, which includes urine toxicology, alcohol levels, iron studies, serum/urine protein electrophoresis, free light chain analysis, and cardiac magnetic resonance imaging.

- Specific etiologies include the following:
    1. Alcoholic cardiomyopathy: Associated with chronic alcohol abuse, characterized by global hypokinesia and concurrent hepatic dysfunction. Management includes alcohol cessation and vitamin supplementation.
    2. Drug-induced cardiomyopathy: Primarily associated with chemotherapeutic agents but potentially caused by various medications. Anthracyclines, human epidermal growth factor receptor-2 (HER2) antagonists, immune checkpoint inhibitors, and select tyrosine kinase inhibitors may be associated with the development of left ventricular (LV) dysfunction and have emerged as an important etiologies of cardiomyopathy. Treatment involves discontinuation of causative agents.
    3. Stimulant-induced cardiomyopathy: Caused by cocaine or amphetamines, characterized by vasoconstriction-mediated ischemia. Management includes benzodiazepines or combined α/β-blockers (carvedilol/labetalol).
    4. Takotsubo cardiomyopathy: Stress-induced condition mimicking acute coronary syndrome, featuring apical ballooning without coronary

occlusion. Self-limiting with beta-blocker benefit for post-discharge mortality [2].

5. Tachycardia-induced cardiomyopathy: Associated with sustained tachyarrhythmias (AF, AVRT, AVNRT). Initial rate control followed by definitive ablation therapy.
6. Giant cell myocarditis: Affects middle-aged adults with rapid cardiac deterioration, arrhythmias, and conduction disorders. Requires immediate high-dose steroid therapy pending biopsy confirmation.
7. Hemochromatosis cardiomyopathy: Presents with conduction defects, fatigue, hepatic dysfunction, and endocrine abnormalities.
8. Cardiac sarcoidosis: Characterized by septal involvement with conduction abnormalities, diagnosed via PET-FDG or cardiac MRI.
9. Peripartum cardiomyopathy: Presents in peripartum or postpartum period, requiring immediate delivery and anticoagulation for LVEF <35%. Future pregnancies are contraindicated with persistent dysfunction.
10. Additional considerations include ischemic heart disease, HIV-associated cardiomyopathy, and eosinophilic myocarditis (characterized by hypereosinophilia, ADHF, and thromboembolism; diagnosed by MRI and treated with corticosteroids).

9.3 Cardiac Amyloidosis [3]

- Cardiac amyloidosis should be suspected in middle-aged or elderly patients presenting with unexplained cardiac dysfunction (predominantly diastolic), accompanied by characteristic echocardiographic findings (speckled myocardium with septal hypertrophy/LVH) and low-voltage electrocardiography. Atrial fibrillation frequently coexists due to atrial enlargement. Cardiac magnetic resonance imaging represents the most sensitive diagnostic modality. Management combines guideline-directed medical therapy with type-specific interventions. Cardiac amyloidosis is more common than we think.
  A. *Light chain (AL) cardiac amyloidosis* is associated with plasma cell dyscrasia, requiring diagnostic workup including serum/urine protein electrophoresis, 24-hour protein collection, and plasma free light chain analysis. Further investigation may require bone marrow or targeted organ/fat pad biopsy. This variant demonstrates increased propensity for cardiac thrombosis [4], and management involves oncology consultation for the underlying plasma cell disorder.
  B. *Transthyretin (ATTR) cardiac amyloidosis* shows higher prevalence in Black populations with TTR gene mutations and presents with concurrent neurological manifestations, including autonomic neuropathy, symmetrical distal neuropathy, and carpal tunnel syndrome. Diagnostic confirmation requires 99m-technetium pyrophosphate scintigraphy, possible endomyocardial biopsy, and TTR gene sequencing. Treatment options include tafamidis (FDA-approved protein stabilizer) and patisiran/inotersen (hepatic transthyretin production inhibitors), requiring specialized cardiology and amyloidosis center referral.

Pearl

Cardiac amyloidosis diagnosis requires either evidence of monoclonal plasma cell disorder or positive 99m-technetium pyrophosphate scintigraphy findings [3]. We should consider cardiac amyloidosis when we see patients with heart failure who have low voltage on ECG, unexplained LV hypertrophy, atrial fibrillation, conduction system disease, or previously diagnosed carpal tunnel syndrome or autonomic neuropathy.

Hospitalist Tip

Treat acute decompensated heart failure according to standard protocols, transition to guideline-directed medical therapy near discharge, avoid digoxin due to potential worsening of diastolic dysfunction, and implement anticoagulation for atrial fibrillation or intracardiac thrombus.

9.4 HOCM [5]

- Hypertrophic obstructive cardiomyopathy (HOCM) represents the most prevalent genetic cardiac condition, predominantly inherited in an autosomal dominant pattern. Clinical suspicion should arise with a family history of early cardiac complications or sudden death in young to middle-aged relatives. Peak presentation typically occurs between ages 30 and 40, and while often asymptomatic, hospitalists frequently encounter symptomatic cases.
- Common presentations in young adults include dyspnea, palpitations, syncope, and sudden cardiac death. Pathophysiology centers on left ventricular outflow tract (LVOT) obstruction due to asymmetric left ventricular hypertrophy and interventricular septal thickening, which results in ischemia, mitral regurgitation, and compromised cardiac output. Diastolic dysfunction manifests through impaired relaxation and increased stiffness. Physical examination typically reveals a dynamic systolic murmur in the parasternal area, exacerbated by preload-reducing maneuvers.
- Diagnostic evaluation includes electrocardiography, which may demonstrate LVH criteria (high-voltage QRS) and diffuse Q waves. Transthoracic echocardiography with Doppler imaging remains the primary diagnostic modality, revealing septal hypertrophy, mitral regurgitation, and LVOT obstruction. Cardiac magnetic resonance imaging offers high specificity and utility in cases of diagnostic uncertainty or suspected infiltrative disease. Inpatient telemetry monitoring is warranted for symptomatic patients to detect potentially lethal arrhythmias. Coronary angiography (CT or invasive) may be indicated when acute coronary syndrome is suspected.

Pearl

HOCM can mimic aortic stenosis but differs through a non-radiating, dynamic murmur, normal pulses, and an earlier age of presentation.

Pearl

Echocardiographic and cardiac MRI findings carry significant prognostic and therapeutic implications, particularly regarding ICD placement.

Pearl

Differential diagnosis includes aortic stenosis, cardiac amyloidosis (characterized by low QRS voltage, advanced age, and systemic manifestations), hypertensive heart disease, athlete's heart (normal function despite LVH), and rare genetic/metabolic conditions. Comprehensive evaluation through history, physical examination, electrocardiography, imaging, and selective additional testing enables appropriate differentiation. Adult-onset genetic conditions mimicking HOCM include Anderson-Fabry disease, Friedreich's ataxia, glycogen storage diseases, and mitochondrial disorders, typically presenting with concurrent neurological and renal manifestations.

- Common complications:
  - (i) Mitral regurgitation (MR)
  - (ii) AF
  - (iii) VT/VF leading to sudden death
  - (iv) CHF

- Treatment objectives in hypertrophic obstructive cardiomyopathy (HOCM) focus on reducing ventricular contractility while maintaining vascular resistance and afterload to optimize ventricular volume. Acute management prioritizes prevention of sudden cardiac death and heart failure manifestations. Inpatient management emphasizes maintenance of euvolemia and appropriate rhythm/rate control. Symptomatic patients with chest pain or dyspnea benefit from cardioselective non-vasodilating calcium channel blockers and beta-blockers (metoprolol succinate or bisoprolol). Acute decompensated heart failure requires cautious diuresis to avoid exacerbating LVOT obstruction through preload reduction. Guideline-directed medical therapy should be initiated upon achieving euvolemia, avoiding afterload-reducing agents. For patients developing systolic dysfunction (LVEF <50%), standard heart failure guidelines should be followed. Management of atrial fibrillation with rapid ventricular response requires aggressive rate control using calcium channel blockers, beta-blockers, and potentially amiodarone, as tachyarrhythmias are poorly tolerated. In cases of significant shock unresponsive to fluid resuscitation, intravenous phenylephrine (increases afterload) or other pure vasoconstrictors, with or without beta-blockade, is indicated. Anticoagulation with direct oral anticoagulants is mandatory for all HOCM patients with atrial fibrillation, regardless of thromboembolic risk scores. Mavacamten represents the only FDA-approved agent for patients with obstructive HCM refractory to first-line therapy. Discharge planning should include counseling regarding activity modification and avoiding extreme exertion while maintaining low to moderate exercise levels to prevent dehydration. Exercise stress testing helps individualize activity recommendations. Genetic counseling referral is essential due to familial implications and the benefits of cascade genetic testing. Long-term interventional management options for medically refractory, symptomatic patients include surgical septal myectomy or alcohol septal ablation. ICD is indicated for the following patients:

A. Previous SCD
B. Sustained ventricular tachycardia
C. Other high-risk patients (sudden death in a first-degree relative, ≥1 episode of arrhythmogenic syncope, LV apical aneurysm, LVEF <50%, LV wall thickness ≥30 mm)

Pearl

Critical management principles in HOCM focus on avoiding three key physiologic derangements: hypovolemia, hypotension/reduced afterload, and tachycardia, as these conditions compromise ventricular filling and exacerbate obstruction.

Pearl

Specific pharmacologic contraindications in HOCM include:
(i) Digoxin in atrial fibrillation, as enhanced contractility exacerbates LVOT obstruction
(ii) Afterload-reducing agents (including amlodipine, nitrates, hydralazine, carvedilol, ACE inhibitors, and ARBs), which may worsen LVOT obstruction through reduced ventricular volume

Pearl

Hypertension management in HOCM patients should emphasize lifestyle modifications combined with selective pharmacotherapy, preferentially utilizing beta blockers and non-dihydropyridine calcium channel blockers.

9.5 Restrictive Cardiomyopathy and Constrictive Pericarditis

- Both were discussed in ▸ Chap. 8, acute pericarditis complications.

References

1. Ferreira A, Ferreira V, Antunes MM, Lousinha A, Pereira-da-Silva T, Antunes D, Cunha PS, Oliveira M, Ferreira RC, Rosa SA. Dilated cardiomyopathy: a comprehensive approach to diagnosis and risk stratification. Biomedicines. 2023;11(3):834. https://doi.org/10.3390/biomedicines11030834. PMID: 36979813; PMCID: PMC10044994.
2. Raposeiras-Roubin S, Santoro F, Arcari L, Vazirani R, Novo G, Uribarri A, Enrica M, Lopez-Pais J, Guerra F, Alfonso F, Pätz T, Fernandez-Cordon C, Montisci R, Corbi-Pascual M, Marchetti MF, Almendro M, Cacciotti L, Vedia O, El-Battrawy I, Blanco-Ponce E, Brunetti ND, Akin I, Martinez-Sellés M, Thiele H, Stiermaier T, Eitel I, Nuñez-Gil IJ, GEIS-TRESEARCHERS. Betablockers and long-term mortality in Takotsubo syndrome: results of the multicenter GEIST Registry. JACC Heart Fail. 2025:S2213-1779(24)00881-3. https://doi.org/10.1016/j.jchf.2024.11.015. Epubaheadofprint.PMID:39918532.
3. Writing Committee, Kittleson MM, Ruberg FL, Ambardekar AV, Branna-gan TH, Cheng RK, Clarke JO, Dember LM, Frantz JG, Hershberger RE, Maurer MS, Nativi-Nicolau J, Sanchorawala V, Sheikh FH. 2023 ACC expert consensus decision pathway on comprehensive multidisciplinary care for the patient with cardiac amyloidosis: a report of the American College of Cardiology Solution Set Oversight Committee. J Am Coll Cardiol. 2023;81(11):1076–126. https://doi.org/10.1016/j.jacc.2022.11.022. Epub 2023 Jan 23. Erratum in: J Am Coll Cardiol. 2023;81(11):1135. https://doi.org/10.1016/j.jacc.2023.02.013. PMID: 36697326.

4. Feng D, Syed IS, Martinez M, Oh JK, Jaffe AS, Grogan M, Edwards WD, Gertz MA, Klarich KW. Intracardiac thrombosis and anticoagulation therapy in cardiac amyloidosis. Circulation. 2009;119(18):2490–7. https://doi.org/10.1161/CIRCULATIONAHA.108.785014. Epub 2009 May 4. PMID: 19414641.
5. Ommen SR, Ho CY, Asif IM, Balaji S, Burke MA, Day SM, Dearani JA, Epps KC, Evanovich L, Ferrari VA, Joglar JA, Khan SS, Kim JJ, Kittleson MM, Krittanawong C, Martinez MW, Mital S, Naidu SS, Saberi S, Semsarian C, Times S, Waldman CB. 2024 AHA/ACC/AMSSM/HRS/PACES/SCMR guideline for managing hypertrophic cardiomyopathy: a report of the American Heart Association/American College of Cardiology Joint Committee on Clinical Practice Guidelines. Circulation. 2024;149(23):e1239–311. https://doi.org/10.1161/CIR.0000000000001250. Epub 2024 May 8. Erratum in: Circulation. 2024;150(8):e198. https://doi.org/10.1161/CIR.0000000000001277. PMID: 38718139.

Perioperative Cardiac Evaluation

Contents

M. Salih, *Practical Hospitalist Guide to Inpatient Cardiology*, https://doi.org/10.1007/978-3-032-03240-9_10

This chapter provides a practical guide for hospitalists on perioperative cardiac risk assessment and anticoagulation management to optimize patient safety during surgery. It outlines a stepwise approach to cardiac evaluation, incorporating clinical risk indices, functional capacity assessment, and targeted diagnostic testing such as ECG, echocardiography, and stress testing. This chapter emphasizes stratifying patients based on cardiovascular risk and the urgency and invasiveness of surgery to guide decision-making. Special focus is given to managing patients on chronic anticoagulation or antiplatelet therapy, balancing thromboembolic risks against bleeding complications, and strategies for perioperative bridging or temporary interruption. It reviews guidelines for common scenarios, including atrial fibrillation, mechanical heart valves, and venous thromboembolism history. Coordination with cardiology, anesthesia, and surgical teams is highlighted to ensure individualized planning. This chapter equips hospitalists with evidence-based tools to reduce perioperative cardiac events and optimize anticoagulation strategies in diverse patient populations.

10.1 How Do You risk Stratify Your Patients? [1]

- Preoperative cardiac risk assessment involves stratifying patients based on comorbidities, surgical urgency, functional capacity, and the presence of acute cardiac conditions.
- The primary determinant is surgical urgency. Low-risk procedures may proceed without additional cardiac evaluation in the absence of acute cardiac issues. Emergent surgeries (involving immediate risk to life or limb) take precedence over cardiac risk factors. For elective procedures, cardiac stability assessment is paramount; acute coronary syndrome, decompensated heart failure, or unstable arrhythmias warrant primary cardiac intervention.
- In non-urgent cases without acute cardiac conditions, perioperative cardiac risk assessment becomes essential. The Revised Cardiac Risk Index (RCRI) provides a validated tool for inpatient risk stratification. Patients with calculated risk below 1% may proceed to surgery without further cardiac evaluation. Functional capacity assessment using metabolic equivalents (METS) guides management for higher-risk patients. Patients demonstrating METS ≥4 may proceed to surgery. In contrast, those with poor functional capacity (<4 METS) may benefit from cardiac stress testing or coronary computed tomography angiography (CCTA), provided that the results would influence surgical timing decisions.
- Routine preoperative invasive coronary angiography is not indicated for perioperative risk modification [7]. Angiography is reserved for acute coronary syndrome or hemodynamically significant left main coronary stenosis ≥50% [1].
- Preoperative biomarker assessment (B-type natriuretic peptide, N-terminal pro-B-type natriuretic peptide, or cardiac troponin) may be appropriate in patients over 65 with a cardiovascular disease history or cardiac symptoms, offering high prognostic and negative predictive value for perioperative cardiac complications [1].

Pearl

Surgical timing classification distinguishes between urgent procedures (requiring intervention within 6–24 hours) and emergent procedures (necessitating intervention within 6 hours) based on imminent risk to life or limb.

Pearl

Indications for preoperative cardiac stress testing parallel those for non-surgical patients. Testing should be pursued based on comprehensive cardiovascular risk assessment rather than solely for perioperative risk stratification. Notably, patients with chronic stable angina may not derive additional benefit from preoperative stress testing [2].

Pearl

The MDCalc application facilitates the calculation of the Revised Cardiac Risk Index (RCRI) and functional capacity assessment. The Duke Activity Status Index (DASI) provides standardized metabolic equivalent (METS) quantification [1]. Special consideration should be given to elderly patients with advanced frailty, impaired functional status, and limited life expectancy, as surgical intervention may offer minimal benefit. In such cases, incorporating goals of care discussions and shared decision-making becomes crucial for preoperative planning. The Clinical Frailty Scale, available through MDCalc, provides an evidence-based assessment tool for frailty evaluation, as endorsed by current guidelines [1].

10.2 Stepwise Approach to Preoperative Cardiac Assessment [1]

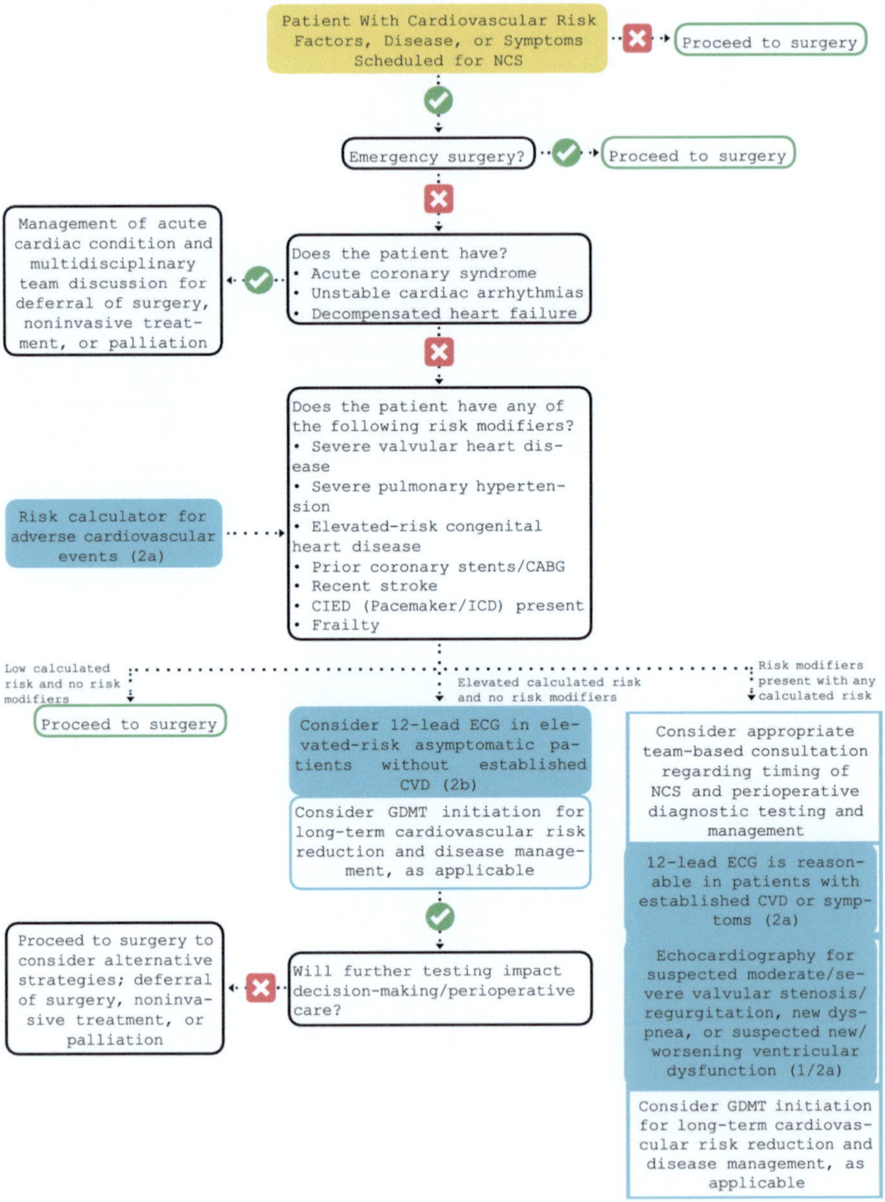

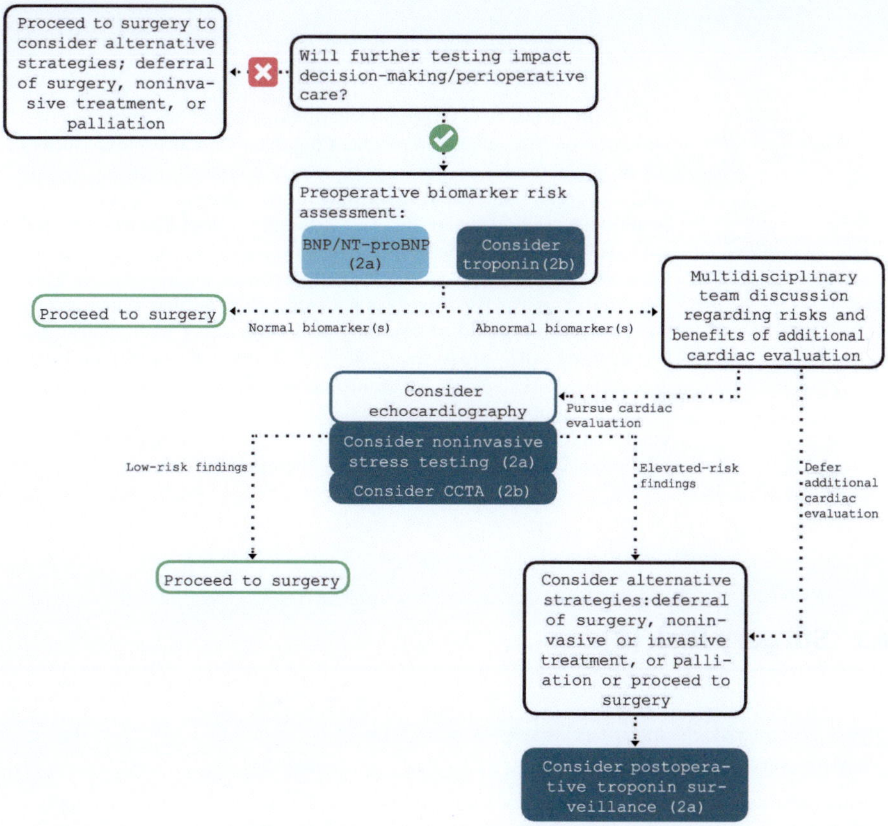

Pearl

Management of patients presenting with acute decompensated heart failure, acute coronary syndrome, or hemodynamically significant arrhythmias requires coordinated multidisciplinary collaboration among hospitalists, cardiology, surgical, and anesthesiology services to optimize cardiovascular status before surgical intervention [1].

Pearl

Significant variation exists among international guidelines regarding preoperative cardiac evaluation. The Canadian Cardiovascular Society (CCS) guidelines reject routine preoperative noninvasive cardiac testing solely for risk stratification, advocating for risk assessment based on age, established cardiovascular disease, Revised Cardiac Risk Index, and B-type natriuretic peptide levels [4]. In contrast, the European Society of Cardiology (ESC) 2022 guidelines endorse stress imaging before high-risk elective noncardiac surgery in patients with poor functional capacity and elevated likelihood of coronary artery disease or high clinical risk [5], aligning with American College of Cardiology/American Heart Association (ACC/AHA) recommendations [1]. Both CCS and ESC guidelines support BNP assessment in high-risk patients and provide limited endorsement for postoperative troponin monitoring (days 1–3) in high-cardiac-risk patients to monitor ischemic events.

10.3 Surgery Risk [2]

Perioperative risk classifications for surgical procedures

Low (<1%)	Intermediate (1%–5%)	High (>5%)
Superficial surgery Breast Dental Cataract Endoscopic Thyroid Gynecologic, minor Orthopedic, minor Urologic, minor (TURP, TURBT) Reconstructive/cosmetic VATS for minor lung resection	Intrathoracic (non major) Intraperitoneal (splenectomy, cholecystectomy, hiatal hernia repair) Carotid, asymptomatic (CEA or CAS) Carotid, symptomatic (CEA) Endovascular aneurysm repair (stents/coils) Head and neck surgery Neurologic or orthopedic, major (hip and spine surgery) Peripheral artery angioplasty Urologic or gynecologic, major Renal transplant	Aortic and major vascular surgery Major abdominal surgery and prolonged blood loss (duodenopancreatic, liver resection, bile duct surgery, perforated bowel, total cystectomy) Esophagectomy Pneumonectomy (VATS or open surgery) Lung, liver, or pancreas transplant Adrenal resection Carotid, symptomatic (CAS) CAS = carotid artery stenting; CEA = carotid endarterectomy; TURBT = transurethral resection of a bladder tumor; TURP = transurethral resection of the prostate; VATS = video-assisted thoracoscopic surgery

Pearl

Perioperative cardiovascular complications demonstrate the highest incidence in the context of major urgent or emergent noncardiac surgical procedures, with particular prevalence in vascular, thoracic, and transplant interventions. Risk stratification follows a direct correlation with comorbidity burden; increased patient comorbidities correspond to elevated risk for perioperative cardiovascular complications [2].

10.4 Clinical Approach and Workup [1]

- Preoperative evaluation requires a comprehensive cardiac history and physical examination, supplemented by selective laboratory and imaging studies and validated risk assessment tools, including the Revised Cardiac Risk Index (RCRI) and Duke Activity Status Index (DASI). Baseline electrocardiography is warranted for patients with established cardiovascular disease or those undergoing intermediate to high-risk procedures [1].
- Perioperative management should emphasize several key interventions: maintenance of normothermia throughout the perioperative period, preoperative iron replacement (oral or intravenous) 1–2 weeks before surgery in iron-deficiency anemia to minimize transfusion requirements, administration of tranexamic acid in procedures with elevated bleeding risk, and implementation of restrictive transfusion protocols with hemoglobin threshold of 8 g/dL for orthopedic surgery patients and those with cardiovascular disease.
- ECHO is needed only when:
  (a) New cardiac symptoms (such as new SOB, chest pain, and ADHF)
  (b) New physical findings (murmur, abnormal new heart sounds, arrhythmias, etc.)
  (c) No recent echo for a patient with a known CHF history within 1 year
- Postoperative surveillance in high-risk patients may include troponin monitoring for 48–72 hours to detect acute coronary syndrome. In cases of postoperative non-ST-elevation myocardial infarction, management should parallel that of spontaneous acute coronary syndrome, with therapeutic modifications accounting for postoperative bleeding risk and hemodynamic status. This decision-making process necessitates collaborative assessment among cardiology, surgery, and primary teams to optimize outcomes while minimizing procedural complications.

Pearl

A comprehensive preoperative assessment must encompass a detailed medication review, evaluation for bleeding diatheses, and documentation of a history of malignant hyperthermia, as these factors significantly influence perioperative management strategies.

Pearl

Laboratory evaluation should follow a targeted approach based on specific clinical indications rather than universal screening protocols. Advanced age alone does not constitute sufficient justification for extensive preoperative laboratory testing.

10.5 Recommended Laboratory Testing Before Elective Noncardiac Surgery [2]

Laboratory test	Indication
Hemoglobin level	Anticipated major blood loss based on type of surgery or symptoms of anemia, known anemia, or liver or kidney disease
Leukocyte count	Symptoms suggesting infection, myeloproliferative disorder, or myelotoxic medications
Platelet count	History of bleeding diathesis, myeloproliferative disorder, or myelotoxic medications; liver disease
Prothrombin time	History of bleeding diathesis, liver disease, malnutrition, recent or long-term antibiotic, warfarin use
Partial thromboplastin time	History of bleeding diathesis, heparin use
Metabolic panel	Known renal insufficiency, hypertension, diabetes, congestive heart failure, liver disease, endocrine dysfunction, dedications, which affect electrolytes

Laboratory test	Indication
Glucose level	Known diabetes or glucocorticoid use
Liver function tests	Cirrhosis
Urinalysis	Symptoms suggestive of urinary tract infection, recent instrumentation of the genitourinary tract
Electrocardiography	Known coronary artery disease, diabetes, uncontrolled hypertension, chronic kidney disease
Chest radiography	Symptoms of examination findings suggestive of active pulmonary disease, active cardiac disease, or recent respiratory infection
Echocardiography	Clinically suspected moderate or severe valvular stenosis or regurgitation if prior echocardiogram >1 year ago or significant change in clinical or physical examination findings Reasonable for noninvasive evaluation of left ventricular function in patients with current heart failure or dyspnea Not recommended in asymptomatic patients having low- or intermediate-risk surgery

Pearl

Smoking cessation for as little as 4 weeks before surgery can decrease postoperative complications. If surgery could be delayed, it is advisable to wait [3].

10.6 Managing Specific Populations and Common Concerns

I. *ADHF/CHF*

- Management of acute decompensated heart failure should precede nonurgent surgical intervention, with restoration to baseline clinical status as a prerequisite. For urgent procedures, careful risk-benefit analysis must guide decision-making. Maintenance of systolic blood pressure ≥90 mmHg is recommended to minimize myocardial injury risk [1].
- Guideline-directed medical therapy should be continued perioperatively without specific contraindications, except sodium-glucose cotransporter-2 inhibitors (SGLT2i). These agents should be discontinued 3–4 days preoperatively to mitigate the risk of perioperative metabolic acidosis.

II. *Patients with a history of CAD* [1]

- Routine cardiac testing or left heart catheterization is not indicated for patients with stable, medically managed coronary artery disease. Stress testing should be pursued only when clinically indicated, independent of surgical planning. In emergent or urgent surgery, procedures should proceed despite the elevated risk of major adverse cardiovascular events (MACE), with risk quantification via the RCRI calculator informing patient and surgical team discussions.
- Elective surgery timing varies based on underlying cardiac conditions: drug-eluting stent placement necessitates a 3–6 month delay; post-acute coronary syndrome with stent placement warrants a 1-year delay; bare metal stent placement requires a 1-month delay due to lower acute thrombosis risk; and post-balloon angioplasty procedures require a minimum 2-week delay. Postoperative cardiac testing should be symptom-driven rather than routine.
- Perioperative medication management includes continuing aspirin throughout procedures, substituting aspirin for discontinued oral anticoagulation when feasible, and maintaining statin and beta-blocker therapy. Initiation of statins and beta-blockers is indicated preoperatively for elevated cardiac risk procedures, with beta-blockers started 1–2 weeks preoperatively to avoid increased stroke and mortality risk [6]. Selective discontinuation of ACE inhibitors/ARBs and diuretics may be necessary. Transfusion thresholds should be modified for type 1 acute myocardial infarction, with more liberal targets of 9–10 g/dL [7].

Pearl

If the antiplatelets are interrupted early before the specified duration, the risk of stent thrombosis might increase.

10.7 Optimal Timing of Elective or Time-Sensitive NCS for Prior PCI Requiring Management of DAPT [1]

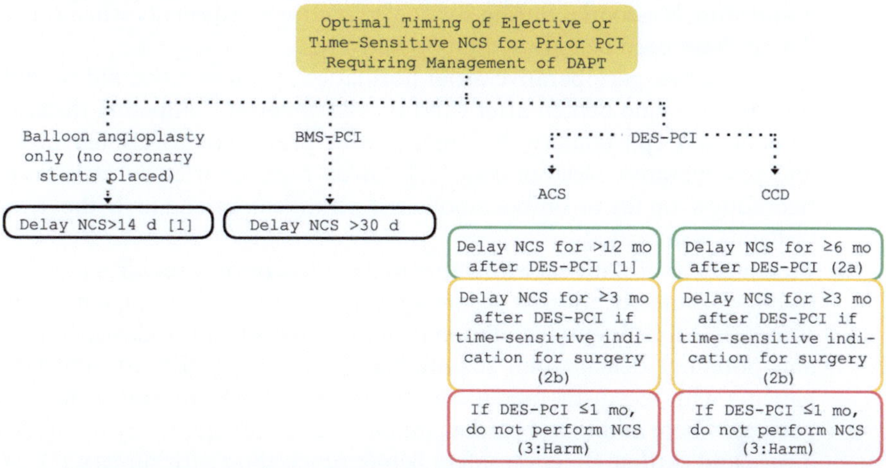

III. *VHD*
- Valvular heart disease (VHD) management in the acute urgent surgical setting requires individualized risk-benefit assessment. If time allows, perioperative transthoracic echocardiography is appropriate for comprehensive evaluation in all surgical candidates.
- Management strategy for nonurgent or elective procedures varies according to symptomatology and disease severity.
  A. *In symptomatic VHD* or significant cardiac dysfunction, valve intervention before noncardiac surgery is preferred, particularly in symptomatic aortic stenosis.
  B. *Asymptomatic patients* may proceed with time-sensitive, low-risk procedures; however, higher-risk patients require careful consideration and explicit risk communication with surgical teams. Cardiology consultation is recommended for preoperative risk stratification, especially in severe valvular disease or planned moderate to high-risk surgical intervention.

IV. *Cardiac arrhythmias*
- Management of acute arrhythmias with hemodynamic compromise takes precedence over surgical intervention, necessitating adherence to Advanced Cardiac Life Support protocols. Patients with established atrial fibrillation or heart failure carry an elevated risk for postoperative arrhythmic complications.

- Perioperative management requires optimizing hemodynamics, volume status, and potential precipitating factors, including infection and pain. Antiarrhythmic therapy should be maintained, particularly in patients with atrial fibrillation or ventricular arrhythmias. Continuous telemetry monitoring is essential during surgical procedures, especially when cardiac devices have been deactivated preoperatively.
- For new-onset perioperative atrial fibrillation, postoperative anticoagulation may provide benefit after careful assessment of competing thromboembolic risk (particularly in patients with prior cerebrovascular events) and perioperative bleeding risk [12]. Given high recurrence rates, outpatient follow-up for thromboembolic risk stratification and arrhythmia surveillance is indicated.
- Management of patients with implanted cardiac devices requires preoperative device interrogation to ensure appropriate function. In urgent surgical scenarios, cardiology consultation facilitates assessment of device function and potential deactivation requirements. This is particularly crucial in patients with recent therapeutic interventions (shocks or anti-tachycardia pacing), where additional cardiac evaluation may be necessary to establish device and cardiac function safety before proceeding with surgery.

Pearl

Perioperative management should prioritize maintenance of euvolemic status while preventing hypotension and significant arrhythmic events.

Pearl

Asymptomatic atrial fibrillation does not warrant additional preoperative evaluation before noncardiac surgery. However, when ventricular rates exceed 110 beats per minute, surgical delay is appropriate to achieve adequate rate control.

V. *Patients with HTN*

- Hypertensive emergency requires stabilization before surgical clearance. In cases of hypertensive urgency, blood pressure reduction below 180/110 mmHg is reasonable before surgical intervention, although supporting evidence for this practice remains limited [1].
- Most antihypertensive medications can be continued perioperatively, with notable exceptions:
  A. Angiotensin-converting enzyme inhibitors and angiotensin receptor blockers warrant specific consideration: continuation is appropriate for heart failure with reduced ejection fraction or poorly controlled hypertension. However, when used solely for hypertension management, these agents may be suspended 24 hours preoperatively due to risks of acute kidney injury and perioperative hypotension. Resumption should occur within 48 hours to avoid increased mortality risk [1]. Persistent perioperative hypertension may justify immediate medication resumption.
  B. Diuretic therapy should be temporarily discontinued on the day of surgery to minimize the risks of hypotension, acute kidney injury, and hypovolemia. Resumption should occur upon achievement of clinical stability.

VI. *Pulmonary hypertension (PHT)*

- Preoperative transthoracic echocardiography is indicated for all patients with established pulmonary hypertension who have not had a recent echocardiographic evaluation to assess right ventricular function.
- Symptomatic pulmonary hypertension, particularly with documented mean pulmonary artery pressure exceeding 40 mmHg on recent or previous echocardiography, necessitates pulmonary hypertension specialist or pulmonologist consultation before surgical intervention, given elevated mortality and morbidity risk and potential requirement for invasive hemodynamic monitoring.
- Management principles emphasize avoiding hypovolemia, which compromises preload in these preload-dependent patients. Additional priorities include optimal blood pressure control to minimize afterload and maintenance of normal sinus rhythm and rate, as tachycardia reduces diastolic filling time, which is critical for cardiac output. Pulmonary vascular targeted therapies should be maintained unless specifically contraindicated by specialist consultation.

Pearl

Given the significant prevalence of undiagnosed obstructive sleep apnea (OSA) in the general population, the American Society of Anesthesiologists (ASA) advocates universal preoperative screening before noncardiac surgery. The STOP-Bang Questionnaire represents the validated screening instrument of choice, with particular emphasis on evaluating patients with elevated body mass index.

VII. *Patients with hip fractures*

- Hip fracture repair or replacement procedures are categorically classified as urgent surgical interventions. Surgical clearance should generally be granted unless contraindicated by acute coronary syndrome or significant hemodynamic compromise (including acute decompensated heart failure, hemodynamically unstable arrhythmias, or severe chronic obstructive pulmonary disease exacerbation).
- Current American Academy of Orthopaedic Surgeons guidelines advocate surgical intervention within 24–48 hours of admission [8]. Surgical delays exceeding 24 hours correlate with increased risk of pulmonary embolism, myocardial infarction, and pneumonia.
- For high-risk patients, surgeons may opt for less invasive approaches such as percutaneous pinning. In cases of prohibitive surgical risk or pre-existing severe functional or cognitive impairment, nonoperative management with a palliative focus may be appropriate [9]. While acute cardiac conditions require expedited evaluation and treatment preoperatively, evidence does not support routine noninvasive cardiac testing in asymptomatic patients [10]. The morbidity associated with surgical delay typically outweighs potential benefits, even in elevated troponin levels [10, 11].
- Preoperative testing should be selective and targeted, with clear potential to impact perioperative management rather than following routine protocols.

10.8 Perioperative Anticoagulant

10.8.1 How to Approach Your Patient [13]

- Perioperative management of antithrombotic therapy requires careful assessment, balancing procedural bleeding risk against patient-specific thrombotic risk. The bleeding risk profile determines the necessity of antithrombotic discontinuation, while thrombotic risk assessment guides bridging decisions (specifically for warfarin therapy). This risk stratification framework generates four distinct clinical scenarios: Critical document review should encompass previous discharge summaries, recent cardiology clinic notes, primary care documentation, and relevant specialty consultation records, enabling a comprehensive assessment of the patient's clinical complexity.

1. Concurrent low bleeding and thrombotic risk: Continuation of antithrombotic therapy is appropriate.
2. Low bleeding risk with high thrombotic risk: Maintenance of antithrombotic therapy is indicated.
3. High bleeding risk with high thrombotic risk: Antithrombotic discontinuation with heparin bridging when feasible.
4. High bleeding risk with low thrombotic risk: Antithrombotic discontinuation without bridging therapy.

10.8.2 Procedure Bleeding Risk [14]

Risk classification for surgery/procedure-related bleeding[a]	
High-bleed-risk surgery/procedure[b] (30-day risk of major bleed ≥2%)	Major surgery with extensive tissue injury Cancer surgery, especially solid tumor resection (lung, esophagus, colon, hepatobiliary, pancreatic) Major orthopedic surgery, including shoulder replacement surgery Reconstructive plastic surgery Major thoracic surgery Urologic or gastrointestinal surgery, especially anastomosis surgery Transurethral prostate resection, bladder resection, or tumor ablation Nephrectomy,kidney biopsy Colonic polyp resection Bowel resection Percutaneous endoscopic gastrostomy placement, endoscopic retrograde cholangiopancreatography Surgery in highly vascular organs (kidneys, liver, spleen) Cardiac, intracranial, or spinal surgery Any major operation (procedure duration >45 minutes) Neuraxial anesthesia[e] Epidural injections
Low/moderate- bleed-risk surgery/procedure[c] (30-day risk of major bleed 0%–2%)	Arthroscopy Cutaneous/lymph node biopsies Foot/hand surgery Coronary angiography by femoral artery approach Gastrointestinal endoscopy ± biopsy[d] Colonoscopy ± biopsy[d] Abdominal hysterectomy Laparoscopic cholecystectomy Abdominal hernia repair Hemorrhoidal surgery Bronchoscopy ± biopsy

Risk classification for surgery/procedure-related bleeding[a]	
Minimal-bleed-risk surgery/procedure[d] (30-day risk of major bleed ~0%)	Minor dermatologic procedures (excision of basal and squamous cell skin cancers, actinic keratoses, and premaligant or cancerous skin nevi) Ophthalmological (cataract) procedures Minor dental procedures (dental extractions, restorations, prosthetics, endodontis), dental cleanings, fillings Pacemaker or cardioverter-defibrillator device implantation Coronary angiography by radial artery approach Selected patients requiring screening gastrointestinal endoscopy and colonoscopy ± biopsy[f]

[a]Adapted from the 2022 CHEST Guidelines

[b]No residual anticoagulant effect at the procedure (i.e., four interruption preprocedure)

[c]Some residual anticoagulant effect allowed (i.e., two to three drug half-life interruption preprocedure)

[d]Procedure can be safely done under full-dose anticoagulation (may consider holding direct oral anticoagulant dose on the day of the procedure to avoid peak anticoagulant effects)

[e]Includes spinal and epidural anesthesia or any other neuraxial (e.g., pain management) intervention; consider not only the absolute risk for major bleeding but also potentially devastating consequences of epidural bleeding and associated lower limb paralysis

[f]Selected patients, especially if talking a vitamin K antagonist and in whom polypectomy is not anticipated, may be classified as minimal-bleed-risk; whether they are classified as low/moderate-bleed-risk (requiring anticoagulant interruption) or minimal-bleed-risk (not requiring anticoagulant interruption) should be based on individual patient characteristics and in discussion with the proceduralist

Pearl

Surgical bleeding risk stratification follows specific temporal and procedural criteria. Low-risk procedures are characterized by an operative duration of less than 1 hour and typically include ambulatory interventions. Conversely, high bleeding risk is associated with procedures exceeding 1 hour in duration or involving neuraxial anesthesia (epidural or spinal approaches).

10.8.3 Primary Thrombotic Risk of the Patient [14]

Risk classification for thromboembolism[a]			
Risk category	Mechanical heart valve	Atrial fibrillation	Venous thromboembolism
High (>10%/year risk of ATE or >10%/month risk of VTE)	Mechanical mitral valve *with* risk factors for stroke[b] Caged ball or tilting disc valve in mitral/ aortic position Recent (<3 months) stroke or TIA	CHA_2DS_2VASc score of ≥7 $CHADS_2$ score of 5 or 6 Recent (<3 months) stroke or TIA Rheumatic valvular heart disease	Recent (<3 months and especially 1 month) VTE Severe thrombophilia (deficiency of protein C, protein S, or antithrombin; homozygous factor V Leiden or prothrombin gene mutation or double-heterozygous for each mutation, multiple thrombophilias) Antiphospholipid syndrome Active cancer associated with high VTE risk[c]
Moderate (4%–10%/year risk of ATE or 4%–10%/month risk of VTE)	Bileaflet AVR *with* major risk factors for stroke[b]	CHA_2DS_2VASc score of 5 or 6 $CHADS_2$ score of 3 or 4	VTE within the past 3–12 months Recurrent VTE Nonsevere thrombophilia (heterozygous factor V Leiden or prothrombin gene mutation) Active cancer or recent history of cancer[d]
Low (<4%/year risk of ATE or <2%/month risk of VTE)	Bileaflet AVR *without* major risk factors for stroke[b]	CHA_2DS_2VASc score of 1–4 $CHADS_2$ score of 0–2 (and no prior stroke or TIA)	VTE more than 12 months ago

[a]Adapted from the 2022 CHEST Guidelines. *ATE* arterial thromboembolism, *AVR* aortic valve replacement, *TIA* transient ischemic attack, *VTE* venous thromboembolism

[b]Includes atrial fibrillation, prior stroke or transient ischemic attack (including during perioperative period), prior valve thrombosis, rheumatic valvular heart disease, hypertension, diabetes, congestive heart failure, age >75 years

[c]Incudes pancreatic cancer, myeloproliferative disorders, primary brain cancer, gastric cancer, and esophageal cancer

[d]Within 5 years if history of cancer, excluding nonmelanoma skin cancer

10.8.4 Approach for Patients Taking Warfarin

- Warfarin discontinuation is indicated 5 days preoperatively for high-bleeding-risk procedures. Bridging therapy is reserved for patients with elevated High thrombotic risk. Upon discontinuation, target INR should approximate the normal range (1.3–1.4) during surgery, with evening resumption at previous dosing. Postoperative bridging is unnecessary for patients without high thrombotic risk when resuming warfarin.

- In cases where warfarin continuation is indicated (low bleeding risk with high thrombotic risk), INR should remain below 3.0.
- Urgent/emergent surgery requiring warfarin reversal necessitates INR reduction below 2.0. Management options include prothrombin complex concentrates (30 IU/kg) for active bleeding or fresh frozen plasma (2–6 units) in non-bleeding scenarios. Elective surgery preparation utilizes oral/intravenous vitamin K (2.5–5 mg).

Hospitalist Tip

Extended interruption beyond 5 days may be necessary for patients with elevated INR or impaired warfarin elimination, including those with chronic kidney disease, advanced age, or hepatic dysfunction.

Pearl

Heparin/low molecular weight heparin bridging (exclusive to warfarin therapy) is indicated when thrombotic risk exceeds bleeding risk, yet surgical bleeding risk necessitates perioperative warfarin interruption.

10.8.5 Approach for Patients Taking DOAC "Direct Oral Anticoagulant" (Eliquis®/Xarelto®)

- For low-risk bleeding procedures, direct oral anticoagulant (DOAC) continuation is appropriate, with morning dose omission to avoid peak drug effect during the procedure.
- Given these medications' approximately 12-hour half-life and 2–3-hour onset of action, high-bleeding-risk procedures require DOAC discontinuation for 2 days (ensuring four half-lives for drug clearance). Standard resumption occurs after at least 24 hours, contingent upon surgical team clearance for high-bleeding-risk cases.
- Bridging therapy is contraindicated with DOACs due to their pharmacokinetic profile, as studies demonstrate increased major bleeding risk without improved thromboembolic prevention [15, 16]. Occasionally, as a hospitalist, when a patient on a DOAC is acutely hospitalized and surgery is anticipated but not yet confirmed, or the bleeding risk is likely to increase, it is reasonable to temporarily hold the DOAC and use unfractionated heparin or LMWH (usually at the next scheduled DOAC dose) until the surgical plan becomes clearer. This approach does not constitute bridging therapy at this stage.

- Urgent/emergent surgery requiring DOAC reversal utilizes prothrombin complex concentrates (30 IU/kg) for active bleeding or emergent surgery. Alternative agents include andexanet-alpha (approved for rivaroxaban and apixaban) or idarucizumab (dabigatran), which is administered as a loading dose with subsequent infusion.

Pearl

DOAC management varies by procedural bleeding risk: continuation for low-risk, 1-day discontinuation for intermediate risk, and 2-day discontinuation for high-risk procedures.

Pearl

Post-procedural DOAC resumption timing varies: approximately 24 hours post-low/moderate-risk procedures and 48–72 hours post-high-risk procedures. During the postoperative holding period, prophylactic low molecular weight heparin may be administered for 48–72 hours in high venous thromboembolism risk surgeries pending DOAC resumption.

Pearl

Routine anti-factor X or DOAC level monitoring is not indicated for perioperative bleeding risk assessment. Such testing should be reserved for time-sensitive surgical cases with specific bleeding concerns. Levels below 30–50 ng/mL do not correlate with increased perioperative bleeding risk [17].

10.8.6 Approach for Patients Taking Antiplatelets [13, 14]

- Perioperative management of antiplatelet therapy for high-bleeding-risk surgery varies by clinical context:
  A. *Single antiplatelet therapy (aspirin or P2Y12 inhibitors)*:

   (i) Discontinuation for a minimum of 4 days preoperatively in stable coronary artery disease without prior revascularization.
   (ii) Continuation recommended for patients with vascular/cardiac stenting, established coronary artery disease, low-bleeding-risk procedures, or acute coronary syndrome within 1 year, subject to surgical team approval.

B. *Dual antiplatelet therapy (DAPT)*:
   (i) Continuation of both agents is appropriate for low-bleeding-risk procedures.
   (ii) For higher bleeding risk, maintain aspirin while discontinuing P2Y12 inhibitors 3–10 days preoperatively (minimum 5–7 days for clopidogrel).
   (iii) Recent drug-eluting stent placement (within 1 month) may warrant DAPT continuation or bridging with short-acting glycoprotein IIb/IIIa inhibitors (tirofiban, eptifibatide) under cardiologist guidance.
   (iv) For CABG candidates, continue aspirin while discontinuing clopidogrel/prasugrel 5 days preoperatively.

Pearl

Aspirin continuation is recommended for low-/intermediate–bleeding-risk procedures, given its association with reduced perioperative major vascular thromboembolism [17]. However, de novo aspirin initiation preoperatively is not indicated.

10.8.7 How Does Bridging Work? [13, 18, 19]

Pearl

Remember to bridge only patients on warfarin when thrombotic risk and bleeding risk are both high. Do not bridge patients on DOAC.

A. *UFH*

- Bridging protocol with unfractionated heparin (UFH) should be initiated according to institutional guidelines when the international normalized ratio (INR) decreases below 2.0. UFH administration should be discontinued 4–6 hours before the scheduled procedure. Post-procedural resumption should occur no earlier than 24 hours following intervention. UFH bridging may be terminated once therapeutic INR levels are achieved.

B. *Therapeutic LMWH/enoxaparin (low molecular weight heparin)*

- The low molecular weight heparin (LMWH) bridging protocol requires discontinuation 24 hours preoperatively, with the final dose administered on the morning of the pre-procedure day. Post-procedural resumption occurs 48–72 hours following intervention. During the interim period between postoperative day 1 and 48 hours, prophylactic enoxaparin (40 mg daily) may be administered.
- Therapeutic LMWH dosing consists of enoxaparin 1 mg/kg twice daily or 1.5 mg/kg daily, initiated when INR decreases below 2.0 (typically 3 days preoperatively). LMWH bridging should be discontinued upon achievement of therapeutic INR.

References

1. Thompson A, Fleischmann KE, Smilowitz NR, de Las Fuentes L, Mukherjee D, Aggarwal NR, Ahmad FS, Allen RB, Altin SE, Auerbach A, Berger JS, Chow B, Dakik HA, Eisenstein EL, Gerhard-Herman M, Ghadimi K, Kachulis B, Leclerc J, Lee CS, Macaulay TE, Mates G, Merli GJ, Parwani P, Poole JE, Rich MW, Ruetzler K, Stain SC, Sweitzer B, Talbot AW, Vallabhajosyula S, Whittle J, Williams KA Sr, Peer Review Committee Members. 2024 AHA/ACC/ACS/ASNC/HRS/SCA/SCCT/SCMR/SVM guideline for perioperative cardiovascular management for noncardiac surgery: a report of the American College of Cardiology/American Heart Association Joint Committee on Clinical Practice Guidelines. Circulation. 2024;150(19):e351–442. https://doi.org/10.1161/CIR.0000000000001285. Epub 2024 Sep 24. Erratum in: Circulation. 2024;150(21):e466. https://doi.org/10.1161/CIR.0000000000001298. PMID: 39316661.
2. Modha K, Whinney C. Preoperative Evaluation for noncardiac Surgery. Ann Intern Med. 2022;175:ITC161–76. [Epub 8 November 2022]. https://doi.org/10.7326/AITC202211150.
3. Thomsen T, Villebro N, Møller AM. Interventions for preoperative smoking cessation. Cochrane Database Syst Rev. 2014;2014(3):CD002294. https://doi.org/10.1002/14651858.CD002294.pub4. PMID: 24671929; PMCID: PMC7138216.
4. Duceppe E, Parlow J, MacDonald P, Lyons K, McMullen M, Srinathan S, Graham M, Tandon V, Styles K, Bessissow A, Sessler DI, Bryson G, Devereaux PJ. Canadian Cardiovascular Society guidelines on perioperative cardiac risk assessment and management for patients who undergo noncardiac surgery. Can J Cardiol. 2017;33(1):17–32. https://doi.org/10.1016/j.cjca.2016.09.008. Epub 2016 Oct 4. Erratum in: Can J Cardiol. 2017;33(12):1735. https://doi.org/10.1016/j.cjca.2017.04.002. PMID: 27865641.
5. Halvorsen S, Mehilli J, Cassese S, Hall TS, Abdelhamid M, Barbato E, De Hert S, de Laval I, Geisler T, Hinterbuchner L, Ibanez B, Lenarczyk R, Mansmann UR, McGreavy P, Mueller C, Muneretto C, Niessner A, Potpara TS, Ristić A, Sade LE, Schirmer H, Schüpke S, Sillesen H,

Skulstad H, Torracca L, Tutarel O, Van Der Meer P, Wojakowski W, Zacharowski K, ESC Scientific Document Group. 2022 ESC guidelines on cardiovascular assessment and management of patients undergoing non-cardiac surgery. Eur Heart J. 2022;43(39):3826–924. https://doi.org/10.1093/eurheartj/ehac270. Erratum in: Eur Heart J. 2023;44(42):4421. https://doi.org/10.1093/eurheartj/ehad577. PMID: 36017553.

6. McKenzie NL, Ward RP, Nagele P, Rubin DS. Preoperative β-blocker therapy and stroke or major adverse cardiac events in major abdominal surgery: a retrospective cohort study. Anesthesiology. 2023;138(1):42–54. https://doi.org/10.1097/ALN.0000000000004404. PMID: 36227278; PMCID: PMC9771981.
7. Portela GT, Carson JL, Swanson SA, Alexander JH, Hébert PC, Goodman SG, Steg PG, Bertolet M, Strom JB, Fergusson DA, Simon T, White HD, Cooper HA, Abbott JD, Rao SV, Chaitman BR, Fordyce CB, Lopes RD, Daneault B, Brooks MM, MINT Investigators. Effect of four hemoglobin transfusion threshold strategies in patients with acute Myocardial infarction and anemia : a target trial emulation using MINT trial data. Ann Intern Med. 2024;177(11):1489–98. https://doi.org/10.7326/M24-0571. Epub 2024 Oct 1. PMID: 39348705.
8. Viamont-Guerra MR, Guimarães R, Bridges C, Antonioli E, Lenza M. Ultra-early versus early surgery for hip fracture. Cochrane Database Syst Rev. 2024;2024(6):CD015697. https://doi.org/10.1002/14651858.CD015697. PMCID: PMC11170678
9. Mand D, Mand D, Kilpatrick L, Probe RA. Orthopedic surgery meets serious illness care: palliative care and advanced care planning for the orthopedic surgeon. JBJS Rev. 2024;12(12):e24. https://doi.org/10.2106/JBJS.RVW.24.00132. PMID: 39626029.
10. Smeets SJM, van Wunnik BPW, Poeze M, Slooter GD, Verbruggen JPAM. Cardiac overscreening of hip fracture patients. Arch Orthop Trauma Surg. 2020;140(1):33–41. https://doi.org/10.1007/s00402-019-03270-z. Epub 2019 Aug 31. PMID: 31471640; PMCID: PMC6942037.
11. Borges FK, Guerra-Farfan E, Bhandari M, Patel A, Slobogean G, Feibel RJ, Sancheti PK, Tiboni ME, Balaguer-Castro M, Tandon V, Tomas-Hernandez J, Sigamani A, Sigamani A, Szczeklik W, McMahon SJ, Ślęczka P, Ramokgopa MT, Adinaryanan S, Umer M, Jenkinson RJ, Lawendy A, Popova E, Nur AN, Wang CY, Vizcaychipi M, Biccard BM, Ofori S, Spence J, Duceppe E, Marcucci M, Harvey V, Balasubramanian K, Vincent J, Tonelli AC, Devereaux PJ, the HIP ATTACK Investigators. Myocardial injury in patients with hip fracture: a HIP ATTACK randomized trial substudy. J Bone Joint Surg Am. 2024;106(24):2303–12. https://doi.org/10.2106/JBJS.23.01459. Epub 2024 Jul 25. PMID: 39052767.
12. Shoamanesh A, Field TS, Coutts SB, Sharma M, Gladstone D, Hart RG, Boriani G, Wright DJ, Sticherling C, Birnie DH, Gold MR, Erath JW, Kutyifa V, Mian R, Benz AP, Granger CB, McIntyre WF, Connolly SJ, Nielsen JC, Alings M, Rivard L, Lopes RD, Healey JS, ARTESiA Study Investigators. Apixaban versus aspirin for stroke prevention in people with subclinical atrial fibrillation and a history of stroke or transient ischaemic attack: subgroup analysis of the ARTESiA randomised controlled trial. Lancet Neurol. 2025;24(2):140–51. https://doi.org/10.1016/S1474-4422(24)00475-7. PMID: 39862882.
13. Douketis JD, Spyropoulos AC, Murad MH, Arcelus JI, Dager WE, Dunn AS, Fargo RA, Levy JH, Samama CM, Shah SH, Sherwood MW, Tafur AJ, Tang LV, Moores LK. Perioperative management of antithrombotic therapy: an American College of Chest Physicians Clinical Practice Guideline. Chest. 2022;162(5):e207–43. https://doi.org/10.1016/j.chest.2022.07.025. Epub 2022 Aug 11. Erratum in: Chest. 2023;164(1):267. https://doi.org/10.1016/j.chest.2023.05.019. PMID: 35964704.
14. Douketis JD, Spyropoulos AC. Perioperative management of anticoagulant and antiplatelet therapy. NEJM Evid. 2023;2(6):EVIDra2200322. https://doi.org/10.1056/EVIDra2200322. Epub 2023 May 23. PMID: 38320132.
15. Sherwood MW, Douketis JD, Patel MR, et al. Outcomes of temporary interruption of rivaroxaban compared with warfarin in patients with non-valvular atrial fibrillation: results from the rivaroxaban once daily, oral, direct factor Xa inhibition compared with vitamin K antagonism for prevention of stroke and embolism trial in atrial fibrillation (ROCKET AF). Circulation. 2014;129:1850–9. https://doi.org/10.1161/CIRCULATIONAHA.113.005754.

16. Garcia D, Alexander JH, Wallentin L, et al. Management and clinical outcomes in patients treated with apixaban vs warfarin undergoing procedures. Blood. 2014;124:3692–8. https://doi.org/10.1182/blood-2014-08-595496.
17. Douketis JD, Spyropoulos AC, Anderson JM, Arnold DM, Bates SM, Blostein M, Carrier M, Caprini JA, Clark NP, Coppens M, Dentali F, Duncan J, Gross PL, Kassis J, Kowalski S, Lee AY, Le Gal G, Le Templier G, Li N, MacKay E, Shah V, Shivakumar S, Solymoss S, Spencer FA, Syed S, Tafur AJ, Vanassche T, Thiele T, Wu C, Yeo E, Schulman S. The perioperative anticoagulant use for surgery evaluation (PAUSE) study for patients on a direct oral anticoagulant who need an elective surgery or procedure: design and rationale. Thromb Haemost. 2017;117(12):2415–24. https://doi.org/10.1160/TH17-08-0553. Epub 2017 Dec 6. Erratum in: Thromb Haemost. 2018;118(9):1679–80. https://doi.org/10.1055/s-0038-1668582. PMID: 29212129.
18. Shah S, Urtecho M, Firwana M, Nayfeh T, Hasan B, Nanaa A, Saadi S, Flynn DN, Abd-Rabu R, Seisa MO, Rajjoub NS, Hassett LC, Spyropoulos AC, Douketis JD, Murad MH. Perioperative management of antiplatelet therapy: a systematic review and meta-analysis. Mayo Clin Proc Innov Qual Outcomes. 2022;6(6):564–73. https://doi.org/10.1016/j.mayocpiqo.2022.09.006. PMID: 36304523; PMCID: PMC9594114.
19. Tan CW, Wall M, Rosengart TK, Ghanta RK. How to bridge? Management of anticoagulation in patients with mechanical heart valves undergoing noncardiac surgical procedures. J Thorac Cardiovasc Surg. 2019;158(1):200–3. https://doi.org/10.1016/j.jtcvs.2018.06.089. Epub 2018 Jul 20. PMID: 30107917.

Adult Congenital Heart Disease (ACHD) Summary

Contents

M. Salih, *Practical Hospitalist Guide to Inpatient Cardiology*, https://doi.org/10.1007/978-3-032-03240-9_11

This chapter addresses *congenital heart disease observed in adults*, such as bicuspid aortic valve, atrial septal defects, and repaired or unrepaired complex lesions, stressing the importance of lifelong surveillance and multidisciplinary care. Diagnostic tools such as echocardiography (including TEE), cardiac MRI, and CT are reviewed alongside indications for surgical or transcatheter interventions. Special considerations are given to anticoagulation, heart failure management, and endocarditis prophylaxis, ensuring that hospitalists and generalists can recognize, risk-stratify, and co-manage these patients in acute and chronic care settings.

11.1 Introduction and Principles [1]

- The adult congenital heart disease (ACHD) population now significantly surpasses the pediatric population due to improved survival rates. Consequently, hospitalists are increasingly encountering patients with ACHD.
- Preoperative consultation with an ACHD specialist is strongly recommended for patients with complex ACHD undergoing elective noncardiac surgery (NCS).
- Transthoracic echocardiography (TTE) is the preferred initial imaging modality. Cardiac magnetic resonance imaging (CMR) is the gold standard for quantifying shunts and assessing right ventricular function. Cardiac computed tomography (CT) may be considered as an alternative if CMR is contraindicated.
- Atrial septal defects (ASDs), patent foramen ovales (PFOS), and ventricular septal defects (VSDs) represent the most prevalent congenital heart defects (CHDs).

Pearl

The most common ACHD conditions include mitral valve prolapse, bicuspid aortic valves, and ASD [2].

11.2 Types and Common Conditions

- Congenital heart defects are broadly classified as cyanotic or non-cyanotic. This discussion will focus primarily on common non-cyanotic conditions, as most cyanotic defects present in early infancy and necessitate specialized, ongoing care.

11.3 Major Complications [3]

(i) *CHF.*
 - Heart failure (HF) constitutes a leading cause of morbidity and mortality in adult congenital heart disease (ACHD). Consultation with a specialist cardiologist is crucial when available. Standard HF therapies are generally effective in managing acute decompensated heart failure (ADHF). Addressing underlying contributing factors, such as obstructive sleep apnea, iron deficiency anemia, thyroid dysfunction (hypothyroidism or hyperthyroidism), and coronary artery disease (CAD), is paramount. In patients presenting with significant cardiogenic shock and pulmonary hypertension (PHT), milrinone or vasopressin are preferred over norepinephrine due to their pulmonary vasodilatory effects. Advanced cases may necessitate consideration of cardiac mechanical circulatory support or cardiac transplantation.

(ii) *Cardiac arrhythmias.*
 - Arrhythmias represent a leading cause of mortality in ACHD, manifesting as sudden cardiac death or heart failure. Detailed treatment guidelines are provided in the 2014 PACES/HRS Expert Consensus Statement on the Recognition and Management of Arrhythmias in ACHD [4]. All reversible causative factors should be addressed. In patients with complex congenital ACHD and atrial flutter or fibrillation, anticoagulation is generally recommended irrespective of low CHA2DS2-VASc scores [5], given the heightened risk of stroke and deep vein thrombosis (DVT) in this population.

(iii) *Systemic infections.*
 - Patients with ACHD exhibit an increased risk of infective endocarditis (IE) and systemic embolic complications, including brain abscesses. A high index of suspicion should be maintained for any patient experiencing rapid clinical deterioration. Infective endocarditis prophylaxis is indicated for dental procedures in patients with a history of IE, unrepaired cyanotic congenital heart disease, prosthetic heart valves, prosthetic material adjacent to shunts, or within 6 months of prosthetic material implantation.

(iv) *Pulmonary complications.*
 - Respiratory complications in ACHD range from circulatory abnormalities to restrictive lung disease and pulmonary hypertension (WHO groups

1 and 2), generally requiring specialist management. Intubation should be avoided whenever possible due to the risk of significant preload reduction and subsequent cardiogenic shock. If intubation is necessary, euvolemia should be maintained with fluid boluses in urgent situations. Propofol and midazolam are preferred sedatives due to their lack of pulmonary vasoconstrictive effects; fentanyl is a suitable analgesic for similar reasons.

(v) *Hematologic complications.*
- Patients with ACHD are at increased risk for hematologic complications, including anemia (predominantly iron deficiency anemia [IDA]), polycythemia, thrombocytopenia, and thrombosis. Anemia is prevalent and may result from acute or chronic blood loss (e.g., from frequent phlebotomy), the effects of anticoagulation or antiplatelet therapy, impaired iron absorption, or increased systemic iron demands. Normocytic anemia, potentially related to iron deficiency, can occur in up to 40% of patients with ACHD [6] and should be considered in all cases of anemia.

(vi) *Hepatic complications.*
- In advanced ACHD, chronic elevation of central venous pressure, secondary to increased right-sided pressures and pulmonary hypertension, can lead to portal hypertension, hepatic fibrosis, and cirrhosis. However, all hospitalized patients with elevated liver function tests (LFTs) require comprehensive evaluation to exclude other etiologies, particularly viral hepatitis, given the potential for prior blood transfusions during childhood.

(vii) *Renal dysfunction.*
- Chronic hypoxia and hyperviscosity in ACHD patients increase the risk of acute kidney injury (AKI) and chronic kidney disease (CKD) [7]. Furthermore, common genetic abnormalities associated with ACHD can also contribute to congenital renal anomalies [7].

(viii) *Neurological concerns.*
- The risk of both hemorrhagic and thrombotic stroke is elevated in ACHD, potentially attributable to polycythemia, effects of anticoagulation, and underlying cardiac anomalies, including atrial arrhythmias.

11.4 ASD

11.4.1 Types and Common Defects [8]

- Atrial septal defect (ASD) is a defect in the atrial septum, resulting in the intermittent shunting of blood from the left atrium (a high-pressure system) to the right atrium (a low-pressure system). While occasionally associated with genetic syndromes such as Down syndrome, this is uncommon. Untreated ASD can lead to pulmonary hypertension and Eisenmenger syndrome. Three types of ASD exist:

A. *Ostium secundum defects (upper septum defect)*. The most common type, often associated with other congenital anomalies, such as hand abnormalities (heart-hand syndrome), and, in cases of advanced pulmonary hypertension, tricuspid regurgitation. Atrial fibrillation (AF) is a frequent complication in adults with this type of ASD.
B. *Ostium primum defects (lower septum defect)*. The second most common type is frequently associated with mitral regurgitation (MR) due to its proximity to the atrioventricular endocardial cushions. It typically presents at a younger age, with left atrial enlargement and atrial fibrillation (AF) often appearing earlier in the disease course compared to ostium secundum defects, which more commonly manifest in adulthood, typically after the age of 40.
C. *Sinus venosus defects*. This less common type involves defects near the superior or inferior vena cava. In the presence of right ventricular volume overload on transthoracic or transesophageal echocardiography (TTE/TEE), without evidence of ASD or pulmonary pathology, a sinus venosus defect should be considered.

11.4.2 Clinical Approach

- In adults, advanced disease typically presents with embolic events or right-sided heart failure. Suspicion should be heightened in young adults with unexplained exertional dyspnea. Early-stage disease is often incidentally discovered, frequently accompanied by right atrial enlargement and atrial fibrillation, a common consequence of atrial dilation. Systemic embolization, migraine-like headaches, and exertional dyspnea may also occur. Physical examination may reveal subtly elevated jugular venous pressure (JVP), right ventricular heave, a tricuspid diastolic flow rumble (indicative of increased flow across a relatively stenotic tricuspid valve), a systolic pulmonary flow murmur, right parasternal heave (in advanced pulmonary hypertension), and a fixed, delayed splitting of the second heart sound (due to increased right ventricular pressure and ejection time). Importantly, the ASD itself may not produce an audible murmur due to its small size [9]. Untreated, common late complications include right heart failure and atrial fibrillation (AF).
- Diagnostic evaluation may reveal electrocardiographic (ECG) findings such as AF, right bundle branch block (RBBB), right atrial (RA) enlargement, and axis deviation (right axis deviation [RAD] in ostium secundum defects, left axis deviation [LAD] in ostium primum defects). Chest X-ray may show prominent pulmonary arteries and right ventricular enlargement. TTE with contrast echocardiography (bubble study or agitated saline) is the diagnostic test of choice, often revealing right heart enlargement; however, pulmonary hypertension and mitral regurgitation are less frequently observed in ostium primum defects. Resting and exercise pulse oximetry is recommended to assess the severity of

shunting in unrepaired ASDs. More advanced imaging techniques (such as TEE, cardiac catheterization, and cardiac MRI) are typically reserved for surgical planning.

11.4.3 Treatment Plan

- Intervention (surgical repair or closure) is indicated for symptomatic patients or asymptomatic individuals with right-sided heart enlargement (right atrium/right ventricle), suggestive of early pulmonary hypertension (PHT) and a significant shunt. In advanced Eisenmenger syndrome, closure is contraindicated due to the risk of hemodynamic instability and increased mortality [10]. Bosentan and PDE5 inhibitors are valid options at this stage. Surgical repair may improve outcomes even in older patients with left to left-to-right shunt cases [8]. In the hospital setting, diuretics are used to manage volume overload, and guideline-directed medical therapy (GDMT) is employed for heart failure (HF) in the absence of significant PHT. Cases with substantial PHT require specialized cardiological management due to increased complexity. When the contribution of an ASD to a patient's symptoms is uncertain, referral to a cardiologist is essential. Patients with advanced PHT should avoid strenuous exercise and pregnancy.

Pearl

Severe pulmonary arterial hypertension, defined as pulmonary artery systolic pressure exceeding two-thirds of systemic pressure or pulmonary vascular resistance exceeding two-thirds of systemic vascular resistance, contraindicates atrial septal defect closure [11].

11.5 PFO

11.5.1 Patent Foramen Ovale (PFO) [8]

- A patent foramen ovale (PFO) persists in approximately 30% of the adult population. Its clinical relevance is primarily in the context of cryptogenic stroke; incidental discovery of a PFO does not require treatment or closure, as it is generally considered benign. Transthoracic echocardiography (TTE) with contrast echocardiography, using agitated saline or a bubble study, is the diagnostic modality of choice, demonstrating right-to-left atrial shunting of contrast material through the PFO.

- PFO is linked to the following complications:
  (i) *Embolic stroke.*
    - For patientsunder 60 years of age presenting with a cryptogenic stroke and a negative workup, PFO closure is recommended if imaging demonstrates a PFO. In patients over 60 years of age with cryptogenic stroke, aspirin monotherapy is indicated without PFO closure [12].
  (ii) *Platypnea-orthodeoxia syndrome.*
    - A significant elevation of right atrial pressure, secondary to right-sided cardiac pathology (e.g., tricuspid regurgitation [TR], inferior myocardial infarction [MI], pulmonary embolism [PE], or pulmonary hypertension [PHT]), can lead to increased right-to- left shunting through a patent foramen ovale (PFO). This results in the passage of deoxygenated hemoglobin into the systemic circulation, causing cyanosis and dyspnea, particularly in the upright position or during exertion.
  (iii) *Migraine.*
  (iv) *Neurological concerns.*
    - The risk of both hemorrhagic and thrombotic stroke is elevated in ACHD, potentially attributable to polycythemia, effects of anticoagulation, and underlying cardiac anomalies, including atrial arrhythmias.

11.6 VSD

11.6.1 Types and Common Defects [8]

- Ventricular septal defect (VSD) is a defect in the ventricular septum, most commonly located in the membranous septum. VSDs may be associated with other ventricular heart defects or genetic syndromes. Significant symptoms typically arise from left-to-right shunting. Small VSDs often close spontaneously and require no intervention. Aortic regurgitation (AR) is sometimes associated with VSDs.

11.6.2 Clinical Approach

- Large, unrepaired VSDs may present with progressive dyspnea and exercise intolerance. Clinical presentation varies with defect size; larger defects carry a greater risk of heart failure (HF) and pulmonary hypertension (PHT). Small VSDs typically produce a loud systolic murmur (due to a significant pressure gradient), whereas larger defects often manifest with a pansystolic murmur at the left lower sternal border. Untreated, advanced VSDs can lead to HF symptoms (including a displaced, hyperdynamic apical impulse) and, in severe cases, PHT (though this is uncommon in adults, as untreated advanced VSDs are often fatal or repaired in infancy).

- Diagnostic testing may reveal right or left ventricular hypertrophy on an electrocardiogram (ECG). Transthoracic echocardiography (TTE) is the primary diagnostic modality for identifying defects and associated complications, such as pulmonary hypertension (PHT). Late complications include infective endocarditis (IE), arrhythmias, and associated valvular heart disease.

Pearl

Most adults with VSD or ASD remain asymptomatic unless significant pulmonary hypertension develops or Eisenmenger syndrome ensues.

Pearl

VSD remains the most common cause of Eisenmenger syndrome [10].

11.6.3 Treatment Plan [8]

- Surgical closure is indicated for VSD in patients with significant pulmonary hypertension (pulmonary-to-systemic blood flow ratio ≥1.5), but contraindicated when shunt reversal has occurred (closure in this setting is associated with worse outcomes due to dependence on right-sided cardiac output). Patients with significant pulmonary hypertension (pulmonary artery pressure >50% of systemic blood pressure) should avoid strenuous exercise, and pregnancy is discouraged. In-hospital management of VSD with associated heart failure mirrors that of acute decompensated heart failure (ADHF), emphasizing diuresis and afterload reduction.

Pearl

Surgical closure is not recommended for small VSDs without pulmonary hypertension (PHT) or large VSDs with advanced PHT (Eisenmenger syndrome).

11.7 COA

11.7.1 Types and Common Defects

- Coarctation of the aorta (CoA) is a congenital narrowing of the aorta, typically distal to the left subclavian artery. A bicuspid aortic valve is present in 50–70% of individuals with CoA. Association with congenital syndromes, particularly Turner syndrome, is observed. Additional anomalies, such as intracranial aneurysms (in approximately 10% of cases), may also be present. Complications include the following:
  (i) HTN
  (ii) CHF
  (iii) Aortic dissections
  (iv) Strokes
  (v) Intracranial aneurysms
  (vi) CAD(considered a common cause of death in adults)
  (vii) VHD
  (viii) IE

11.7.2 Clinical Approach

- In adults, coarctation of the aorta (CoA) often presents as uncontrolled hypertension, particularly in young adults, when other secondary causes are unlikely. Reduced perfusion distal to the stenosis may cause leg cramping (claudication) and weakness. Given the high prevalence of bicuspid aortic valve (present in >50% of cases), signs and symptoms of aortic stenosis are frequently observed. Physical examination may reveal higher systolic blood pressure (SBP) in the arms compared to the legs, delayed or absent femoral pulses, a loud S2 heart sound, and a continuous systolic murmur at the left lower sternal border, which is often due to collateral circulation.

- Diagnostic evaluation includes measuring blood pressure in both upper and lower extremities, which demonstrates a pressure gradient. Echocardiography (echo) is the primary diagnostic test, visualizing the coarctation, potential bicuspid aortic valve, and left ventricular (LV) hypertrophy. A chest X-ray may show an enlarged ascending aorta and rib notching (resulting from collateral vessels). ECG may demonstrate LV hypertrophy secondary to increased afterload. Computed tomography (CT) angiography and cardiac magnetic resonance imaging (MRI) are occasionally employed for further clarification, primarily when surgical intervention is considered [13].
- Screening for coronary artery disease (CAD) is crucial in adults with CoA due to its significant contribution to mortality. Screening for intracranial aneurysms using CT or MR angiography is also recommended [14].

11.7.3 Treatment Plan

- Treatment for coarctation of the aorta (CoA) is primarily surgical, with younger age at intervention associated with improved outcomes. Indications for intervention include a significant systolic blood pressure gradient between the upper and lower extremities (≥20 mmHg), uncontrolled hypertension, declining left ventricular function, significant aortic valvular stenosis or regurgitation, and imaging demonstrating severe stenosis [13]. Medical management with antihypertensive medications is employed for patients awaiting surgery or those not requiring intervention; most patients, even post-surgery, require continued antihypertensive therapy to manage persistent hypertension. Aggressive modification of all cardiovascular risk factors is crucial. In the inpatient setting, established cases of CoA are more likely to be encountered post-surgical repair.
- Pre-pregnancy counseling by a cardiologist is essential, as pregnancy is discouraged in patients with advanced CoA.

11.8 PDA

11.8.1 Main Types [8]

- Persistent left superior vena cava (PLSVC) is a congenital anomaly characterized by a persistent connection between the aorta and the left pulmonary artery. If left untreated, this connection can lead to pulmonary hypertension (PHT) in young adults. Complications include infective endocarditis (IE), left-sided heart failure, and, in advanced stages, PHT with subsequent right-sided heart failure. Maternal rubella infection during pregnancy is a known risk factor. Normally, the connection closes shortly after birth.

11.8.2 Clinical Approach [8]

- Persistent left superior vena cava (PLSVC) should be suspected in the presence of a continuous murmur in the left upper chest, unexplained left-sided heart enlargement, and a wide pulse pressure (e.g., 140/50 mmHg) [15]. The clinical presentation, including symptoms of hyperdynamic circulation and pulmonary hypertension (PHT), may mimic aortic regurgitation (e.g., a displaced apical impulse, wide pulse pressure or a collapsing pulse, and bounding peripheral pulses). A palpable thrill is typically present in the second left intercostal space, accompanied by a characteristic continuous "machinery" murmur. Advanced disease can lead to Eisenmenger syndrome, which sometimes manifests with preferential clubbing of the toes, due to relatively lower oxygen saturation in the lower extremities.
- Transthoracic echocardiography (TTE) with contrast echocardiography, using agitated saline or a bubble study, is the diagnostic test of choice for visualizing the aortopulmonary connection. Electrocardiography (ECG) may reveal left-sided heart enlargement, evidence of pulmonary hypertension (PHT), and features of right ventricular hypertrophy.

Hospitalist Tip

In adults, a major concern with PDA is IE and septic emboli.

Pearl

A hyperdynamic circulation, characterized by a bounding pulse and wide pulse pressure, is a common finding in both aortic regurgitation and patent ductus arteriosus (PDA). Other conditions that may present with similar findings include ventricular septal defect (VSD) and pulmonary arteriovenous fistula.

11.8.3 Treatment Plan [8]

- Given that surgical closure of patent ductus arteriosus (PDA) typically occurs early in life, adult presentations to hospitalists are uncommon. Intervention is indicated when symptoms develop, such as left atrial (LA) or left ventricular (LV) enlargement with a significant left-to-right shunt, indicating chronic left-sided volume overload. The timing of intervention is crucial; significant pulmonary hypertension (pulmonary systolic pressure >50% of systemic systolic blood pressure) is associated with poorer outcomes following closure. Percutaneous closure is the preferred method. Inpatient management focuses on standard acute decompensated heart failure (ADHF) treatment, including diuresis and afterload reduction.

11.9 PS

11.9.1 Types and Common Defects

- Pulmonary valve stenosis (PS) is typically a congenital or syndromic valvular lesion, often associated with conditions such as tetralogy of Fallot or Noonan syndrome. It results in elevated right ventricular pressure and hypertrophy, mimicking the effects of aortic stenosis on the left ventricle. Consequently, patients often present with features of pulmonary hypertension. Rare adult-onset causes include carcinoid syndrome and radiation-induced injury. Importantly, rheumatic heart disease (RHD) rarely affects the pulmonary valve.

Pearl

(PR) pulmonary regurgitation is mostly secondary to pulmonary hypertension.

11.9.2 Clinical Approach

- Symptoms of pulmonary valve stenosis (PS) reflect the underlying pulmonary hypertension (PHT), including exertional dyspnea and, in advanced cases, right-sided heart failure with volume overload. Physical examination may reveal a systolic ejection murmur at the left upper sterna border (pulmonary area) and a delayed or absent second heart sound (S2).
- Transthoracic echocardiography (TTE)) is the primary diagnostic modality used to demonstrate the pressure gradient across the pulmonary valve. Sup-

porting electrocardiographic (ECG) findings may include right atrial (RA) enlargement, right axis deviation (RAD), right bundle branch block (RBBB), and right ventricular (RV) hypertrophy.

11.9.3 Treatment Plan

- Intervention is indicated for symptomatic patients or asymptomatic individuals with severe pulmonary stenosis. Balloon valvuloplasty is the preferred treatment, with surgical intervention reserved for specific circumstances. Pulmonary regurgitation represents a potential complication of valvuloplasty.

11.9.4 Tetralogy of Fallot (TOF)

- Tetralogy of Fallot (TOF) is the most common cyanotic congenital heart defect, typically corrected in childhood; therefore, adult presentations are largely related to the consequences of previous surgical interventions rather than the initial disease itself. The classic features of TOF include a large ventricular septal defect (VSD), overriding aorta, pulmonary stenosis (PS), and right ventricular hypertrophy. Genetic associations, such as with Down syndrome, exist.
- Adult presentations often involve atrial and ventricular dilation with associated arrhythmias, frequently attributable to chronic pulmonary regurgitation (PR) following surgical repair. Patients presenting with a history of TOF and symptoms such as shortness of breath or chest pain should undergo transthoracic echocardiography (TTE). A chest X-ray and electrocardiogram (ECG) may reveal cardiomegaly and a right bundle branch block (RBBB), respectively. Advanced imaging techniques, such as cardiac CT/MRI or cardiac catheterization, may be necessary for surgical planning.
- Intervention is indicated for significant pulmonary hypertension (PHT) secondary to advanced PR, or in the presence of symptoms or arrhythmias. Pulmonary valve replacement is the primary treatment modality. Patients should avoid strenuous exercise. Genetic screening for 22q11.2 deletion is recommended for individuals with TOF considering pregnancy due to the increased risk of inheritance.

11.10 Eisenmenger Syndrome

11.10.1 Presentation and Mechanism [8]

- Eisenmenger syndrome represents severe pulmonary hypertension (PHT) with a reversed right-to-left shunt, a consequence of long-standing, untreated congenital heart defects (most commonly ventricular septal defect [VSD], atrial septal defect [ASD], and patent ductus arteriosus [PDA]).

- Symptoms include exertional dyspnea, edema, palpitations (often due to arrhythmias), and syncope. Hyperviscosity, secondary to erythrocytosis, may manifest as headaches, thromboembolic events, confusion, and epistaxis. Physical examination reveals signs of PHT, including finger clubbing and cyanosis; the original murmur associated with the underlying shunt is typically absent at this stage.
- Significant complications include stroke, deep vein thrombosis/pulmonary embolism (DVT/PE), anemia, gout (due to hyperuricemia), renal failure (with proteinuria), and hyperviscosity syndrome due to chronic hypoxia and Iron deficiency (RBCs becoming stiffer and more likely to block small vessels). The median age of death is between 30 and 50 years [16].

Pearl

Common physical examination findings suggestive of pulmonary hypertension include a loud P2 heart sound (palpable as a pulsation in the left upper intercostal space in severe cases), a right ventricular heave (a palpable lift of the chest wall during systole), a diastolic pulmonary regurgitation murmur (Graham-steel murmur), a tricuspid regurgitation murmur, and elevated jugular venous pressure (JVP).

Hospitalist Tip

Symptoms of hyperviscosity syndrome can include, but are not limited to, headache, tinnitus, visual disturbances, fatigue, dizziness, vertigo, stroke, and gastrointestinal bleeding.

11.10.2 Diagnostic Workup

- The diagnosis of Eisenmenger syndrome typically begins with a transthoracic echocardiography (TTE) examination. Electrocardiography (ECG) may reveal right atrial enlargement, right ventricular hypertrophy (RVH), and arrhythmias. A chest X-ray or computed tomography (CT) scan of the chest may reveal enlargement of the pulmonary arteries. Complete blood count (CBC) typically shows erythrocytosis, a compensatory response to chronic hypoxia. Right heart catheterization may be performed for both diagnostic and prognostic purposes.
- Given the central role of pulmonary hypertension (PHT) in Eisenmenger syndrome, other potential causes of PHT should be considered and excluded, including sleep-disordered breathing (OSA/OHS) via polysomnography and chronic thromboembolic pulmonary hypertension (CTEPH) via ventilation/perfusion (V/Q) scan.

11.10.3 The Primary Treatment Point as a Hospitalist

- Management of Eisenmenger syndrome focuses on maintaining euvolemia and preventing dehydration, particularly in the context of hyperviscosity [8]. All intravenous (IV) fluids should be administered through microfilters to minimize the risk of paradoxical embolism. Deep vein thrombosis (DVT) prophylaxis is recommended for hospitalized patients, although long-term anticoagulation is generally not indicated. Infective endocarditis prophylaxis is crucial before any invasive dental procedure. Supplemental oxygen is often necessary due to the propensity for hypoxia and cyanosis; a 6-minute walk test or home oxygen assessment is helpful before discharge. Therapeutic phlebotomy may be considered for symptomatic hyperviscosity with hemoglobin levels exceeding 20 g/dL [17]. Iron replacement is essential, given the high prevalence of iron deficiency. Transferrin saturation is the best marker for assessing iron deficiency in Eisenmenger syndrome. Values below 20% warrant consideration of iron supplementation [17].
- The significant comorbidity burden associated with Eisenmenger syndrome necessitates lifestyle modifications, including avoidance of strenuous exercise, minimization of physiological stress, and restriction of pregnancy. Patients with advanced disease require specialized cardiological consultation, as they may benefit from pulmonary vasodilator therapy or lung/heart transplantation. Advanced right ventricular failure portends a poor prognosis. Preoperative cardiac evaluation by an experienced cardiologist or referral to a specialized center is essential before any noncardiac surgery.

Pearl

Overall, pregnancy is not advised in all patients with Eisenmenger syndrome

References

1. Thakkar AN, Chinnadurai P, Lin CH. Adult congenital heart disease: the magnitude of the problem. Curr Opin Cardiol. 2017;32(5):467–74. https://doi.org/10.1097/HCO.0000000000000429. PMID: 28617685
2. Ashley EA, Niebauer J. Cardiology Explained. London: Remedica; 2004. Chapter 14: Adult Congenital Heart Disease. Available from: https://www.ncbi.nlm.nih.gov/books/NBK2212/

3. Kendsersky P, Krasuski RA. Intensive care unit management of the adult with congenital heart disease. Curr Cardiol Rep. 2020;22(11):136. https://doi.org/10.1007/s11886-020-01389-9. PMID: 32910318; PMCID: PMC7481759
4. Khairy P, Van Hare GF, Balaji S, Berul CI, Cecchin F, Cohen MI, Daniels CJ, Deal BJ, Dearani JA, Groot Nd, Dubin AM, Harris L, Janousek J, Kanter RJ, Karpawich PP, Perry JC, Seslar SP, Shah MJ, Silka MJ, Triedman JK, Walsh EP, Warnes CA. PACES/HRS expert consensus statement on recognizing and managing arrhythmias in adult congenital heart disease: developed in partnership between the Pediatric and Congenital Electro-physiology Society (PACES) and the Heart Rhythm Society (HRS). Endorsed by the governing bodies of PACES, HRS, the American College of Cardiology (ACC), the American Heart Association (AHA), the European Heart Rhythm Association (EHRA), the Canadian Heart Rhythm Society (CHRS), and the International Society for Adult Congenital Heart Disease (ISACHD). Can J Cardiol. 2014;30(10):e1–e63. https://doi.org/10.1016/j.cjca.2014.09.002.
5. Khairy P, Aboulhosn J, Broberg CS, Cohen S, Cook S, Dore A, Fernandes SM, Fournier A, Kay J, Levesque S, Macle L, Marcotte F, Mondésert B, Mongeon FP, Opotowsky AR, Proietti A, Rivard L, Ting J, Thibault B, Zaidi A, Hamilton R. Anticoagulation therapy in congenital heart disease (TACTIC) investigators and the Alliance for adult research in congenital cardiology (AARCC). Thromboprophylaxis for atrial arrhythmias in congenital heart disease: a multicenter study. Int J Cardiol. 2016;223:729–35. https://doi.org/10.1016/j.ijcard.2016.08.223. Epub 2016 Aug 13. PMID: 27573597
6. Gaeta SA, Ward C, Krasuski RA. Extra-cardiac manifestations of adult congenital heart disease. Trends Cardiovasc Med. 2016;26(7):627–36. https://doi.org/10.1016/j.tcm.2016.04.004. Epub 2016 Apr 21. PMID: 27234354
7. Dimopoulos K, Diller GP, Koltsida E, Pijuan-Domenech A, Papadopoulou SA, Babu-Narayan SV, Salukhe TV, Piepoli MF, Poole-Wilson PA, Best N, Francis DP, Gatzoulis MA. Prevalence, predictors, and prognostic value of renal dysfunction in adults with congenital heart disease. Circulation. 2008;117(18):2320–8. https://doi.org/10.1161/CIRCULATIONAHA.107.734921. Epub 2008 Apr 28. PMID: 18443238
8. Stout KK, Daniels CJ, Aboulhosn JA, Bozkurt B, Broberg CS, Colman JM, Crumb SR, Dearani JA, Fuller S, Gurvitz M, Khairy P, Landzberg MJ, Saidi A, Valente AM, Van Hare GF. 2018 AHA/ACC Guideline for the Management of Adults With Congenital Heart Disease: Executive Summary: A Report of the American College of Cardiology/American Heart Association Task Force on Clinical Practice Guidelines. J Am Coll Cardiol. 2019;73(12):1494–563. https://doi.org/10.1016/j.jacc.2018.08.1028. Epub 2018 Aug 16. Erratum in: J Am Coll Cardiol. 2019 May 14;73(18):2361. https://doi.org/10.1016/j.jacc.2019.03.017. PMID: 30121240
9. Menillo AM, Alahmadi MH, Pearson-Shaver AL. Atrial Septal Defect. [Updated 2025 Jan 21]. In: StatPearls [Internet]. Treasure Island (FL): StatPearls Publishing; 2025 Jan-. Available from: https://www.ncbi.nlm.nih.gov/books/NBK535440/
10. Basit H, Wallen TJ, Sergent BN. Eisenmenger Syndrome. [Updated 2023 Feb 13]. In: StatPearls [Internet]. Treasure Island (FL): StatPearls Publishing; 2025 Jan-. Available from: https://www.ncbi.nlm.nih.gov/books/NBK507800/
11. Jain S, Dalvi B. Atrial septal defect with pulmonary hypertension: when/ how can we consider closure? J Thorac Dis. 2018;10(Suppl 24):S2890–8. https://doi.org/10.21037/jtd.2018.07.112. PMID: 30305949; PMCID: PMC6174154
12. Farjat-Pasos JI, Chamorro A, Lanthier S, Robichaud M, Mengi S, Houde C, Rodés-Cabau J. Cerebrovascular events in older patients with patent foramen ovale: current status and future perspectives. J Stroke. 2023;25(3):338–49. https://doi.org/10.5853/jos.2023.01599. Epub 2023 Sep 26. PMID: 37813671; PMCID: PMC10574307
13. Law MA, Collier SA, Sharma S, et al. Coarctation of the Aorta. [Updated 2024 Dec 11]. In: StatPearls [Internet]. Treasure Island (FL): StatPearls Publishing; 2025 Jan-. Available from: https://www.ncbi.nlm.nih.gov/books/NBK430913/

14. Pickard SS, Prakash A, Newburger JW, Malek AM, Wong JB. Screening for intracranial aneurysms in coarctation of the aorta: a decision and cost-effectiveness analysis. Circ Cardiovasc Qual Outcomes. 2020;13(8):e006406. https://doi.org/10.1161/CIRCOUTCOMES.119.006406. Epub 2020 Jul 30. PMID: 32762482; PMCID: PMC7442667
15. Gillam-Krakauer M, Mahajan K. Patent Ductus Arteriosus. [Updated 2023 Aug 8]. In: StatPearls [Internet]. Treasure Island (FL): StatPearls Publishing; 2025 Jan-. Available from: https://www.ncbi.nlm.nih.gov/books/NBK430758/
16. Kaemmerer H, Mebus S, Schulze-Neick I, Eicken A, Trindade PT, Hager A, Oechslin E, Niwa K, Lang I, Hess J. The adult patient with Eisenmenger Syndrome: a medical update after Dana point, part I: epidemiology, clinical aspects, and diagnostic options. Curr Cardiol Rev. 2010;6(4):343–55. https://doi.org/10.2174/157340310793566154. PMID: 22043211; PMCID: PMC3083816
17. Oechslin E, Mebus S, Schulze-Neick I, Niwa K, Trindade PT, Eicken A, Hager A, Lang I, Hess J, Kaemmerer H. The adult patient with Eisenmenger syndrome: a medical update after Dana point part III: specific management and surgical aspects. Curr Cardiol Rev. 2010;6(4):363–72. https://doi.org/10.2174/157340310793566127. PMID: 22043213; PMCID: PMC3083818

Palliative Cardiology

Contents

M. Salih, *Practical Hospitalist Guide to Inpatient Cardiology*, https://doi.org/10.1007/978-3-032-03240-9_12

This chapter explores the role of palliative care in the management of patients with advanced cardiovascular disease, emphasizing symptom relief, quality of life, and holistic patient-centered care. It highlights common symptoms such as dyspnea, pain, fatigue, and psychosocial distress and offers practical strategies for their assessment and management in heart failure, refractory angina, and end-stage cardiomyopathies. The chapter underscores the importance of early integration of palliative principles alongside curative treatments, effective communication about prognosis and goals of care, and shared decision-making with patients and families. It also addresses advanced care planning, ethical considerations, and coordination with multidisciplinary teams to navigate complex interventions such as device deactivation and transplant candidacy. This guidance equips hospitalists to deliver compassionate, comprehensive care that aligns with patients' values and improves quality of life in advanced cardiac illness.

12.1 What Are the Main Objectives of Palliative Care in Cardiology-Related Cases? [1]

(i) Reducing physical symptom burden
(ii) Managing emotional and spiritual distress
(iii) Providing sufficient support for caregivers
(iv) Assisting patients in making decisions that coincide with their goals of care

12.2 Prognostic Approach

- The short- and long-term prognosis of a heart failure (HF) patient can be determined based on symptom severity, frequency of hospitalizations, biomarker levels, medication burden, and the presence of comorbidities. Predictive models, such as the Seattle Heart Failure Model, can help estimate life expectancy and provide valuable insights to guide discussions about clinical prognosis with patients.
- For patients with advanced heart failure, it is essential to evaluate the need for palliative care and hospice both before hospital discharge and during subsequent follow-up visits. Addressing these considerations early in patients with severe HF ensures comprehensive care planning and supports informed decision-making regarding treatment goals and quality of life [2].

Pearl

Palliative care should not be misconstrued as the abandonment of the patient or the limitation of medical interventions. On the contrary, it represents a comprehensive approach that provides resources, support, and symptom-focused treatment tailored to the patient's needs rather than employing a one-size-fits-all strategy. Integrating palliative care specialists into the care team for all patients with complex, chronic illnesses is strongly recommended, regardless of their preferences regarding the continuation of disease-directed therapies, consideration of hospice care, or the decision to transition exclusively to comfort-focused measures. This approach ensures patients receive holistic, patient-centered care that aligns with their unique clinical and personal circumstances.

Pearl

Hospice care encompasses the cessation of life-sustaining interventions for individuals with a terminal prognosis of 6 months or less. In this context, curative treatments are generally discontinued, except therapies that provide demonstrable palliative benefits. A validated clinical assessment tool for determining hospice candidacy involves the "surprise question" methodology: clinicians should consider whether they would be surprised if the patient expired within the next 6 months. A negative response to this query indicates the appropriateness of initiating hospice care discussions. Notably, research demonstrates that patients with advanced heart failure who elect hospice care do not experience reduced survival rates compared to their non-hospice counterparts [3].

Hospitalist Tip

In cases where a patient enters the terminal phase of illness with an anticipated life expectancy of hours to days, it is appropriate to transition to comfort care protocols. The therapeutic focus shifts to optimizing comfort measures, primarily through targeted symptomatic management utilizing appropriate pharmacological interventions while simultaneously addressing psychosocial and spiritual needs. This patient-centered approach emphasizes alleviating distressing symptoms and providing comprehensive end-of-life support to ensure dignity and quality of life during the terminal phase.

12.3 Patients with Cardiac Devices

- Pacemakers (PM) and implantable cardioverter-defibrillators (ICD) should be adjusted according to patient symptomatology and care goals. In dying patients, ICDs may be deactivated to prevent distressing shocks in alignment with patient and family preferences. However, pacemakers can remain active to provide symptomatic benefits.
- For patients with advanced heart failure, cardiac resynchronization therapy (CRT) plays a crucial role in improving symptoms and should remain active, even if the ICD function is turned off. This approach helps maintain optimal cardiac function and quality of life in patients nearing end-of-life care [4].

> **Pearl**
>
> In PM-dependent patients, death will follow shortly after terminating PM therapy.

12.4 Role of Palliative Pharmacotherapy [1]

- Palliative pharmacotherapy in heart failure aims to enhance the quality of life by alleviating symptom burden while maintaining physical and cognitive function. Common treatment goals include reducing pain, dyspnea, fatigue, mood disturbances, insomnia, and appetite loss. Treatment should be individualized based on the patient's specific needs and preferences. Primary medication options include the following:
  (a) Cardiovascular drugs (optimized to balance symptom control and avoid unnecessary burden)
  (b) Opioids (for refractory dyspnea and pain relief)
  (c) Antidepressants (to manage mood disorders and improve overall well-being)
- To minimize unnecessary or harmful medications, the American Geriatrics Society's Beers Criteria can guide deprescribing. According to these guidelines, certain cardiovascular medications should be avoided in older adults or those in palliative care, including the following:
  (a) Peripheral α-1 blockers (terazosin, doxazosin) and central α-agonists (clonidine) for hypertension

(b) Antiarrhythmic agents (dronedarone, immediate-release nifedipine)
(c) Specific anticoagulants/antiplatelet drugs (dabigatran, prasugrel, ticagrelor)
(d) Medications that may exacerbate heart failure, such as cilostazol and non-dihydropyridine calcium channel blockers (diltiazem, verapamil)

- Ultimately, deprescribing decisions should be shared between the patient and healthcare provider, ensuring that medication choices align with the patient's goals, prognosis, and quality of life considerations.

12.5 Selected Common Symptoms and Their Palliative Treatment Effects on the Heart [1]

Pain	NSAIDS may worsen heart failure by retaining fluids and increasing BP
	Gabapentin and pregabalin may lead to fluid retention and lower limb edema with HF exacerbation.

Depression, insomnia, and anxiety	Sertraline is considered safe as it has the lowest QT-prolonging effects. Mirtazapine is another good option because of its sleeping effects and it is an appetite stimulant.
	MAO and TCA have the worst side effects, including arrhythmias, hypotension, and HTN.
	Psychostimulants are best for advanced hospice patients with depression, as they work fast, within 1–2 days. Unfor-tunately, it has significant cardiac side effects, such as HTN and arrhythmia.
	Trazodone, melatonin agonist, and mirtazapine are the best option for insomnia the safest.

Dyspnea	Treat advanced congestion with diuretics.
	Opioids for advanced cases with refractory dyspnea (modify perceptions of breathlessness and the urge to breathe). Used in patients with maximized GDMT and still has class IV NYHA symptoms. Oral low-dose morphine 2.5 mg scheduled or as needed is considered the standard dose and may escalate accordingly.
	Fan pointing to the face is a good non-pharmacological treatment for dyspnea awareness.

Fatigue	Adjust B-blocker dose and diuretics or switch to nighttime dosing.
	Correction of iron deficiency anemia with high-dose IV iron showed improved functional status, quality of life, and reduced hospi-talizations among patients with HF [5].
	Occupational and cardiac therapy is useful as an additional support.

GI symptoms and Anorexia (common in cardiac cachexia)	For nausea and vomiting, useful lifestyle changes include eating more frequent, smaller meals, avoiding spicy and high-fat foods, and sitting upright while eating. Antiemetic medication is use-ful but should be monitored for prolonged QT effects.
	For constipation, stimulant laxatives and osmotic laxatives are suggested in addition to lifestyle changes, including increased consumption of high-fiber foods and water.
	For anorexia, options to use include mirtazapine, as it also helps with sleeping and mood. Steroids, megestrol, and dronabinol are second-line options in advanced cases or patients with cancer treatment.

Hospitalist Tip

It is crucial to acknowledge that some individuals may perceive deprescribing as a sign of "giving up," potentially leading to increased emotional distress. In such cases, prioritizing medication safety is essential for the effective managementof polypharmacy. This can be achieved through a thoughtful prescribing approach, which involves selecting the most appropriate therapy based on the patient's diagnosis, prognosis, and treatment goals while continuously monitoring outcomes. There is no absolute right or wrong decision; rather, it is imperative to align clinical choices with the patient's objectives and overall well-being.

I. *Palliative pharmacotherapy in CHF*

- The approach to guideline-directed medical therapy (GDMT) in palliative care remains a common consideration. If GDMT effectively maintains symptom control, such as preserving euvolemia and cardiac output, it is reasonable to continue therapy even when the primary goal is no longer life prolongation. However, this can be challenging in hospice patients, particularly when insurance coverage limits access to costly medications. In such cases, transitioning to a more affordable alternative within the GDMT framework may be appropriate, provided it continues to support symptom management. The overarching objective is not to extend life but to ensure a comfortable, symptom-free lifespan.

▪ Selected Common Medication Use in CHF Palliative Patients [1]

Medication	Palliative or hospice goal
Loop diuretics	Reasonable to use orally/IV/subcutaneously to manage hypervolemia and congestive symptoms such as edema and pulmonary edema with SOB. Torsemide and bumetanide have better oral bioavailability and are preferred if furosemide is not helpful. If the patient is diuretic refractory with significant symptomatic pleural effusion or ascites, indwelling pleural and peritoneal catheters are good options.
All GDMT	If helping with the patient's distressing symptoms, it is reasonable to continue if possible. Always keep in mind the cost and pill burden.
β-Blockers	Are usually withheld due to side effects, which include extreme fatigue, worsening edema, and congestion in advanced low-cardiac-output heart failure. If not exerting symptomatic benefits, it should be discontinued slowly and tapered over time (to prevent withdrawal HTN and high output failure leading to more distressing symptoms).

Medication	Palliative or hospice goal
Inotropes	Are usually not used, except in palliative care patients not eligible for heart transplants or assisted devices, consistent with their goals to *improve advanced heart failure symptoms*. Patients and families should understand the risks, which include arrhythmias, infection from an indwelling venous catheter, cost, the burden of living with a continuous intravenous infusion, and early death. Another concern is that insurance may deny coverage post-discharge if the patient is in hospice.
NSAIDS	Should be avoided because of the increased risk of fluid retention, bleeding, and AKI.

II. *Palliative pharmacotherapy in coronary heart disease (CHD)*

■ Selected Common Medication Use in CHD Palliative Patients [1]

Medication	Palliative or hospice goal
Antianginal (blockers, CCB, nitrates, ranolazine)	May continue them if they are helping with symptoms.
Statin treatment	If causing significant myopathic symptoms, should be avoided
Antiplatelets/anticoagulant	May discontinue them if comfort or hospice care, especially if there is increased risk of bleeding.

III. *Palliative pharmacotherapy in pulmonary arterial hypertension (PAH)*

- Most therapies for pulmonary arterial hypertension (PAH) effectively reduce symptom burden and preserve quality of life and can be continued as long as their benefits outweigh patient-specific risks. If discontinuation is necessary, a gradual tapering process is essential to mitigate the risk of significant symptom recurrence.

IV. *Palliative pharmacotherapy in arrhythmias*

- In general, if a medication effectively alleviates distressing palpitations and dyspnea, its continuation may be appropriate. These medications primarily regulate heart rate or rhythm, including beta-blockers, calcium channel blockers, and most class I-IV antiarrhythmic agents. The decision to continue therapy should be guided by carefully balancing risks, benefits, potential side effects, and symptomatic relief. Discontinuation should be considered if the medication causes significant adverse effects or contributes to patient distress.

Medication	Palliative or hospice goal
Digoxin	May continue for patients with HF (as it lowers hospitalization rate) and control AF rate with symptom relief. Should be monitored in patients with palliative disease-oriented care goals as it has a narrow therapeutic window.
Anticoagulant	May be continued for patients depending on goals of care discussion. The discussion is tailored to the patient's goals, condition, and understanding of his condition. It may continue if the patient has a long life expectancy with palliative disease-oriented care. Otherwise, if the patient is terminally ill with a hospice goal, it may be discontinued. Some patients may elect to continue them even when sick terminally to avoid severe disabilities that complicate strokes. There is no right or wrong answer, but the patient or family should understand the implications and financial costs that come with it (as insurance may decline it in patients with hospice goals).

Pearl

This chapter's key takeaway is recognizing early warning signs of patient decompensation, including refractory symptoms, increased healthcare utilization, and frequent hospital admissions. When these indicators arise, it is essential to initiate discussions about care goals with the patient or their advocates, facilitate advance directive planning, consult a palliative care specialist, and consider intensifying palliative pharmacotherapy to optimize symptom management and quality of life.

References

1. DiPalo KE, Feder S, Baggenstos YT, Cornelio CK, Forman DE, Goyal P, Kwak MJ, McIlvennan CK, American Heart Association Clinical Pharmacology Committee of the Council on Clinical Cardiology and Council on Cardiovascular and Stroke Nursing. Palliative pharmacotherapy for cardiovascular disease: a scientific statement from the American Heart Association. Circ Cardiovasc Qual Outcomes. 2024;17(8):e000131. https://doi.org/10.1161/HCQ.0000000000000131. Epub 2024 Jul 1. PMID: 38946532.
2. Diop MS, Bowen GS, Jiang L, Wu WC, Cornell PY, Gozalo P, Rudolph JL. Palliative care consultation reduces heart failure transitions: a matched analysis. J Am Heart Assoc. 2020;9(11):e013989. https://doi.org/10.1161/JAHA.119.013989. Epub 2020 May 27. PMID: 32456514; PMCID: PMC7428983.
3. Gelfman LP, Barrón Y, Moore S, Murtaugh CM, Lala A, Aldridge MD, Goldstein NE. Predictors of hospice enrollment for patients with advanced heart failure and Effectson health care use. JACC Heart Fail. 2018;6(9):780–9. https://doi.org/10.1016/j.jchf.2018.04.009. Epub 2018 Aug 8. PMID: 30098966; PMCID: PMC6119083.
4. Wan EY, Rogers AJ, Lavelle M, Marcus M, Stone SA, Ottoboni L, Srivatsa U, Leal MA, Russo AM, Jackson LR 2nd, Crossley GH, American Heart Association Electrocardiography and Arrhythmias Committee of the Council on Clinical Cardiology, Council on Cardiovascular and

Stroke Nursing, Council on Cardiovascular Surgery and Anesthesia, Council on Peripheral Vascular Disease. Periprocedural management and multidisciplinary care pathways for patients with cardiac implantable electronic devices: a scientific statement from the American Heart Association. Circulation. 2024;150(8):e183–96. https://doi.org/10.1161/CIR.0000000000001264. Epub 2024 Jul 10. PMID: 38984417.
5. Graham FJ, Pellicori P, Kalra PR, Ford I, Bruzzese D, Cleland JGF. Intra- venous iron in patients with heart failure and iron deficiency: an updated meta-analysis. Eur J Heart Fail. 2023;25:528–37. https://doi.org/10.1002/ejhf.2810.

Pregnancy and the Heart

Contents

M. Salih, *Practical Hospitalist Guide to Inpatient Cardiology*, https://doi.org/10.1007/978-3-032-03240-9_13

This chapter addresses the unique cardiovascular adaptations and challenges during pregnancy, focusing on evaluating and managing pregnant patients with preexisting or newly diagnosed heart disease. It reviews physiological changes, such as increased blood volume, cardiac output, and heart rate, and their implications for conditions like congenital heart disease, valvular disorders, cardiomyopathies, and arrhythmias. This chapter highlights risk stratification tools to predict maternal and fetal outcomes, discusses management of common complications including preeclampsia and peripartum cardiomyopathy, and outlines safe pharmacologic and procedural considerations during pregnancy. Emphasis is placed on multidisciplinary care involving obstetrics, cardiology, and anesthesia to optimize maternal-fetal health. This chapter equips hospitalists with essential knowledge to recognize, evaluate, and manage cardiovascular issues in pregnancy, ensuring timely intervention and improved outcomes for both mother and baby.

13.1 Physiological Consideration [1]

- As gestational age advances, blood volume, and all blood components increase progressively. Heart rate and cardiac output rise from baseline, whereas systemic vascular resistance declines. However, blood pressure remains largely unchanged.
- Common clinical findings include a soft systolic murmur due to increased blood flow and a third heart sound. Additional findings may include a full carotid pulse, a mildly displaced apex beat, lower extremity varicose veins, and edema.
- A 12-lead electrocardiogram (ECG) may reveal nonspecific ST-segment changes in the left leads and minor axis shifts, predominantly toward left axis deviation (LAD).

Pearl

Fatigue, mild dyspnea, ankle edema, and occasional dizziness are common benign symptoms during normal pregnancy. However, more severe symptoms may indicate an underlying pathology [2]. Abnormal clinical findings, such as a loud fourth heart sound (S4), a prominent systolic murmur, a loud diastolic murmur, or a fixed split of the second heart sound (S2), are typically suggestive of pathological conditions and warrant further evaluation.

13.2 Assessing Pregnancy Risk with Cardiovascular Conditions

- Various classification systems assist in assessing pregnancy-related cardiovascular risk, and the system choice depends on institutional preference and convenience. Commonly used classifications include the WHO classification,

CARPREG I and II, and the Zahara risk model. The most critical risk factors include a history of cardiac prostheses, pulmonary hypertension, advanced symptomatic heart failure or cyanosis, left ventricular outflow obstruction, and prior arrhythmias.

- Patients classified as high risk, such as those in Modified WHO Risk Class IV, are generally advised to avoid pregnancy. However, if pregnancy occurs, comprehensive management by a multidisciplinary team is essential to optimize outcomes.
- The mode of delivery should be determined based on the severity of the underlying cardiac condition. In cases of significant cardiovascular compromise, a cesarean section is preferred. This decision should be made collaboratively by an experienced cardiologist and obstetrician. Indications for cesarean delivery typically include severe congestive heart failure, severe pulmonary hypertension, and the presence of preterm labor in patients on warfarin therapy [3].

13.3 Clinical Considerations

- Significant cardiac symptoms, particularly in the postpartum period, should alert physicians to potential cardiovascular complications. The diagnostic workup should be tailored to the suspected underlying condition.
- Management of these patients requires specialized care that considers the bidirectional impact of pregnancy on cardiac function and vice versa. A specialist should assess the patient's preexisting cardiac conditions, risk factors, and mortality risk while optimizing physiological parameters and medications to ensure the best possible outcomes for both the mother and fetus. To minimize complications, a multidisciplinary team including an obstetrician, cardiologist, and nursing staff experienced in high-risk pregnancies is essential, especially given that most cardiovascular complications arise during the peripartum or postpartum period.
- It is important to note that most cardiac medications cross the placenta and are present in breast milk. No medication is entirely risk-free during pregnancy; therefore, treatment decisions should always involve carefully assessing the potential risks and benefits based on the clinical context.
- When anticoagulation is required during pregnancy, the only approved options are warfarin (at a therapeutic dose of less than 5 mg to minimize fetal harm in the first trimester), low molecular weight heparin (LMWH), and unfractionated heparin (UFH). Since LMWH and UFH do not cross the placenta, they are preferred in acute settings, near delivery, or when warfarin doses exceed 5 mg. However, no anticoagulant is entirely risk-free. Warfarin, for example, is associated with an increased risk of fetal loss and complications, making risk-benefit assessment crucial [4]. In general, LMWH and UFH pose higher risks to the mother, whereas warfarin carries greater fetal risks. If a patient on therapeutic vitamin K antagonist (VKA) therapy enters labor or requires urgent delivery, a cesarean section should be performed following anticoagulation reversal [5]. For non-urgent deliveries, transitioning to UFH is recommended,

with administration paused 4–6 h before delivery [5]. Switching to LMWH or UFH at least 1 week before the anticipated delivery is generally advisable to optimize peripartum anticoagulation management [6].

Pearl

The following commonly used cardiac medications should be avoided during pregnancy due to potential fetal harm: angiotensin-converting enzyme (ACE) inhibitors, angiotensin receptor blockers (ARBs), amiodarone (consider alternatives such as sotalol, flecainide, or procainamide if needed), aldosterone antagonists, sacubitril-valsartan, statins, and ivabradine. Additionally, there is insufficient data to support the routine use of clopidogrel during pregnancy. Direct oral anticoagulants (DOACs) should generally be avoided. Always consult reliable medical resources before prescribing any medication to a pregnant patient—tools such as *Epocrates® Interaction Check* can be useful for evaluating drug safety.

Pearl

Warfarin teratogenicity is associated with fetal warfarin syndrome, characterized by nasal hypoplasia and bone dysplasia. These complications are more commonly observed with warfarin doses exceeding 5 mg/day [4].

Hospitalist Tip

DOACs should not be used in pregnancy, as they are not approved for this population.

Hospitalist Tip

When necessary, low-dose/radiation contrast CT scans can be performed with caution due to the potential risks of fetal hypothyroidism and radiation exposure. Institutional protocols should be followed to minimize fetal exposure. When protective shielding is used, X-rays are generally considered safe in appropriate clinical scenarios. MRI is typically safe during pregnancy and can be considered when needed [7].

13.4 Considerable Cardiac Complications to Mention

(i) Peripartum cardiomyopathy [8]: PPCM is a diagnosis of exclusion characterized by new-onset heart failure occurring in the last trimester of pregnancy or up to 6 months postpartum. Risk factors include preeclampsia, a history of cardiomyopathy, African descent, and multiparity. Key differential diagnoses include stress cardiomyopathy, viral myocarditis, and ischemic heart disease (IHD) due to coronary dissection. In acute settings, PPCM should be managed similarly to acute decompensated heart failure (ADHF). Patients with advanced disease should be referred to specialized centers, as some may require heart transplantation or a ventricular assist device (VAD). In critically ill patients, delivering the baby is crucial, regardless of gestational age. The post-acute phase is managed similarly to chronic heart failure (CHF), with the exclusion of teratogenic drugs. Anticoagulation may be considered in patients with an ejection fraction (EF) <35%, typically using warfarin, as directed by a cardiologist. Some patients may progress to dilated cardiomyopathy (DCM). Prognosis depends on heart failure severity; those with severely reduced EF have worse outcomes, though most patients experience recovery.

(ii) CHF: CHF in pregnancy presents similarly to ADHF, with elevated BNP levels (notably, BNP is never normal in pregnant patients) [9]. Standard ADHF treatment includes digoxin, nitroglycerin (NTG), hydralazine, beta-blockers, and diuretics while avoiding previously mentioned teratogenic medications. Cesarean delivery is recommended in advanced heart failure cases [3].

(iii) Acute pericarditis [10]: Acute pericarditis should be managed similarly to nonpregnant patients, with caution regarding medication safety. Aspirinand NSAIDs should be avoided after 20 weeks of gestation due to the risk of fetal renal impairment. Steroids, acetaminophen, and colchicine are relatively safe throughout pregnancy.

(iv) ACS [11]: Spontaneous coronary artery dissection (SCAD) is the most common cause of pregnancy-related ACS, typically occurring in late pregnancy or the postpartum period. SCAD is associated with fibromuscular dysplasia, making a history of uncontrolled hypertension an important consideration. Initial management is conservative, with percutaneous coronary intervention (PCI) reserved for cases where conservative treatment fails [12]. For ST-elevation myocardial infarction (STEMI), PCI is the preferred treatment, with appropriate fetal shielding. Dual antiplatelet therapy (DAPT) is required, but clopidogrel should be held for 7 days before a scheduled delivery. Statins may be considered for secondary prevention postpartum.

(v) SVT: Acute SVT should be managed similarly to nonpregnant patients. Beta-blockers and calcium channel blockers (CCBs) are reasonable for recurrent SVT. Electrical cardioversion is safe if required.

(vi) VHD [1]: An experienced cardiologist should manage patients with symptomatic VHD. Maintaining euvolemia is crucial. Treatment options include diuretics or afterload reduction in cases of volume overload, beta-blockers (except atenolol, which is linked to low birth weight), digoxin, or selective cardiac calcium channel blockers for atrial fibrillation (AF) rate control. In advanced cases, intervention may be required [1].

(vii) Pulmonary HTN: PH is considered a very high-risk condition in pregnancy. Patients should be followed closely by an experienced maternal cardiologist. Pulmonary vasodilators, except for endothelin receptor antagonists, should be continued, as the latter are contraindicated due to their teratogenic potential [13].

(viii) HTN: Acceptable antihypertensive medications during pregnancy include labetalol, nifedipine, hydralazine, and nitrates. Chronic hypertension should be managed with a goal blood pressure of <140/90 mmHg [14].

References

1. Nanna M, Stergiopoulos K. Pregnancy complicated by valvular heart disease: an update. J Am Heart Assoc. 2014;3(3):e000712. https://doi.org/10.1161/JAHA.113.000712. PMID: 24904015; PMCID: PMC4309052.
2. Choi HS, Han SS, Choi HA, Kim HS, Lee CG, Kim YY, Hwang JJ, Park JB, Shin HH. Dyspnea and palpitation during pregnancy. Korean J Intern Med. 2001;16(4):247–9. https://doi.org/10.3904/kjim.2001.16.4.247. PMID: 11855154; PMCID: PMC4578053.
3. Hill NE, Granlund B. Anesthesia for labor, delivery, and cesarean section in high-risk heart disease. [Updated 2023 Feb 21]. In: StatPearls [Internet]. Treasure Island (FL): StatPearls Publishing; 2025.
4. Vitale N, De Feo M, De Santo LS, Pollice A, Tedesco N, Cotrufo M. Dose-dependent fetal complications of warfarin in pregnant women with mechanical heart valves. J Am Coll Cardiol. 1999;33(6):1637–41. https://doi.org/10.1016/s0735-1097(99)00044-3. PMID: 10334435.
5. Otto CM, Nishimura RA, Bonow RO, Carabello BA, Erwin JP 3rd, Gentile F, Jneid H, Krieger EV, Mack M, McLeod C, O'Gara PT, Rigolin VH, Sundt TM 3rd, Thompson A, Toly C. 2020 ACC/AHA guideline for the management of patients with valvular heart disease: executive summary: a report of the American College of Cardiology/American Heart Association Joint Committee on Clinical Practice Guidelines. Circulation. 2021;143(5):e35–71. https://doi.org/10.1161/CIR.0000000000000932. Epub 2020 Dec 17. Erratum in: Circulation. 2021 Feb 2;143(5):e228. doi: 10.1161/CIR.0000000000000960. Erratum in: Circulation. 2021 Mar 9;143(10):e784. doi: 10.1161/CIR.0000000000000966. PMID: 33332149.
6. Lindley KJ, Bairey Merz CN, Asgar AW, Bello NA, Chandra S, Davis MB, Gomberg-Maitland M, Gulati M, Hollier LM, Krieger EV, Park K, Silversides C, Wolfe NK, Pepine CJ, American College of Cardiology Cardiovascular Disease in Women Committee and the Cardio-Obstetrics Work Group. Management of women with congenital or inherited cardiovascular disease from pre-conception through pregnancy and post-partum: JACC Focus Seminar 2/5. J Am Coll Cardiol. 2021;77(14):1778–98. https://doi.org/10.1016/j.jacc.2021.02.026. PMID: 33832605; PMCID: PMC8061781.
7. Yoon I, Slesinger TL. Radiation exposure in pregnancy. [Updated 2023 May 1]. In: StatPearls [Internet]. Treasure Island (FL): StatPearls Publishing; 2025. Available from: https://www.ncbi.nlm.nih.gov/books/NBK551690/.

8. Cho L, Davis M, Elgendy I, Epps K, Lindley KJ, Mehta PK, Michos ED, Minissian M, Pepine C, Vaccarino V, Volgman AS, ACCCVD Womens Committee Members. Summary of updated recommendations for primary prevention of cardiovascular disease in women: JACC State-of-the-Art Review. J Am Coll Cardiol. 2020;75(20):2602–18. https://doi.org/10.1016/j.jacc.2020.03.060. PMID: 32439010; PMCID: PMC8328156.
9. Tanous D, Siu SC, Mason J, Greutmann M, Wald RM, Parker JD, Sermer M, Colman JM, Silversides CK. B-type natriuretic peptide in pregnant women with heart disease. J Am Coll Cardiol. 2010;56(15):1247–53. https://doi.org/10.1016/j.jacc.2010.02.076. PMID: 20883932.
10. Brucato A, Pluymaekers N, Tombetti E, Rampello S, Maestroni S, Lucianetti M, Valenti A, Adler Y, Imazio M. Management of idiopathic recurrent pericarditis during pregnancy. Int J Cardiol. 2019;282:60–5. https://doi.org/10.1016/j.ijcard.2019.02.003. Epub 2019 Feb 6. PMID: 30773267.
11. Smilowitz NR, Gupta N, Guo Y, Zhong J, Weinberg CR, Reynolds HR, Bangalore S. Acute myocardial infarction during pregnancy and the puerperium in the United States. Mayo Clin Proc. 2018;93(10):1404–14. https://doi.org/10.1016/j.mayocp.2018.04.019. Epub 2018 Jul 18. PMID: 30031555; PMCID: PMC6173614.
12. Saw J, Aymong E, Sedlak T, Buller CE, Starovoytov A, Ricci D, Robinson S, Vuurmans T, Gao M, Humphries K, Mancini GB. Spontaneous coronary artery dissection: association with predisposing arteriopathies and precipitating stressors and cardiovascular outcomes. Circ Cardiovasc Interv. 2014;7(5):645–55. https://doi.org/10.1161/CIRCINTERVENTIONS.114.001760. Epub 2014 Oct 7. PMID: 25294399.
13. Zhang X, Huangfu Z. Management of pregnant patients with pulmonary arterial hypertension. Front Cardiovasc Med. 2022;9:1029057. https://doi.org/10.3389/fcvm.2022.1029057. PMID: 36440029; PMCID: PMC9684470.
14. Brown CM, Garovic VD. Drug treatment of hypertension in pregnancy. Drugs. 2014;74(3):283–96. https://doi.org/10.1007/s40265-014-0187-7. PMID: 24554373; PMCID: PMC4558097.

Cardiac Data Collection

Contents

M. Salih, *Practical Hospitalist Guide to Inpatient Cardiology*, https://doi.org/10.1007/978-3-032-03240-9_14

This chapter outlines a systematic approach to collecting and interpreting cardiac data essential for effectively evaluating and managing patients with cardiovascular disease. It emphasizes comprehensive history taking focused on symptoms such as chest pain, dyspnea, palpitations, syncope, and risk factors including hypertension, diabetes, and family history. Physical examination techniques targeting cardiovascular signs, murmurs, jugular venous pressure, and edema are detailed. This chapter guides hospitalists in selecting and interpreting key diagnostic tools and approaching difficult cases. It highlights integrating clinical findings with diagnostic data to formulate differential diagnoses and guide management. The approach prioritizes patient-centered care, risk stratification, and timely collaboration with cardiology and other specialties. This chapter equips hospitalists with practical skills to efficiently assess cardiac patients, enabling accurate diagnosis and optimized treatment plans in the inpatient setting.

14.1 EMR and the Cardiac Patient

- Initial data collection should begin with a review of emergency department documentation and laboratory findings, facilitating preliminary differential diagnosis formulation before patient encounter.
- Critical document review should encompass previous discharge summaries, recent cardiology clinic notes, primary care documentation, and relevant specialty consultation records, enabling a comprehensive assessment of the patient's clinical complexity.
- This preliminary information synthesis allows for focused patient evaluation, with history and physical examination directed by predetermined diagnostic considerations.
- This systematic approach to pre-encounter preparation, while requiring only 3–5 min, significantly enhances the efficiency and effectiveness of subsequent patient evaluation through informed clinical reasoning and targeted assessment.

14.2 Cardiac Medical History Art

- Clinical data collection should employ standardized frameworks such as OPQRST for pain evaluation or SOCRATES for non-pain symptoms. The interview should progress from open-ended to focused questioning, ensuring comprehensive symptom characterization. Particular attention should be directed toward associated cardiovascular and respiratory manifestations, including angina, dyspnea, orthopnea, paroxysmal nocturnal dyspnea, cough, sputum production, hemoptysis, wheezing, stridor, dizziness, and syncope.
- Past medical history documentation should encompass cardiac and systemic conditions, including surgical interventions, heart failure, diabetes mellitus, hypertension, myocardial infarction, coronary interventions, cerebrovascular

events, and peripheral vascular disease. Critical attention must be paid to cardiac device history (pacemakers, ICDs) and revascularization procedures.

- Family history should emphasize sudden cardiac death, premature cardiovascular events, and atherosclerotic disease patterns. Social history must document tobacco use, alcohol consumption, lifestyle factors, dietary patterns, psychosocial stressors, and occupational exposures.
- Medication reconciliation requires particular attention, acknowledging potential discrepancies between patient reporting and medical records. Universal screening for recreational substance use is indicated regardless of demographic factors. Sexual history may be relevant in specific contexts, such as HIV-associated cardiomyopathy or syphilitic aortitis.
- A systematic review of systems should identify additional symptoms that may refine differential diagnosis. This should proceed anatomically, encompassing neurological (headache, syncope, seizures, sensory/motor changes), psychiatric, gastrointestinal (dysphagia, abdominal pain), constitutional (weight changes, fever), dermatologic, and musculoskeletal manifestations. This comprehensive approach often reveals diagnostic clues in atypical presentations.

Pearl

Patients receiving chemotherapy or immunotherapy warrant particular attention due to potential cardiovascular complications. Careful review of agent-specific adverse effect profiles is essential for appropriate risk assessment and management.

14.3 Effective CVS Examination

Checklist	Comments
Does the patient look ill?	Indicates significant distress if looks sick. Check for cyanosis in the face, extremities, and tongue.
Hands	Look for clubbing, signs of IE, cyanosis (may indicate severe hypoxia/ACHD/severe PHT), warm/cold (indicate poor perfusion if cold), capillary refill time (>2 s indicates poor perfusion, and is an early sign of shock).

Pearl

DD of clubbing in cardiac patients includes IE, myxoma, and ACHD (cyanotic).

Radial and brachial pulses	Check for regularity or irregularity (AF), poor pulsation in AS, or poor perfusion.
	The brachial pulse is medial to the biceps tendon and helps assess volume status and check the collapsing pulse in AR or MR.
Face	Check for cyanosis and conjunctival pallor for anemia.

Checklist	Comments
Jugular venous pressure	If elevated (3 cm from the angle of Louis or visible pulsation in front of the right ear), it indicates CHF with volume overload.
Carotid palpation	Helps synchronize the murmur with the pulsation; if it is systolic, it usually coincides with the pulsation.
	Most important determinant on CPR.
Heart palpation	If the apex is displaced laterally, it indicates a dilated heart with LVH, more common in severe DCM, MR, or AR, with a heaving apex (your finger will be pushed vertically away from the chest).
	Thrill indicates an underlying murmur (usually AS).
	Left parasternal heave (placing your hand on top of the sternum, where you will feel a pulsation and lifting, which should not be there) indicates PHT and right ventricular hypertrophy.

Heart auscultation	S1 is louder at the base of the heart, while S2 is louder near the aortic and pulmonary areas. Listen to the murmur and follow where it is loudest for radiation. Check whether the carotid pulsation is synchronous with the pulsation while listening to the difference. Do maneuvers accordingly to resonate the sounds of the murmur; remember inspiration makes the right heart murmur louder, while expiration resonates the left side murmur more.
	Physical examination correlation between carotid pulse palpation and cardiac auscultation provides valuable diagnostic information; murmurs coinciding with carotid pulsation typically represent a systolic murmur.
Chest auscultation	Check for pleural effusion and basal crackles in CHF.
Abdominal palpation	Look for enlarged liver and ascites in right-sided failure.
	An obvious abdominal pulsation could indicate an aortic aneurysm.
Leg exam	Feel for edema in CHF, also pulses for PVD or acute ischemia event.

Pearl

Keep the patient at 45° to check the internal JVP. Turn the neck slightly to the left side (avoid tensing neck muscles); you can see faint pulsation up to the mid-neck, which is normal. Any pulsation seen in front of the ear is likely elevated JVP. Pulsation anterior to the ear is not arterial. The external jugular vein (it will cross the sternocleidomastoid muscle superficially) could correspond with the internal jugular vein if it is pulsating (which indicates a connection to the intrathoracic pressure). You do not usually need to do the other maneuver except if it is completely unseen and doubtful of the volume status; in this case, apply mild but firm pressure in the middle/right upper quadrant for a few seconds and keep looking to the internal JV rising only for 1–2 s. If seen, it may indicate the volume status is euvolemic. Another helpful technique, if JVP is elevated but would like to make sure it is not carotid, is to try to milk the vein from the top of the neck going to the neck base reaching the collar bone; if the pulsation, which was evident, disappears, it indicates the JVP was elevated.

14.4 Example of a Case Writing Summary

- The example below is my typical case summary of the initial admission note. It is intended to be comprehensive but succinct and optimized.
- A 65-year-old male patient with a history of aortic stenosis (AS), coronary artery disease (CAD) status post coronary artery bypass grafting (CABG), heart failure with reduced ejection fraction (HFrEF) at 40%, paroxysmal atrial fibrillation (AF), diabetes mellitus (DM), hypertension (HTN), and chronic obstructive pulmonary disease (COPD) on 2 L oxygen presented to the hospital with severe chest pain rated 9/10. The pain is described as dull, located on the left side of the chest, and began 2 h ago. It is unremitting and not alleviated even by sublingual nitroglycerin. The patient reports the pain radiating to the left shoulder and being aggravated by deep breaths and exertion. He also experienced shortness of breath when exerting himself for the past few days. Still, he denies any other respiratory symptoms, syncope, fever, cough, GERD, abdominal complaints, recent heart attacks, or acute decompensated heart failure (ADHF). The patient has a notable cardiac history, including CAD with CABG in 2008, and is on Plavix. He was diagnosed with HFrEF in 2014, with the most recent ejection fraction at 40%, and is managed on guideline-directed medical therapy by his cardiologist. He is known to have AF and is on Eliquis, with moderate AS that is asymptomatic. His last cardiologist visit was a month ago, with no new events reported. He denies recent acute coronary syndrome (ACS) or ADHF events and does not have any pacemaker, ICD, or stents. Upon presentation to the emergency department, the patient's vitals were stable, and he was afebrile on his baseline 2 L oxygen. The emergency department examination revealed basal crackles and a systolic murmur at the right upper sternal border. The workup in the ED was unremarkable, with no acute changes in the EKG, normal troponin levels, and non-contributory CBC and CMP. A chest X-ray showed nonspecific infiltrates suggestive of pulmonary edema. My examination assessment was consistent with the ED findings, with the additional observation of bilateral pedal edema at +2.

Hospitalist Tip

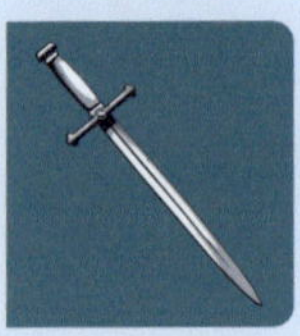

Your case writing is the most important puzzle to organize, as it will help you and other providers build your DD and assessment/plan workflow.

14.5 Differential Diagnosis Art

- The diagnostic approach should prioritize Occam's razor principle, emphasizing the consideration of common etiologies based on epidemiological factors and individual patient context before pursuing rare diagnoses.
- Clinicians must maintain awareness of cognitive biases, particularly confirmation and anchoring biases, which can significantly impact diagnostic accuracy. Recognition of these inherent cognitive limitations is essential for maintaining diagnostic rigor.
- When conventional differential diagnoses fail to fully explain the clinical presentation, systematic expansion to rare conditions becomes necessary. This process is optimized by focusing on unique or distinguishing clinical features to narrow the differential diagnosis. For instance, in a presentation of abdominal pain with eosinophilia, building the differential diagnosis around eosinophilia (the more specific finding) before incorporating the less specific symptom of abdominal pain can enhance diagnostic precision.
- In cases of persistent diagnostic uncertainty, a structured literature review utilizing Boolean operators to combine key symptomatic findings, laboratory abnormalities, and physical examination findings in academic databases (e.g., "Eosinophilia" AND "Abdominal pain" OR "GI symptoms") provides a systematic approach to rare disease identification. This algorithmic approach to diagnosis demonstrates high utility in resolving complex clinical presentations.

Supplementary Information

M. Salih, *Practical Hospitalist Guide to Inpatient Cardiology*, https://doi.org/10.1007/978-3-032-03240-9

Index

A

D

E

F

G

H

I

L

M

N

O

P

Q

R

S

T

U

V

W

MIX
Papier aus verantwortungsvollen Quellen
Paper from responsible sources
FSC® C105338

If you have any concerns about our products,
you can contact us on
ProductSafety@springernature.com

In case Publisher is established outside the EU,
the EU authorized representative is:
Springer Nature Customer Service Center GmbH
Europaplatz 3, 69115 Heidelberg, Germany

Printed by Libri Plureos GmbH
in Hamburg, Germany